D0327643

Oxford Medical Publications

THE ECONOMICS OF
INFECTIOUS DISEASE

THE ECONOMICS OF INFECTIOUS DISEASE

Edited by

JENNIFER A. ROBERTS

Emeritus Professor of Economics of Public Health and
Director of the Collaborative Centre for Economics of
Infectious Disease
London School of Hygiene and Tropical Medicine, UK

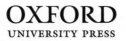

OXFORD
UNIVERSITY PRESS

OXFORD

UNIVERSITY PRESS

Great Clarendon Street, Oxford OX2 6DP

Oxford University Press is a department of the University of Oxford.
It furthers the University's objective of excellence in research, scholarship,
and education by publishing worldwide in

Oxford New York

Auckland Cape Town Dar es Salaam Hong Kong Karachi
Kuala Lumpur Madrid Melbourne Mexico City Nairobi
New Delhi Shanghai Taipei Toronto

With offices in

Argentina Austria Brazil Chile Czech Republic France Greece
Guatemala Hungary Italy Japan Poland Portugal Singapore
South Korea Switzerland Thailand Turkey Ukraine Vietnam

Oxford is a registered trade mark of Oxford University Press
in the UK and in certain other countries

Published in the United States
by Oxford University Press Inc., New York

British Library Cataloguing in Publication Data

Data available

Library of Congress Cataloging in Publication Data

The economics of infectious disease / edited by Jennifer A. Roberts.
  Includes bibliographical references and index.
    ISBN-13: 978–0–19–851621–7 (Hbk.: alk. paper)
    ISBN-10: 0–19–851621–5 (Hbk.: alk. paper)
    ISBN-13: 978–0–19–851622–4 (pbk.: alk. paper)
    ISBN-10: 0–19–851622–3 (pbk.: alk. paper)   1. Communicable disease—
    Economic aspects.   2. Communicable diseases—Prevention—Costs.
    [DNLM: 1. Communicable Disease Control—economics.
  2. Communicable Diseases—economics. WA 110 E19 2006]   I. Roberts, Jennifer A.
    RA643.E26 2006   362.196'900681—dc22   2006000901

Typeset by Newgen Imaging Systems (P) Ltd., Chennai, India
Printed in Great Britain
on acid-free paper by
Biddles Ltd., King's Lynn

ISBN 978–0–19–851622–4 (Pbk.: alk. paper)   978–0–19–851621–7 (Hbk.: alk. paper)
ISBN 0–19–851622–3 (Pbk)   0–19–851621–5 (Hbk)

10 9 8 7 6 5 4 3 2 1

Foreword

Professor Barry Cookson

> Prediction is very difficult, especially about the future.
> *Niels Bohr*

I was delighted when Jenny Roberts asked me to write a foreword to this very important and thought provoking book. I have worked with Jenny for many years and this volume reflects the modern multi-disciplinary approach to infectious disease we have adopted. As a medical microbiologist and infection control doctor I have seen this multi-disciplinary approach blossom and evolve along side the increasing complexity of healthcare delivery, the drive to improve clinical governance and apply cost effectiveness techniques to infection and its control. We now face new challenges from newly emerging diseases and the resurgence of diseases we thought were conquered, in addition we face the threat of bioterrorism. The complexity of the issues that arise in this area continue to excite me and, indeed, make me want to read this book. I am sure others will feel the same.

It provides an introduction for economists to the major challenges of work in infectious disease, whilst also describing for the professions involved in infectious disease prevention and control, the concepts, terminology and methodological approaches that economists may bring to bear on the evaluation and planning of infectious disease control. This is achieved by bringing together many illustrative examples from professionals who have been researching the relevant aspects of infectious disease.

The volume addresses many important infectious diseases that plague developed and developing countries. Issues relating to tuberculosis, antimicrobial resistance, malaria, HIV, animal health and food safety are included. The use of modelling techniques are well illustrated. Governance issues in the context of infectious disease are explored. This concept led to the introduction of clinical governance in the UK. It is now adopted in many other countries. It is perhaps the most important driver to produce improvements in the quality of patient care.

Healthcare associated infections and the related issues of antimicrobial resistance, my own areas of major interest, are addressed in several chapters.

Policy makers and politicians paid little attention to such infections for many years but are now aware of the importance of their prevention and control. The reasons for this are complex, but include a realisation that standards in infection control reflect the whole health care organisation and can be powerful tools in the hands of inspecting and review bodies. Our major assessment of the socio-economic impact of hospital acquired infections alluded to in these chapters was used extensively by the National Audit Office (NAO), whose reports stimulated action throughout the NHS. At a recent WHO meeting politicians and policy makers emphasised that they wanted similar assessments performed in their own countries, realising that the findings had to be applied to their own, rather others', healthcare delivery systems. Patient advocates, the electorate and the media are now aware of the burden of such infections, although the threat of antimicrobial resistance which looms large, is perhaps uppermost in their minds? Antimicrobial resistance has two chapters devoted to it and the issues raised by the most widely known antibiotic resistant organism MRSA is addressed in the Epilogue.

Readers might, like myself, be tempted to 'graze' through this fascinating book. I would recommend reading it in a more orderly fashion, at least start with the introduction where important concepts are described very clearly and concisely. The historical background is also well covered and may surprise many readers. Each chapter has appropriate descriptions of the methodologies used, and the authors assume little prior knowledge amongst their readers; this is a reflection of a good brief provided by the editor no doubt.

Economic approaches to infectious disease are, for very good reasons, becoming embedded in many areas of our work and cannot be ignored. The National Institute for Clinical Excellence in the United Kingdom, for example now requires economic assessments included in guidelines. Specifications for grants to assess interventions used to prevent or control infections now often include economic assessments.

This book combines the work of outstanding investigators in several related disciplines. I anticipate that it will become essential reading for those wishing to locate information and references and others wanting to learn about the approaches to the various issues relating to the economics of infectious disease. I expect that other editions or volumes will follow, as contributors are invited to update their chapters and others provide additional contributions as the state of the art develops further and new challenges such as the threatened pandemic of Avian flu H5N1, now relentlessly moving westwards affecting wild birds, runs its course. It is impossible to predict whether or when a pandemic might occur but the Epilogue shows how economic analysis might be utilized in modifying its impact.

Professor Barry Cookson
Director, Laboratory of Healthcare Associated Infection
Centre for Infections

Acknowledgements

The idea for a book of readings was stimulated by the papers presented at the first and second International Conference on Economics of Infectious Disease sponsored by the Collaborative Centre for Economics of Infectious Disease, at the London School of Hygiene and Tropical Medicine in 2000 and 2001. Some chapters have developed from contributions made at these meetings updated to take into account subsequent developments. I would like to thank those attending the meetings for their stimulating contributions and enthusiasm. Other papers have been developed from major research projects relating to hospital-acquired infection, hepatitis C, intestinal infectious disease in England, Wellcome-funded studies on flu and pneumonia, the Economic and Social Science Research Council study on risks, managed markets and infectious disease, and graduate research projects. I would like to thank colleagues on these projects for sharing their knowledge of infection and the sponsors for funding the research. In particular, I would like to thank colleagues Pauline Allen, Jean Buzby, Barry Cookson, Ben Cooper, Geoff Dusheiko, Nick Graves, Elizabeth Haworth, Chris Kibbler, Punam Mangtani, Ros Plowman, Tanya Roberts, Laura Rodrigues, Paul Sockett, Sheldon Stone, Linda Taylor; Karen Alford and colleagues at the National Audit Office; colleagues at the Health Protection Agency; and Michael Miles and students studying on the masters course Control of Infection Disease that we jointly coordinated at the London School of Hygiene and Tropical Medicine. I would like to thank contributors and Oxford University Press for patience during the unexpected delay in completing the volume.

Contents

Chapter 1

Introduction to the economics of infectious disease

Jennifer A. Roberts

Introduction

Infection is an ever-present threat to the health of populations. Its control is of the utmost importance. Scarce resources are used to care for those who are sick and to prevent or control the transmission of infection. Productive capacity is constrained by infection, and trading relationships are disrupted. Thus, infection poses an economic problem that needs to be addressed. The characteristics of infectious disease raise important issues for economists seeking to apply their tools in this area.

This book provides an opportunity to bring economics to bear on complex issues surrounding the prevention of infectious disease and its control. It begins by addressing issues that arise in the application of economic evaluative techniques to infectious disease and its control, and the modelling approaches that have been used to evaluate interventions. It moves on to consider issues of governance, including risk, agency and contracting, and regulations that are encountered in the implementation of infection control programmes. The book has two objectives: to introduce economic analysis and its application to those who are involved in infectious disease and its control; and to introduce economists to infectious disease and the challenges that it raises.

This introduction provides a background to infectious diseases. It includes a brief historical account of the economic impact of infectious disease, outlines the burden of certain diseases today and highlights new threats. The economic characteristics of infectious disease and its control are described and compared with normal goods and services. The application of economic evaluation and theories of governance to infectious disease management is discussed. This chapter concludes by describing the contents of the book.

Background

There is increasing concern about infectious diseases and the ability of states to control them. This concern arises not only because of the deaths and morbidity attributed to infectious disease but also from fears that it might become difficult and costly to control. Threats are posed by the emergence of new and the resurgence of old pathogens and by the growing resistance of organisms to prophylactic therapies and antibiotics. Added to this is the spectre of bio-terrorism. These concerns call for an economic assessment of infectious disease and its control.

There is nothing new about using the economic calculus to assess the impact of infections on the economy (see Fein 1971). In the seventeenth century, Petty suggested moving people from the City of London to Hampstead, then a rural area on high ground a few miles away, to save them from the plague (Petty 1888). This policy he concluded would be worthwhile, as it would save lives of productive labourers. Thus, although the technique of cost-benefit analysis (CBA) was not refined, economic rationale was used to support interventions to prevent the ravages of disease. The estimates of the burden of illness were used to justify sanitary improvements in the nineteenth century when benefits were expressed as years of life saved and the value of such years to the economy. Chadwick (1842) recommended sanitary improvements: 'well executed measures, directed by engineering science' that would reduce the burden of 'excessive mortality'. In the USA, Shuttuck's report in 1850, on the conditions in Massachusetts, was similarly evangelical, 'The state suffers, from imperfect sanitary conditions, an unnecessary annual loss of more than $7.5 m and this arises, partly at least, from the non-adoption of a measure which will cost but about $3000' (Shuttuck 1948). The appointment of William Farr as superintendent of the Statistical Department of the Registrar General's Office in England heralded a period of active research into morbidity and mortality. Farr (1885) provided estimates of the values of lives lost that ranged from £5 at birth to £246 at 30; the value then declined to £138 at 55 and £1 at 70 years of age. The maintenance costs for those over 70 outweighed their productive value. He used these estimates to assess the costs of disease such as cholera and consumption (see Fein 1971). Not only did infection affect the labour force but some epidemics were so extensive that structural changes have been attributed to them. The plague in England depleted the labour force to such an extent that it propelled changes in methods of agriculture (McNeill 1989).

Infectious disease has played a part in political and military events (Ward 1952). It helped small European armies conquer the Americas by weakening native populations who had no immunity to the infections introduced by the invaders. Infection thus contributed to the fall of the Aztec and Incan empires. Later, smallpox prevented the American army from capturing Canada. Price-Smith (2002) cites many events such as these and examines the impact of infection on the security of the state.

Forty-one per cent of the global disease burden has been attributed to infections. The World Health Organization (2002) has estimated that there are about 9 million new cases of tuberculosis (TB) each year and 2 million annual TB deaths, including those also infected with human immunodeficiency virus (HIV)/acquired immune deficiency syndrome (AIDS) whose depleted immune system provides a receptive host for TB. TB remains a scourge in deveoping countries, is common in countries of the former Soviet Union, and has re-emerged in developed western countries that have been relatively free of this disease for decades. AIDS wrecks havoc across Africa and Southeast Asia; some 41 million are infected and, as few drugs are available, these people will die prematurely. As the group most affected is of working age, the economies suffer and many communities have to cope with orphan children many of whom have the disease. A total of US$1.6 billion was spent on treat-ment, care and orphan support in 2002. This is an enormous burden yet fewer than 20% of those at risk have access to programmes to prevent the disease. (World Health Organization 2002).

Those with other blood-borne infections, such as hepatitis B and C, have a 20-fold higher risk of primary liver cancer than the rest of the population. Antiviral drugs that can clear the infection in some cases are available. An effec-tive vaccine is available for hepatitis B. Transmission of hepatitis C through sexual intercourse is less than for HIV or hepatitis B, but hepatitis C has the highest transmission rate via blood and blood products. Hepatitis C is thus a problem for those with haemophilia and for intravenous drug users. The trans-mission amongst addicts in prisons is very high (Weild 2002). As the clinical path of disease is long, most studies use modelling techniques to predict the impact of the various stages of the illnesses over 30 or 40 years (Dusheiko and Roberts 1995; Grieve and Roberts 2003; see also Grieve Chapter 5).

Leprosy is the archetypal example of an infectious disease with long-term sequelae. More recently, Guillain–Barre syndrome has been associated with *campylobacter*, Epstein–Barr virus with cancers, human papilloma virus 16 with cervical cancer, and *Chlamydia pneumoniae* with heart disease.

The mosquito takes its toll. Malaria claimed the lives of 1.1 million in 2001, 963 million of whom were from Africa (World Health Organization 2002). It accounts for 10% of the disease burden in sub-Saharan Africa. Vector-borne diseases, such as malaria, are not passed on by person-to-person contact but the blood of an infected person is a reservoir of infection that is spread by mosquitoes. Individuals can protect themselves by using bed-nets or taking prophylactic drugs. Action of a more communal kind is needed to control the breeding areas of the mosquitoes. Even malaria, that has been present for thousands of years, does not stay constant but evolves and adapts to changes in the environment and to interventions that threaten it. The effectiveness of prophylactic regimes is reduced as malaria acquires resistance to sulfadoxine-pyrimethamine (SP) and chloroquine. These issues of dynamic change are addressed by Goodman *et al.* in Chapter 2. Outbreaks of West Nile fever in New York and the Eastern sea-board of the USA have been seen as evidence of the extension of the mosquito vector in the northern hemisphere possibly caused by climate change.

Dengue haemorrhagic fever, another mosquito-borne disease, is endemic in southern Asia and countries of the South Pacific including many parts of northern Australia, the eastern coast of Africa and the Gulf States. The World Health Organization (2002) estimates that dengue kills 10 000 children per year and Japanese encephalitis 8000 children per year. Leishmaniasis, a disease spread by sand flies, is fatal unless treated. It occurs in rural parts of the tropical and sub-tropical countries of Asia, the Middle East, sub-Saharan Africa and central and southern America. Tick-borne diseases continue to cause encephalitis in Russia, other European countries and in North America.

Zoonotic transmission of disease to humans is an important disease vector. A number of pathogens affect human health. One is brucellosis, a debilitating disease in cattle that transmits infection to humans in contact with infected animals or consuming unpasteurized milk or milk products. This disease is controlled in Western Europe but remains a problem in countries of the former Soviet Union where vetinarary practice has broken down, and in the Middle East. *Escherichia coli* O157, relatively harmless to animals, is a life-threatening illness in humans. It is passed on via the food chain in meat that is not well cooked and in milk that is unpasteurized or where pasteurization has failed, and environmentally by contact with animals or contaminated surfaces and by water that has run off pasture (Roberts and Upton 1999). TB, in the form of *Mycobacterium bovis*, the bovine tubercle bacillus, is a problem in some areas if milk is unpasteurized.

New zoonotic infections have emerged. Bovine spongiform encephalopathy (BSE) that can cross the species barrier and cause new variant Creutzfeldt–Jakob disease (vCJD), a rare incurable neuro-degenerative condition, caused a major health scare in the UK. Severe acute respiratory syndrome (SARS) caused a crisis in 2003 when it spread rapidly in the Far East and reached Canada, threatening a pandemic. Human proximity to animals and poultry affects the ease with which viruses from animals and birds might 'reassort' with other viruses, such as influenza, to cause an antigenic shift that produces a novel subtype that might prove dangerous as populations will have no immunity. An outbreak of avian flu in the Far East in 2003 led to the culling of 100 million poultry. The disease was probably widespread before it was identified, thus there is a risk that the virus will 'reassort' with other viruses to produce a highly virulent strain. The World Health Organization has produced a plan of action to be used in the event of a flu pandemic (World Health Organization 2004) and the financial needs have been estimated (World Bank 2005, Roberts Chapter 19). Riviere-Cinnamond discusses animal and human health systems in Chapter 12.

Many common-place infections, such as intestinal infections, continue to be a problem in both developed and developing countries (see Food Standard Agency 2000). These include *Salmonella enteritidis* that was widespread in the late 1980s. It was spread by the consumption of, or contamination from, infected chicken and eggs (see Buzby *et al.* Chapter 16, for the economic assessment of intervention strategies). Intestinal infection is the second most common cause of child deaths. It is responsible for 12% of deaths of children under five in developing countries–a total of 1.3 million deaths each year. Although in richer areas with appropriate interventions there are far fewer deaths, intestinal illnesses are still the most important cause of childhood admissions to hospitals.

Respiratory tract infections are a major cause of death amongst the young, the old and immune-compromised people. It has been estimated that 2 million children under five die every year from acute respiratory infections. An epidemic of influenza in 1989 in England and Wales caused the deaths of over 25 000 people, 20 000 of whom were over the age of 75. Vaccination can reduce the impact of influenza (see Mangtani and Shah Chapter 9).

Poor developing countries still struggle to combat common childhood infections for which vaccinations are available and widely used in the developed world. Vaccines are costly and out of the reach of many. The situation has deteriorated in some areas. In Nigeria, only 25% of children were vaccinated in 2002 compared with 50% 10 years earlier. There have been successes. The Global Polio Eradication Initiative reported 2000 cases in 2002 compared with 350 000 in 1988, with fewer countries experiencing endemic polio: seven compared with 125 in 1988.

Antimicrobial resistance has emerged as a new threat to infection control. Methicillin-resistant *Staphylococcus aureus* (MRSA) is endemic in many hospitals and increasingly in the community. It is difficult and expensive to treat and leads to increased morbidity and mortality (see Roberts Chapter 19). *Staphylococcus aureus* is not the only resistant organism. The Public Health Laboratory Service (2002) [now incorporated in the Health Protection Agency (HPA)] in the UK reported that 55% of cases of bacteraemia caused by *E.coli* were resistant to ampicillin/amoxycillin and 30% to trimethoprim (see Laxminarayan Chapter 3; Coast *et al.* Chapter 11). Resistant strains of TB are proliferating because of the shortage of drugs or non-compliance with treatment regimes. Treatment of resistant strains of TB is expensive as combined therapy with up to five drugs may be needed, and even such intense treatment does not always clear the organism successfully (Costa *et al.* Chapter 7).

The story in the developed world, however, is far from gloomy. 'In 1901, the death rate from infections in England was 369 per 100,000; a century later, it was 9 per 100,000. It is estimated that infection accounts for 70,000 deaths each year in England and Wales. The improvement was due to a higher standard of living, strong public health regulations and the adoption of vaccination for common infections of childhood and the success of antibiotics' (Department of Health 2002). Thus, infectious disease has been low down the policy agenda of health care systems in the rich developed economies. The major scares, e.g. AIDS, Ebola and the recent outbreak of SARS, that disrupted large cities, i.e. Toronto and Beijing, and wrecked havoc on international travel and trade, have revived awareness of infection (Roberts Chapter 19). Thus fear of infection associated with new virulent organisms, the re-emergence of old diseases, the growth of resistant forms of infection and bio-terrorism have ensured infectious disease is now high on the public health policy agenda.

The impact of infection on economy

Outbreaks of infection can have a considerable impact on economies. The botulinum infection in Canadian salmon in the 1980s had disastrous effects on the industry. Large government grants were needed to revive the industry (Sockett 1993). The discovery of *S.enerididis* in eggs in the UK in the late 1980s devastated the egg-producing industry and cost the minister responsible her job (HMSO 1989). The zoological disease BSE found to be capable of crossing the species barrier devastated the beef industry in the UK. Fears of the infection led to bans on British beef imports to Europe and many other countries. The bans were lifted only after extensive animal culling and the introduction of documentation stating the place of birth and subsequent movement of each animal prior to slaughter: giving each animal a passport. BSE led to labelling of surgical equipment to facilitate tracing and the introduction of disposable equipment at great cost to the National Health Service (NHS). Bans on the use of blood products from British residents are in place. In the UK, persons who have had blood transfusions since 1980 are banned from donating blood (Department of Health 2004). France and the USA will not accept blood donations from people who have lived in Britain. Similar bans imposed in Ireland led to severe blood shortages as so many citizens had spent time in Britain.

Though the large or unusual outbreaks make headlines, there are numerous more commonplace outbreaks that affect producers. Producers may take products off the market as a precaution because they fear losing market share or because they are ordered to. They may or may not receive compensation. Investigation and control of outbreaks are very important and require an adequate infrastructure (see Jamasji-Pavri Chapter 14).

Infection can result in death, pain, long-term sequelae, and loss of work and leisure time. Estimates of the costs of many infections have been made but are of limited value as they differ in the methods used to cost the infection and do not reflect the value placed on the preventive interventionsm (see Plowman Chapter 8). Whilst infection can affect the economy, economic conditions can also influence the prevalence of infection.

The impact of the economy on infection

The wealth of an economy and the state of its infrastructure, e.g. water, education and transport, affect the prevalence of infectious disease. Vulnerability to infection is determined by the immune systems of the person, their proximity to transmission routes and the virulence of the organism (Benenson 1994).

The immune status can be affected by living conditions, by the quality and quantity of food consumed and by access to clean water. 'Unsafe water and sanitation, and indoor air pollution are also strongly associated with absolute poverty. For unsafe water and sanitation, the relative risks for those in households with an income of less than $1 per day, as compared to households with an income greater than $2 per day ranged from 1.7 (WPR-B) to 15.1 (EMR-D)' (World Health Organization 2002). The most common and serious vector-borne diseases are transmitted by mosquitoes that breed in standing water. Cleaning up and draining require action by individuals, communities and governments.

Poor nutrition increases the vulnerability to infection: '50–70% of the burden of diarrheal diseases, measles, malaria and lower respiratory infections in childhood is attributable to under nutrition', and 'the risk of intestinal infectious disease is highest amongst the poor' (World Health Organization 2002). Social class gradients in the USA have been shown to have significant effects on the risk of rotavirus and risk of cases being hospitalized. A recent study in the UK found a strong association with accommodation—living in public housing with fewer than five rooms was a significant risk factor (Food Standard Agency 2000; Sethi et al. 2001).

This brief sketch has shown the importance of infectious disease. In the next section, the characteristics of infection and its control will be considered and compared with other goods and services produced in the economy.

Economic aspects of infectious disease

Market forces determine the value of a commodity. Trade for mutual advantage occurs when those who wish to buy and those who wish to sell come together to exchange goods or services for value. Buyers and sellers in perfectly competitive markets can both 'walk away' if the product or the price is not to their liking. This ability to walk away ensures that via competition the firms will sell at market price and will produce the products that people value most highly. Markets that fulfil these conditions ensure optimization: the point beyond which there are no further opportunities for mutually beneficial exchange. Not all goods are suitable for market production and delivery. It is difficult to establish efficient exchanges amongst those exposed to infectious agents and those whose actions put them at risk or offer them protection. The problems occur on both the demand and supply side of the trading relationships. Whilst the demand is beset by information problems and externalities, supply is beset by coordination and integration problems. Thus there are likely to be missing markets for infection control, i.e. no suppliers available or no identifiable buyers.

Even when markets exist, they can fail if there are externalities, public goods, lack of information or information imbalances and uncertainty. The market will not provide efficient answers. Infectious disease control exhibits many features commonly associated with market failure. The task for the economic analyst is to understand how organizations cope with the properties associated with infectious disease and to determine whether they have the most appropriate governance structure (market or public provision or finance) for the task in hand.

If an individual has an infected wound, she will seek treatment to cure it. This can be obtained by a transaction between the person and providers—pharmacists, nurses or doctors. The cure cannot be resold or exchanged as it is embodied in the person: its market exchange will be attenuated but a market solution will exist. If the wound becomes infected with an organism that can be transmitted to others (especially if the organism has acquired resistance to antibiotics, e.g. MRSA), it may be expensive to treat and to control. These spillover effects on others are called externalities. In this case, the externality imposes a cost to the patient to whom the infection may be transmitted and to the health sector. Yet it is difficult to 'internalize' this eternality by charging or compensating the parties involved. The market will fail.

There may also be external benefits. Individuals can protect themselves from illness by vaccination. Vaccination may appear to be a simple market transaction, but vaccination affects both those who are vaccinated and those whom they might have affected. Vaccination of a proportion of the population will benefit the rest: herd immunity will occur. Herd immunity is a spillover effect that reduces the risk to those not vaccinated; but the vaccination imposes risks and burdens on those who are vaccinated. Perceived benefits may become very small as prevalence falls, and private individuals may not buy the vaccine at any price. This may give rise to failure of prevention and the re-emergence of disease if the vaccination rate falls below that required for herd immunity (Philipson 1996). Philipson attempts to determine the prevalence-elasticity of demand for prevention: the response of demand at different levels of prevalence. Econometric techniques have been used in conjunction with robust epidemiology to model optimal vaccination strategies (Philipson and Posner 1993; Philipson 1996; Gerovitz and Hammer 2004). The value of eradication tends to be greatest for future generations who are protected but whose values cannot be assessed nor extracted. There will be missing markets between the generations (see Coast *et al*. Chapter 11).

Quarantine has been used for centuries as a way of limiting the spread of infection and so protecting society. It was used in the recent SARS outbreak. Penalties (sometimes severe) for not complying were imposed. Whilst containing the infection, quarantine attenuates the rights of individuals and exposes them to increased risks of infection and death. Compliance is often enforced.

Some externalities are dealt with by public provision: supplying condoms, clean needles and other paraphernalia to reduce infection with AIDS amongst drug users. Efficient public provision may be cost-effective if it reduces infection and transmission rates.

Infection control activities have features of a 'public good'. A public good is a good that is provided or consumed in common. It has two important features: it is non-excludable and non-rival. One person's consumption may not reduce the amount available to others, i.e. non-rival, and it may be difficult to exclude anyone from the benefits, i.e. non-excludable. Properties of public goods raise problems for the funding of services. If no one can be excluded, who will pay? There will be a temptation to 'free ride'. However, if one person's consumption does not deplete that available to others, then that person's marginal benefit will have no marginal cost; it will thus be inefficient to impose a charge. If the good is to be produced, some other means of financing has to be found; it is often funded directly from tax-based state funds.

Recent work on public goods suggests that communities may provide some goods having public good attributes for themselves. Experiments in economic psychology show that, in the absence of a market, groups will come together to pay for and provide public goods especially if there is a continuing relationship and there are penalties for non-compliance. The formation of 'clubs' is an attempt to produce 'public goods' for members of the club. Residents of an area may secure for themselves clean water or sanitation or access to gyms or swimming pools. Such 'clubs' may not be adequate, however, to protect people from all vectors of infection, e.g. air-borne organisms and viruses. Exclusion from the public bad—infection—is often very difficult.

Differences between infection control and other goods can be explored by considering the property rights pertaining to them. Property rights are the rights to use, change, exchange or destroy the good. Without property rights, trade cannot take place because interest in the good cannot be assigned. Property rights to infection control are largely held in common, affected by regulatory frameworks and cultural norms.

It is difficult to allocate rights to shared but exhaustible resources: 'When many people have the right to use a single shared resource, there is an incentive for the resource to be overused and, correspondingly, when many people share the obligations to provide some resource, it will be under supplied. When the residual returns to an asset are widely shared, no one person has a sufficient interest to bear the costs of maintaining and increasing its value'. This dilemma is sometimes referred to as the 'tragedy of the commons'. Although not all infection control has the features of a public good, the 'tragedy of the commons' is displayed frequently when infection control procedures are neglected because the benefits are widely dispersed and failure cannot be attributed.

Protecting the public requires the development of a governance system that aligns the interests of agents and the public's health. The agency relationships in infectious disease control are multiple and complex. The implementation of policies intended to protect public health often depend on networks of relationships amongst professionals and agencies that share resources and knowledge because there are mutual gains from pooling. 'The entangling strings of reputation, friendship, interdependence and altruism become integral parts of relationships' (Powell 1991). They may be supportive and productive if professionals share expertise to solve a problem, such as identifying a SARS virus, but they can be fragmented by organizational and structural changes (see Davis and Lederman 2000; Roberts and Haworth 2003). Networks can also collude against the public health interest (see Jamasji-Parvi Chapter 14; Narasimhan Chapter 18).

Information imbalance is suggested to be a reason why markets in health care may not be efficient. Information technology (IT) has reduced the information gap between the agent providing the service and those who seek care. The information about the chances of being infected, the implications of the infection and the effectiveness of drugs or other interventions will aid decision taking. However, much remains unknown, and patterns of infectious disease and its virulence change.

Uncertainty, unlike risk for which a probability cannot be calculated, is not amenable to estimation. Control agencies have little forewarning of new organisms emerging or of old ones mutating into something more virulent. Even when probabilities are known, there is often asymmetry in the response by individuals and organizations confronted with risks of saving or losing lives. One factor identified as explaining the apparent inconsistency or non-rational behaviour is our propensity to pay excessive attention to low-risk high-impact outbreaks of infections and overlook continuous sources of more common infections that may have similar or greater overall mortality or morbidity (Kahneman and Tversky 1979). Some explain asymmetry by pointing to peoples' risk aversion, but experiments have shown that when the outcome is specified as a loss, i.e. deaths rather than lives saved, people were prepared to take a risk to avoid this loss rather than face the prospect of a sure loss. Tverski and Kahneman (1986) explain the asymmetry by the human propensity to hate loss. Perhaps the most interesting proposition offered to explain this is regret theory that suggests that decisions are based on the potential for regret that will be experienced if something avoidable occurs (see Loomes and Sugden 1983). Possibly, it is to avoid 'regret' that many politicians and governments espouse the precautionary principle: 'all that can be done should be done to prevent infection'.

Precautionary principle is not always the motivating factor. Where disclosure of an infection is likely to be accompanied by an economic loss, governments may conspire with producers or medical establishments to conceal a problem. Networks can cooperate or collude against the public health interest (Jamasji-Pavri Chapter 14). Even diseases that are notifiable under international agreements may go unreported by countries to protect their national interests. Infection can be used as an excuse to impose restrictions on trade and retain the restrictions long after the public health threat has been resolved (Kumaranayake Chapter 17; Narasimhan Chapter 18).

Professionals perceive risks differently depending upon whether they are affected, i.e. personally accountable or personally at risk, or whether the organization for which they work is at risk of losing its reputation or funds, or whether the publics' health is at risk (Archibald 2001). The professionals and organizations can be called to account if their actions are negligent or reckless of other persons' welfare.

Equity is also an issue for infection and its control. Whilst most societies make provision for the health care of the poor or seek to reduce inequalities in access to health care in the case of infection, it may be imperative to protect the poor as those too poor to protect themselves may be a reservoir infecting others. There is a significant externality associated with inequality in the context of infectious disease.

For all these reasons, externalities, public goods, uncertainty and equity, the market may not produce the most appropriate level of infectious disease control and some form of intervention may be required. Evaluating such interventions is a central task for economists wanting to contribute to the adoption of efficient policies to control infection, but economic evaluations are not sufficient. Economists wanting to contribute to efficient policy formation must contribute to the governance debate and indicate the effects of different forms of governance of infectious disease. But before tackling governance factors that affect infectious disease control, economic evaluation will be considered.

Economic evaluation

There is a rich literature on economic evaluations, and each chapter dealing with economic evaluation in this volume contains a brief resume of the technique whilst illustrating its policy application (Drummond *et al.* 2005). Thus, in this chapter, only a brief description of the types of economic evaluation and an outline of some features of infectious disease that have a bearing on evaluation will be provided.

CBA is the traditional method of evaluating projects that cannot easily be evaluated by market processes. It attempts to identify and evaluate costs and benefits wherever and whenever they occur. CBA seeks to answer questions such as, 'Does the intervention represent a rate of return equal to that which could be earned elsewhere in the economy?' For example, does a hospital infection control team yield as much benefit as a new screening programme or a new road scheme? A full CBA will have embodied within it an analysis of the alterative ways of producing the goods and it will identify the most efficient way of producing them.

Cost-effectiveness studies seek not to see if the project is worthwhile but to determine the most economically efficient way of producing it. This technique compares products having the same effect to determine which method uses resources most efficiently, i.e. produces the product at least cost or enables the greatest amount to be produced from a given budget. Malaria prophylaxis, for example, may be considered worthwhile but it may not be clear which amongst the alternative products is the most cost-effective. In order to compare the products using cost-effectiveness analysis, there should be just one output, cases avoided for example. Usually different alternatives affect a number of dimensions that have to be compared one with another. One method may prevent more cases but cause more side effects or more pain than another. These different dimensions have to be evaluated. Health economists have developed scales that attempt to measure the health impact of interventions. Perhaps the best known scales are quality adjusted life year (QALY) and disability adjusted life year (DALY). Attitudes towards these measures differ. Some economists rely upon them and have advocated their use on moral as well as economic grounds, e.g. Williams (1985), whilst others consider they are too narrow to encompass all health-related facets that are valued. Attempts to overcome these difficulties have led some researchers to adopt what they have labelled a 'cost-consequences approach' that specifies, and when possible quantifies, the additional features. Neither the health status measures nor the cost-consequence approach allow the return from projects to be compared with that from other goods and so are of limited use in determining the optimum amount of resources that should be invested in health care or infection control.

Cost of illness (COI) or burden of illness studies are often called for by policy makers wishing to understand the implications of an illness on the use of resources. COI studies, if care is taken to measure economic costs derived from underlying production processes, can be useful for management purposes. A recent hospital-acquired infection study undertaken in England is a good examples of a COI study that influenced policy (see Plowman *et al.* 2000; Alford *et al.* 2001; Graves and Weinhold Chapter 6; Plowman Chapter 8). COI studies may, however, over- or underestimate the benefits or value of the resources used (Mishan 1971). Also, as Philipson (1985) has pointed out, they often neglect to assess the costs or value of actions to reduce the burden of the illness.

Many economists prefer to measure benefits by assessing the population's willingness to pay (WTP). This technique allows benefits to be stated in money terms, so allowing the rate of return of the investment to be compared with other investment projects. Although WTP studies have much to offer, they are notoriously difficult to construct. There are a number of problems. WTP is affected by the information available about the disease: the probability of acquiring the infection, its severity and likely impact on everyday life. The status of the persons affected, their responsibilities to family or work and their concerns about transmitting the infection may all influence their WTP. The views expressed may be influenced by whether respondents believe that the results might lead to the introduction of charges or removal of a service. Those used to free at point of use services, common in Western European health systems, may feel aggrieved to have been asked, and fear it is a precursor of charges (see Mangtani and Shah Chapter 9). Such fears can lead to distortions.

It has been possible in a few studies to assess WTP in a situation where it is also possible to observe what was actually paid (see Bhatia and Fox-Rusby Chapter 10). A WTP study should also estimate what people would accept to forgo a service, possibly a more difficult task. It might be expected, given the discussion of uncertainty above, that there will be some asymmetry between values placed on gains and losses, and some individuals are likely to be more risk averse than others (see Mangtani and Shah Chapter 9).

The basis for costing should be the underlying production function that describes the ways in which resources are combined to produce output. All the inputs should be identified and the relationships amongst them established if possible. The production should be technically efficient: no more resources than necessary should be used to produce a given output. As well as being technically efficient, it should be economically efficient: the combination of resources chosen should be that which ensures that the relative contribution of the inputs is equal to the relative price of the inputs. The production processes that underlie the costs should be explored for possible economies of size and scope. Joint production is a common feature in infection control: actions undertaken together may yield more or be cheaper than if done separately. Inputs may not have a stable relationship to output. Sometimes an organism's antibacterial resistance to a drug will change: there may not be a monotonic function of input to output; the intransivity rule may appear to be violated. Thus 'if X is preferred to Y it will not continue to be so preferred'; cycling can occur where 'Y is also sometimes preferred to X'. Therefore, switching inputs may have a beneficial impact upon resistance. This cycling phenomena is discussed by Kumaranayake *et al.* in Chapter 4 and Laxinarayan in Chapter 3.

Empirical cost and cost-effectiveness analyses are sometimes carried out without regard to whether production is carried out efficiently. Little attention is paid to the relationships amongst variables or the effect of size, scale or scope on costs. Some studies rely on a top-down approach dividing various input components, e.g. staff or drugs, by the number included in the study. This gives little information about the inter-relationships amongst inputs, scale or scope and may provide inaccurate estimates (see Whynes and Walker 1995).

Economic evaluations require a great deal of data. This includes the epidemiology of the disease: the incidence of the disease, its spread, the trend over time and the risk factors associated with its spread. It is important to know the clinical path of the disease and to assess the impact on the individual of the different phases of the disease, especially if the disease has a long gestation period, e.g. cancer in those with hepatitis B and C. Each stage would have different resource implications (see Grieve Chapter 5).

Often randomized control trials and clinical trials of efficacy and economic evaluations take such care to have a precise case definition that they exclude a great number of cases, thus making generalizability of subsequent findings problematic. Kumaranayake *et al.* in Chapter 4 address the generalizability issue. Another failure with many studies is the lack of attention to alternatives available. Costing in many studies assumes that technology will remain unchanged. For many diseases that develop over a long period, this assumption is untenable (see Grieve Chapter 5).

Production costs are not the only costs that need to be considered. Different forms of governance incur different costs of coordinating activities or transactions. It is crucial that an appropriate form of governance is chosen to ensure that costs are minimized.

Governance

Governance is the system by which organizations coordinate their activities. The choice of governance structures depends upon the nature of the product being produced and the economic environment of the organization. In deciding which governance system to adopt, i.e. hierarchies, markets or some hybrid form, the costs of loss of control over interactions between principals and agents determines whether a far-sighted entrepreneur would choose to produce a good or service or buy it from others.

Traditional economic analysis uses the price system to signal values and costs, and assumes costless transaction arrangements, a 'frictionless system' of trading. Williamson (1985) refers to this as 'bliss'. Often, however, there will be costs of trading. These costs are referred to as transaction costs. 'Broadly conceived, transaction costs refer to any use of resources required to negotiate and enforce agreements, including the cost of information needed to facilitate a bargaining strategy, the time spent higgling, and the costs of preventing cheating by the parties to the bargain' (Cooter 1990, p. 65).

In competitive market transactions, we expect nothing more than that we can exchange goods at mutually satisfactory rates. There is no scope for parties to the transaction to manipulate the arrangements in their own interests, i.e. behave 'opportunistically'. Transaction costs can occur in any organization but, whilst firms operating in the market place may be disciplined by competitive or contestable markets, other organizations, including public bureaucracies, may be resistant to change and can be subjected to political pressures. The minimization of transaction costs involves the selection of the appropriate governance. Buckley and Chapman (1997, p. 136) comment that 'transaction costs are funny things: the most important of them exist not in reality but in realities that have been avoided, in worlds that have not come to be'. This characterizes infection control nicely, as that too is about ensuring that some worlds 'do not come to be'.

Williamson (1996) suggests that three factors are likely to cause problems for contracting and give rise to opportunism: bounded rationality, uncertainty and asset specificity. Simon (1957) defines bounded rationality: 'behaviour is intendedly rational, but only limitedly so'. Both the bounded nature of the rationality (recognition that we have limited ability or knowledge to behave rationally) and the 'intended rationality' (that keeps behaviour within the maximizing framework of economics) are important. Some theorists do not separate production and transaction costs but see them as inter-related. They see different organizational arrangements as solutions to problems of coordination and motivation (Milgrom and Roberts 1992, p. 294). Coordination costs take different forms in different organizational structures. As there may not be complete information, attention is given to devising mutually acceptable terms that will not be undermined by fears of opportunistic behaviour.

Assets that are specific have low opportunity costs, i.e. their return in the next best alterative use is low, e.g. kits or machinery to perform specific auto-mated tests. Thus, losses will be large if the original transaction is terminated. 'Bygones are forever bygones' but one would like to prevent them occurring. 'Hold-ups' can occur if one party has power because the asset he owns is of strategic importance to the other party. In these circumstances, continuity of the relationship is valued. If trusting relationships do not exist, the relation-ship may change from a market to a hierarchy: integration or internal gover-nance may be preferred.

In contractual situations in which there is bounded rationality, uncertainty or asset specificity, it will not be so easy to achieve a mutually satisfactory contract or to 'walk away'. Even 'high-minded honest' economic organizations will be easily 'invaded and exploited' by other agents who do not possess these qualities. Moral hazard is possible during the execution of the contract. The high transaction costs involved in scrutinizing agents as they implement contracts and the problems of attributing blame for adverse outcomes make it possible for standards to be eroded during the execution of the contract—cutting corners to save either time or money (see Jamasji-Pavri Chapter 14). In situations such as these, the maintenance of ongoing relations are import-ant and adjustments to the contract will be a feature of the relationship. Contracts that are obligational relationships involve high trust and continued involvement. Not all agents are motivated by self-interest. When investigating an outbreak of *E.coli* O157 in children, all those involved gave up their time to control the infection and treat the cases (Roberts and Upton 2000). In another study, we found that cleaners were bringing in their own materials because contractors were not providing enough. They seemed to have felt obliged to act not in the interests of the immediate principal, the contracted cleaning company, but in the interests of the NHS or the patients (see Le Grand 1997; Crawshaw and Roberts 2000; Allen and Croxson Chapter 15).

Regulation can be seen as a method of dealing with potential transaction costs. Regulations in the form of standard setting, guidelines as well as legally enforceable regulations are common methods of improving governance in the control of infectious disease (see Buzby *et al*. Chapter 16). Regulations are often introduced for the purpose of improving the safety or preventing fraudulent practices; they have a welfarist base. Regulators and those they regulate may, however, develop a close relationship that may at times amount to 'regulatory capture' as the regulators become intimately involved with the firms or industries they regulate (Cullis and Jones 1992). They can, however, be used to protect an industry from external trade pressures; hence the need for some international intervention to set and monitor regulations (see Kumaranayake Chapter 17 and Narasimhan Chapter 18).

The complex interactions between multiple agents and principals, and the special features of infectious disease, make it a fruitful area for economists to hone their skills and provide guidance for policy makers and managers to provide effective and efficient control programmes.

The organization of the book

The book begins with a series of chapters that use forms of economic evaluation to explore the control of infectious disease. In Chapter 2, Goodman *et al*. outline methodological and contextual issues that arise in framing the analysis and the range of costs and benefits that need to be considered in the use of first-line antimalaria therapy given the growth of resistance. The potential contribution and limitations of such models for policy makers are discussed, and suggestions for their further development proposed.

Economic issues related to antimicrobial resistance are considered by Laxminarayan in Chapter 3, who addresses issues that arise as antimicrobial resistance gains a hold. He considers the drugs as both fixed and renewable assets and explores the potential trade-offs from cycling drug use to retain their potency. He discusses the incentives faced by patients, physicians and hospital administrators in choosing antibiotics and the strategies pharmaceutical companies adopt. He continues to work in this area since his conference presentation in 2001 reported here (see Laxminarayan 2003).

Generalizability is an important attribute of economic evaluations, as they are expensive and time consuming, so to provide information that can be used in other settings is valuable. Kumaranayake *et al.* in Chapter 4 consider the growth of cost-effectiveness studies on AIDS/HIV, survey studies that have been undertaken, and, using dynamic models and varied time dimensions, address issues of attribution and the lack of generalizability of the largely contextual findings.

Chapter 5 contributed by Grieve shows how technological changes affect the evaluation of interventions for long-term infections using the example of hepatitis C. In this case, changes in the intervention, the delivery of care and the treatment of sequelae occur with attendant problems for evaluation.

Graves and Weinhold in Chapter 6 consider the underlying production function and the problems of attributing costs to a hospital-acquired infection. Attribution is a serious problem for empirically based studies. They consider the biases that might be involved in different methods of attribution and conclude that estimations using instrumental variables and probit analysis are likely to be the most accurate way of attributing costs.

In Chapter 7, Costa *et al.* provide details of their study of TB in San Salvador. Choice of strategy to ensure the greatest compliance with TB treatment is modelled. It indicates that in the context of San Salvador, contract tracing and follow-up for treatment is crucial to the control of disease. Plowman in Chapter 8 critically reviews estimates of the costs of infection and evaluative studies that have assessed the cost-effectiveness of an intervention based on COI estimates of infections avoided. The study described in Chapter 9 by Mangtani and Shah evaluates a flu and pneumonia intervention in the UK. This study combines a detailed COI study with estimates of the WTP derived from the same sample. Bhatia and Fox Rushby in Chapter 10 discuss the theoretical background to WTP studies and report the results of both the amounts people said they were willing to pay for bed-nets with the amount they were observed paying.

There is a close relationship between animal and human infections, yet little attention has been given to this in spite of the problems of food-borne infections and new infections such as BSE, SARS and avian flu. Riviere-Cinnamond addresses some parallels and differences in animal health systems and human health in Chapter 12

The issue of risk is addressed in Chapter 13 by Tanya Roberts in the context of the USDA food protection. In this chapter, governance issues are linked to hazard analysis and critical control points (HACCP), a technique that assesses the critical control points in the control of an outbreak that have to be managed effectively if the disease trajectory is to be controlled. In spite of the best control policies, outbreaks will happen. Jamasji-Pavri in Chapter 14 discusses the management of outbreaks using the framework of new institutional economics and public choice theory of agency. New institutional economics is drawn upon by Allen and Croxson in Chapter 15 to examine the place of contracts as a way of providing services for the control of infectious disease in the context of the purchaser—provider split in the NHS in the UK.

In the context of market failure, regulations come into play. Regulations have an increasingly important role in the control of infections. Buzby *et al.* outline the implications of regulations at the national level exploring the issue of food safety—*salmonella* in eggs and *listeriosis*. The framework for international action following the introduction of the World Trade Organization is outlined by Kumaranayake who considers the use of regulations in the global market in Chapter 17. Narasimhan outlines the impact of infections on national markets and the need for international action in Chapter 18.

These chapters together illustrate ways in which economics can be used to understand processes and contribute to the control of infectious diseases. The final chapter is used to explore control of two infections of contemporary concern: MRSA and Avian Flu. This epilogue offers suggestions for economic studies that might be useful in managing these infections and others that undoubtedly will emerge.

References

Alford, K., Plowman, R. *et al.* (2001) *The Way Ahead: Progress Towards the Control of Hospital Acquired Infection.* National Audit Office, London.

Allen, P. (1999) Contracts in the National Health Service internal market. *Modern Law Review* **58**, 321–342.

Archibald (2001) *Professionals Perceptions of Risk.* First International Conference on the Economics of Infectious Disease. Collaborative Centre for Economics of Infectious Disease, London School of Hygiene & Tropical Medicine, London,

Bartlett, W., Roberts, J. *et al.* (1998) *A Revolution in Social Policy: Quasi-market Reforms in the 1990's.* The Policy Press, Bristol.

Benenson, A. (1994) *Control of Infectious Disease Manual,* 16th edn. American Public Health Association, Washington, DC.

Bernstein, P. (1996) *Against the Gods: The Remarkable Story of Risk.* Wiley, New York.

Buchanan, J. M. (1965) An economic theory of 'clubs'. *Economica* **32**, 1–14.

Buckley, P. J. and Chapman, M. (1997). The perception and measurement of transaction costs. Cambridge Journal of Economics, vol **21**, 136.

Chadwick, E. (1842) *The Sanitary Conditions of the Labouring Population.*

Cooter, R. (1990) The coase theorem. In: Eatwell, J., Milgate, M. Newman, P. (eds), *Allocation, Information and Markets.* The New Palgrave, Macmillan, London.

Crawshaw, S. and Roberts, J. (2000) Managing the risk of infectious disease: the context of organizational accountability. *Health, Risk and Society* **2**, 125–141.

Cullis, J. and Jones, P. (1992) *Public Finance and Public Choice Analytical Perspectives.* McGraw-Hill, London.

Davis, J. and Lederman, J. (2000) *Public Health Systems and Emerging Infections. Assessing the Capabilities of the Public and Private Sectors.* National Academy Press, Washington, DC.

Defoe, D. (1969) *A Journal of the Plague Year.* Oxford University Press, Oxford.

Department of Health (2002) *Getting Ahead of the Curve. A Strategy for Combating Infectious Diseases (Including Other Aspects of Health Protection).* A report of the Chief Medical Officer. Department of Health, London.

Department of Health (2004) *Transfusion Service.* Department of Health, London.

Drummond, M., Sculpher, M. *et al.* (2005). *Methods of the Economic Evaluation of Health Care programmes.* Oxford University Press, Oxford.

Dusheiko, M. and Roberts, J. (1995) Treatment of chronic type B and C hepatitis with interferon alfa: an economic appraisal. *Hepatology* **22**, 1863–1872.

Farr, W. (1885) Vital statistics. In: Humphreys, N. *A Memorial Volume of Selections from the Reports and Writings of Willam Farr.* Offices of the Sanitary Institute, London, pp. 313–314.

Fein, R. (1971) On measuring economic benefits of health programmes. Hospitals, N.P. *Medical History and Medical Care: A Symposium of Perspectives.* Oxford University Press, Oxford, pp. 181–217.

Food Standards Agency (2000) *Intestinal Infectious Disease in England.* The Stationery Office, London.

Grieve, R. and Roberts, J. (2002) Proceedings of the Belgian Hepatitis C Day. *Acta Gastroenterologica Belgica.*

House of Lords Select Committee on Science & Technology (1998) *7th Report.* The Stationery Office, London.

Kahneman, D. and Tversky, A. (1979) *Prospect Theory: An Analysis of Decision under Risk.* Econometrica 1979, **47**, 313–327.

Le Grand, J. (1997) Knights, knaves or pawns? Human behaviour and social policy. *Journal of Social Policy* **26**, 149–169.

Laxminarayan, R., (2003) Battling Resistance to Antibiotics and Pesticides: An Economic Approach. Resources for the Future Press. Washington.

Loomes, G. and Sugden, R. (1983) Regret theory and measurable utility. *Economic Letters* **12**, 19–21.

McNeill, W. (1989) *Plagues and People.* Doubleday, London.

Milgrom and Roberts (1992) Economics ownership and management. *Efficient Incentives, Contracts and Ownership.* p. 294.

Mishan, E. (1971) *Cost Benefit Analysis.* Penguin, London.

Petty, W. (1888) *Essays Mankind and Political Arithmatic.* Cassell's National Library, London.

Philipson, T. (1995) The welfare loss of disease and the theory of taxation. *Journal of Health Economics* **14**, 386–396.

Philipson, T. (1996) Private vaccination and public health: an empirical examination for US measles. *Journal of Human Resources* **31**, 611–630.

Plowman, R., Graves, N. *et al.* (1999) *The Socio-economic Burden of Hospital Acquired Infection.* PHLS, London.

Price-Smith, A. (2002) *The Health of Nations, Infectious Disease, Environmental Change and their Effects on the National Security and Development.* MIT Press, Cambridge, MA.

Roberts, J. and Upton, P. (2000) *E.coli O157. An Economic Assessment of an Outbreak.* Lothian Health and London School of Hygiene & Tropical Medicine, Edinburgh.

Sethi, D., Cumberland, P. A., Hudson, M. J., Roberts, J. A., Rodrigues, L. C., Wheeler, J. G., Cowden, J. M., Tomkins, D. S., Roderick, P. J. (2001) The study of infectious intestinal disease in England: Risk factors associated with Group A Rotavirus infection in children. *Epidemiology and Infection* **126**: 63–70.

Shuttuck, L. (1948) *Report on the Sanitary Commission of Massachusetts.* Cambridge, MA.

Simon, H. (1957) *Models of Man.* Wiley, New York.

Sockett, P. (1993) *The Economic and Social Impact of Human Salmonellosis in England and Wales.* PhD thesis. University of London, London.

Todd, E. (1985) Economic loss from foodborne disease and non-illness related recalls because of mishandling of food processors. *Journal of Food Protection* **48**, 621–633.

Ward, C. (1952) *The War of the Revolution.* Macmillan, London.

Weild (2000) *Communicable Disease and Public Health*, Vol. **3**, No. 2. PHLS, London.

Weild (2002) *Prevalence of HIV, Hepatitis B and Hepatitis C Antibodies in Prisoners in England and Wales: A National Survey.*

Whynes, D. and Walker, A. (1995) On approximations in treatment costing. *Health Economics* **4**, 31–39.

Williams, A. (1985) Economics of coronary artery bypass grafting. *British Medical Journal* **291**, 326–329.

Williams, F. (2003) *Financial Times.*

Williamson, O. (1985) *The Economic Institutions of Capitalism.* New York Free Press, New York.

Williamson, O. (1996) *The Mechanisms of Governance.* Oxford University Press, New York, Press.

World Bank (2005) Avian and Human Influenza: financing needs and gaps.

World Health Organization (2002) *World Health Report.* WHO, Geneva.

World Health Organization (2004) *Avian Flu.* WHO, Geneva.

Chapter 2

Choosing the first-line drug for malaria treatment—how can cost-effectiveness analysis inform policy?

Catherine Goodman, Salim Abdulla, Paul Coleman, Godfrey Mubyazi, Nassor Kikumbih, Tuoyo Okorosobo and Anne Mills

Introduction—the problem of antimalarial drug resistance in Africa

Malaria drug policy in Africa is frequently argued to be in, or fast approaching, crisis (Attaran *et al.* 2004; Institute of Medicine 2004). Malaria is already responsible for over 10% of the total disease burden in sub-Saharan Africa, and its impact is increasing as a result of antimalarial drug resistance. For decades, most countries have relied on chloroquine as their first-line drug for treating uncomplicated malaria, benefiting from its effectiveness, low price and good safety profile. Those days are over because chloroquine resistance is already high in many African countries and growing fast in others (Bloland *et al.* 1998; EANMAT 2003). This is a cause of great concern as, if not effect-ively treated, uncomplicated malaria may progress to the severe form of the disease, with symptoms such as convulsions, coma and severe acidosis, and a significant risk of neurological sequelae in survivors. The in-patient case fatality rate is high, but in many settings the bulk of patients cannot access hospital care, leading to an even higher risk of death. High levels of chloroquine resist-ance have been associated with a high case fatality rate for malaria admissions in Kenya (Zucker *et al.* 1996), and with a dramatic increase in community-based measures of malaria-related mortality in Senegal (Trape *et al.* 1998).

After taking chloroquine for granted for so many years, ministries of health are now engaged in urgent debates over the questions: 'Should we change the first-line drug?' and, if so, 'What should the replacement be?' The answers are far from clear-cut because so many factors have to be taken into account, encompassing drug efficacy and safety, the likely growth of drug resistance, acceptability and use, cost, and even political considerations, as malaria policy is often a high profile issue. Moreover, drug policy in low income countries is not merely a domestic matter, but is also influenced by the policies and funding decisions of donors and international agencies (Shretta *et al.* 2001). As of December 2004, more than a third of African countries continued to use a 3 day treatment with oral chloroquine as their first-line therapy, but the majority had switched to other drugs (World Health Organization RMB 2004). Several replaced chloroquine with sulfadoxine-pyrimethamine (SP), another relatively cheap and safe therapy, given in a single dose. Others replaced chloroquine with a combination of drugs, such as chloroquine and SP, or amodiaquine and SP. There has been growing pressure for countries to adopt artemisinin-based combination regimens (ACTs) to improve treatment efficacy and slow the development of resistance to both component drugs, despite their higher cost and more complex dosing regimens (White 1999; Attaran *et al.* 2004). By early 2005, five African countries had adopted ACT, and a further 15 planned to do so. However, the total costs are high, necessitating a considerable increase in external funding, mainly sourced from the Global Fund for AIDS, Tuberculosis and Malaria.

There have been repeated requests for cost-effectiveness analyses (CEAs) of these drug policy questions, to guide national and international policy makers on when and how to change treatment regimens. CEA can provide a useful framework for synthesizing data on the wide range of epidemiological, behavioural and economic factors concerned. However, in a setting of growing drug resistance, a CEA of drug policy change is more complex and challenging than analyses for many other health care interventions. In particular, framing the question to be addressed is far from straightforward because it is not clear how the comparators should be defined. In addition, the analysis requires prediction from current resistance levels to final health outcomes, both now and in the future as resistance increases. As a result, the analysis requires a dynamic perspective and is subject to particularly high levels of uncertainty.

In this chapter, we begin by outlining the range of costs and benefits that need to be considered in such a CEA. (Unless otherwise stated, all prices have been converted to 1999 US$.) Methodological issues involved in the framing of the analysis are explored, and a CEA of changing first-line drug in Tanzania is presented as an example. Finally, the potential contribution and limitations of such models for policy makers are discussed, and suggestions for their further development proposed.

The costs and benefits of drug policy change

The incremental costs of change

The two key incremental costs of drug policy change are any increase in the costs of the drugs themselves, and the costs of the other activities required to implement the policy change. To predict the change in drug costs, accurate information is needed on the cost and quantities required for the new first-line therapy. Similar data are also needed for the second-line therapy, which is often changed as well, and is provided to patients who have failed with the first line or for whom the first line is contra-indicated. Even this first step may involve practical challenges for many programme managers, as basic data on the number of first and second line treatments required, or the price of different drugs, are often not readily available.

Figure 2.1 shows the average cost per adult treatment with a selection of anti-malarial drugs, based mainly on prices from The International Drug Price Indicator Guide (Management Sciences for Health 1999), a good source of information on recent prices of many generic drugs bought in bulk. ACT prices are drawn from a World Health Organization (WHO) source (World Health Organization RMB 2003) (Another useful source of drug price information is the World Health Organization/RBM, UNICEF, PSI and MSH 2004.). In tablet form, chloroquine and SP are the cheapest, at an average of US$0.10 per adult treatment (all prices include an extra 20% on top of the FOB price to cover shipping). Amodiaquine tablets are 50% more at US$0.15. Quinine and meflo-quine tablets are substantially more costly, at US$1.56 and US$2.17, respectively. The price of ACT ranges from US$1.56 for artesunate plus amodiaquine to US$2.88 for artemether-lumefantrine. Future prices are more difficult to predict. In particular, it is difficult to estimate how ACT prices will change as both demand increases and production capacity is scaled up.

The average cost per treatment depends not only on the choice of drug, but also on the formulations used. In injection or syrup form, the cost of chloro-quine exceeds that of SP and amodiaquine tablets. A course of chloroquine injections costs US$0.66 (including the cost of the syringe), and treatment with chloroquine syrup, the formulation of preference for young children, costs US$0.99. The impact on the drugs budget of changing first-line treat-ment will therefore depend on the balance of formulations used with the current drug and proposed replacement. For example, as SP syrup is rarely used, changing from chloroquine to SP may significantly reduce the average cost per oral treatment, as the proportion of cheaper tablet formulations is likely to rise. On the other hand, for patients unable to take oral preparations, the lack of SP injectables will necessitate the replacement of chloroquine

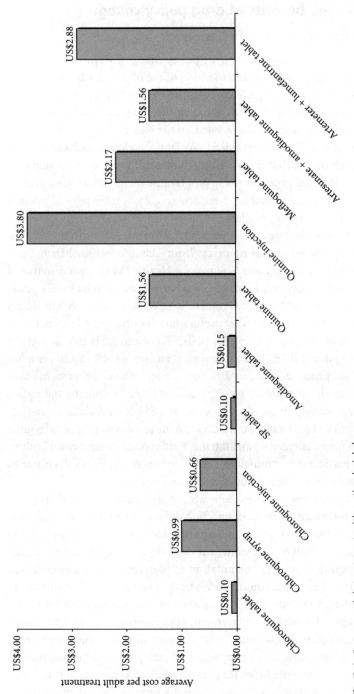

Fig. 2.1 Cost per adult treatment with antimalarial drugs.

Source: International Drug Price Indicator Guide (Management Sciences for Health, 1999) and WHO 2003 (World Health Organization RMB, 2003). Doses were based on an average weight of 60 kg. Twenty per cent was added to the FOB price to cover shipping.

injections with another injectable product, such as quinine, which is substantially more expensive.

In addition to incremental drug costs, there are costs involved with making the policy change. Implementation requires consultation, consensus building and policy formulation, revision and production of treatment guidelines, training of public and private sector health workers, and finally communication and publicity. Both the managerial capacity requirements and financial costs of these activities are significant.

Estimating the health benefits of change

The health benefits of a more effective first-line drug should be wide ranging, including a reduction in treatment failures, severe cases, neurological sequelae, cases of chronic anaemia, low birth weight and deaths. The magnitude of these effects is very difficult to predict from an assessment of drug resistance data alone. First, comparative data on drug resistance are often available only from a few scattered sites across a country, which may not be representative of the national situation. Secondly, they are collected under very controlled conditions where the intake of drugs is carefully monitored, and do not capture effectiveness under operational conditions where non-compliance may be common. Compliance is likely to vary between drugs, depending on factors such as their dosing regimen, minor side effects and taste. The limited evidence available shows that full compliance with multiple dose regimens is often very low. For example, in Malawi, prompt, correct administration of the 3 day chloroquine treatment was reported for only 14% of children at clinics, and 12% at other treatment sources (Slutsker et al. 1994). Compliance with single dose therapies, such as SP, would be expected to be higher, but again good evidence is lacking. In predicting the health impact of a change in drug, the way drugs are actually taken must be considered, and ideally some estimation made of the health impact of under- and overdosing.

A further problem with available efficacy measures is that they are generally expressed in terms of failure rates alone. Policy makers need to predict the impact of these failures on final health outcomes, such as severe disease and mortality, in order to assess their public health significance and the cost-effectiveness of drug policy change. Extrapolating from failure rates to final health outcomes is complicated and inevitably speculative, requiring assumptions about clinical parameters, such as the probability of developing severe malaria after treatment failure, and case fatality rates with and without in-patient care. The influence of behavioural variables on health outcomes is equally important, such as treatment-seeking decisions in response to treatment failure and severe disease.

Finally, only current and historical estimates of drug efficacy are available, but policy makers need to know how resistance will change in the future. In particular, they are interested in whether resistance to some regimens will grow faster than to others. This is perhaps the most uncertain area of all. Only very limited historical time series data are available, and their extrapolation across epidemiological and socio-economic settings is highly problematic. Using models to predict resistance trends requires consideration of not only the characteristics of the drugs and level of malaria transmission, but also of the volume of use, drug quality and compliance. Furthermore, it cannot be assumed that the growth of drug resistance will depend on the role of the drug in official policy alone. It has been estimated that between 40 and 60% of anti-malarials in sub-Saharan Africa are distributed through formal and informal private providers, such as clinics, pharmacies, shops and traders (Foster 1991). Whilst models of resistance evolution are under development, we currently remain largely dependent on the very limited historical empirical data, and ball-park estimates.

The potential for treatment cost savings

Policy makers will also be keen to know whether they can expect significant cost savings arising from the health benefits of introducing a more effective first-line drug. Reductions in the number of treatment failures should reduce the number of repeat visits and the number of cases becoming severe, which could lead to important cost savings in out-patient and in-patient treatment. The reduced health burden could also lead to improved quality of care and reduced costs to patients. However, these cost savings are difficult to predict because they depend on the proportion of people with treatment failure who make repeat visits to formal facilities, which is likely to be well below 100%. For example, when treatment failure with chloroquine in Zambia was around 40%, only 15% of children under five who visited a clinic for fever or convulsions did so more than once (Barat et al. 1998; Baume and Macwan'gi 1998). Moreover, the potential economic benefits from reducing the number of cases treated cannot be assumed to equal current expenditure on malaria treatment, as some proportion of the costs will be fixed, meaning that they will not vary with the number of patients. Examples include buildings and equipment, supervision and training, and most staff costs, at least in the short term. Reducing patient numbers should reduce the demand for drugs, but if drug stock-outs are common, the main impact may be to make drug supplies last longer each month, rather than to produce significant financial savings.

The need for a dynamic perspective

A key feature of the drug costs, health benefits of change and potential treatment cost savings is that they are all a function of resistance to the first-line drug. Resistance changes over time, so we need to evaluate these costs and benefits over time, and any CEA of drug policy change therefore requires a dynamic perspective. For example, if we were to compare chloroquine and SP as first-line drugs at current levels of resistance, an immediate switch would look clearly cost-effective, as they are similar in price, and SP is more effective in nearly all settings. However, this would ignore the concern that SP resistance will rapidly increase after the switch. For example, in Thailand, SP replaced chloroquine as the first-line treatment in 1973, and although morbidity and mortality fell over the next 7 years, by 1981 there were reports of diminishing efficacy, and in 1983 a new first-line drug was introduced in some areas (World Health Organization 1994). Rapid growth in SP resistance has also been observed more recently in some areas of Eastern Africa (EANMAT 2003). It is therefore essential that any evaluation includes not only current costs and benefits, but also their magnitude in years to come.

Framing the analysis

Specifying the alternatives

In designing or framing any CEA, a key step at the outset is to define clearly the question to be addressed. A CEA involves the consideration of the incremental costs and health effects of implementing an intervention, compared with some alternative; either the status quo, a different intervention or the null set (no intervention) (Murray *et al.* 2000). In selecting suitable options, any analyst should consider questions of efficacy, safety, availability and feasibility of implementation. For drug policy change in a setting of growing resistance, it is not clear what the relevant alternatives should be. A policy maker considering the introduction of SP as first line could make a comparison with the costs and effects of continuing with chloroquine. Alternatively, they could compare changing immediately to SP with changing after a delay of, say, 3 or 5 years. SP could be compared with other replacement regimens, such as amodiaquine, or a combination regimen. If the comparison involved combination therapy, the combination could be compared with a single monotherapy, or with sequential monotherapy with each combination drug. Framing the question that the CEA is supposed to answer is therefore a key first step to the analysis, and is not straightforward.

Choice of timeframe

As the analysis involves the consideration of trade-offs in costs and benefits over time, the timeframe of evaluation has an important impact on the results. A second key step in framing the analysis is to choose whether the costs and effects should be considered over 5, 10 or even 20 years. If a longer timeframe is chosen, it will be very difficult to predict the availability and efficacy of potential therapies. If we choose a shorter timeframe, we risk placing inadequate weight on the long-term consequences of policy decisions. In addition, within the chosen timeframe, we need to decide how to weight costs and outcomes occurring now relative to those occurring far into the future. It is common practice in economic evaluations to discount costs and benefits over time to reflect the preference of individuals and governments to receive the benefits of improved health earlier rather than later (time preference), and to reflect the increased uncertainty about receiving predicted benefits further into the future (risk premium) (Gold *et al.* 1996; Cairns 2001). Using a positive discount rate will make regimens with better health outcomes and/or lower costs in the short to medium term look relatively more attractive.

Incorporating uncertainty

As described above, there are a wide range of costs and health outcomes to consider, and considerable uncertainty surrounding their magnitudes. Key uncertain factors include the change in drug efficacy over time, and the impact of drug resistance on treatment-seeking behaviour and health outcomes. In contrast, policy makers need to feel very confident that they are making the right choice before implementing a decision, which is not only of vital importance for effective primary health care, but also highly visible to the general public and politically sensitive. A CEA must therefore strike a balance between the need to produce results that are understandable and provide some policy guidance, and the need to explore and express the high levels of uncertainty involved.

Changing the first-line drug in Tanzania

As an example of a framework to explore the above issues, the methods and results are presented below of a study to assess the cost-effectiveness of changing the first-line drug in Tanzania. The study was commissioned by the National Malaria Control Programme (NMCP) of the Tanzanian Ministry of Health, in order to feed into the policy debate on the choice of first-line drug. The cost-effectiveness model had been designed by a team at the London School of Hygiene and Tropical Medicine (Goodman *et al.* 2001), and was developed and adapted for use in the local policy context, in collaboration with researchers in Tanzania. The model was used to compare chloroquine and SP as first-line drugs, reflecting the policy choice faced by the Tanzanian government at the time. Full details of the model design, input parameters and results are presented in Abdulla *et al.* (2000).

Background

Malaria is a leading cause of the burden of disease in Tanzania. A third of all out-patient visits and in-patient admissions, and a quarter of in-patient deaths, are attributed to malaria (Ministry of Health 1998), which is also an important cause of chronic anaemia in children and pregnant women, neurological impairment and low birth weight, and increases the severity of other diseases. Until 2001, the official first-line treatment for uncomplicated malaria was chloroquine, which was the only antimalarial available in most health centres and dispensaries. In the late 1990s, considerable debate took place in Tanzania about whether the first-line drug should be replaced due to the high level of chloroquine resistance, which on average across the nation's sentinel sites had a probability of total treatment failure (TTF) of 50% in 1999 (Ministry of Health 1999) [defined as clinical failure and parasitaemia by day 14 following treatment (World Health Organization/CTD 1996)]. SP was proposed as an alternative, which at the time had an average TTF of 14%.

The following choices were made in framing the Tanzanian CEA. The alternatives compared were the existing regimen (chloroquine as first line and SP as second line) and the proposed alternative regimen (SP as first line and amodiaquine as second line) with quinine as the treatment for severe malaria under both alternatives. These alternatives were chosen on the basis that over the coming decade they would be technically acceptable in terms of efficacy, compliance and safety, feasible to implement through the current health system and financially affordable for the Tanzanian government. Timeframes of 5 and 10 years were considered, to reflect the number of years over which outcomes could be predicted with some confidence. In line with standard practice in economic evaluations, a 3% discount rate was used for costs. No discount rate was applied to health outcomes, as it was felt that local policy makers would consider this inappropriate and difficult to interpret. To balance the need for policy guidance with the inherent uncertainty involved, a base case was modelled, complemented by considerable use of simple one-way and multiway sensitivity analysis.

The Tanzanian model

A first step in developing the model was to predict the growth rates of drug resistance over time, bearing in mind that this would depend on the characteristics of the drug, the epidemiological setting and treatment-seeking behaviour. In the absence of good data or reliable resistance models, the growth rate of chloroquine resistance if retained as first-line drug was predicted by extrapolating from a logistic growth function fitted to rough historical estimates from Tanzania over the last 50 years (Ministry of Health 1999). Estimates were made of the relative growth rates of resistance to the other drugs, based on the characteristics of each drug, such as their half-lives, and their role in the official regimen. There is general consensus that resistance to SP as a first-line drug grows more rapidly than chloroquine resistance, because of differences in the mechanisms by which resistance develops, and because SP persists longer in a patient's blood (White and Olliaro 1996). However, it is difficult to predict how much faster. In the base case, it was assumed that once adopted as first line, resistance to SP would grow twice as fast as resistance to chloroquine, an assumption which was varied in the sensitivity analysis. Figure 2.2 shows the historical estimates and fitted function for chloroquine resistance in children under five, assuming chloroquine was maintained as first line, and the estimated function for SP resistance,

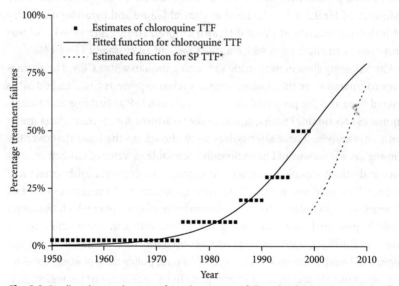

Fig. 2.2 Predicted growth rates of total treatment failure (TTF) in patients under five with chloroquine or SP as first-line drug: historical estimates and fitted function for chloroquine TTF (assuming it was maintained as first-line drug) and estimated function for SP TTF, assuming SP was introduced as first-line drug in 2000.

* SP TTF was estimated using the base case assumption that growth rate of resistance to SP is twice the growth rate of resistance to chloroquine.

assuming that SP was adopted as first line in 2000. The function predicted that average chloroquine TTF in children under five would be 53.1% in the year 2000, and that if the chloroquine regimen were maintained, chloroquine TTF would increase to 65% in 2004 and 77% in 2009. In the base case, the SP TTF for children under five was predicted to be 15% in 2000, and if SP were introduced as first-line drug in that year, its TTF was predicted to increase to 32% in 2004 and 61% in 2009.

A decision tree model was then used to extrapolate from resistance levels to health and utilization outcomes, using estimates of compliance, treatment-seeking behaviour, the probability of developing severe disease and case fatality rates (see Fig. 2.3). The starting population was all people presenting at an out-patient facility with suspected uncomplicated malaria. Due to the use of clinical diagnosis alone in most facilities, a large proportion of these patients may not actually be suffering from malaria. The outcomes for these false-positive cases were not calculated as they were assumed to be unaffected by a change in the antimalarial used. Of those who were suffering from malaria, the probability of operational failure with an out-patient drug was defined as:

$$\text{Probability of operational failure} = 1 - (\text{cure rate} \times \text{probability of compliance})$$

where the cure rate is defined as (1 − TTF). Compliance was defined as receiving at least the minimum required dose. Allowance was made for the possibility of drug stock-outs, and efficacy in some cases of minor under-dosing. The decision tree traces the possible paths a presenting patient could follow, with probabilities attached to each option or branch of the tree. For example, for a patient with treatment failure, probabilities are assigned to reflect the likelihood of remaining with uncomplicated malaria or developing severe disease. If the latter, probabilities are estimated for the likelihood of seeking admission to hospital, and the case fatality rate with and without in-patient treatment.

For a given level of treatment failure with the first-line drug, the model predicted the numbers of operational treatment failures, severe malaria episodes, in-patient admissions and deaths for patients initially presenting at an out-patient facility (outcomes for patients obtaining drugs purely through outlets such as shops or drug vendors were not incorporated). Estimates were made separately for patients over and under 5 years of age, assuming that 40% of out-patients with suspected malaria were under five (Ministry of Health 1998). Costs were also attached to the tree to predict the expected cost per patient. A provider costing perspective was used as the main incremental

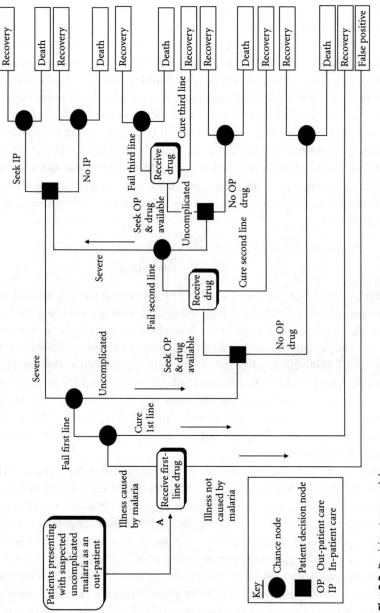

Fig. 2.3 Decision tree model.

Table 2.1 Input variables used in the decision tree model

Model input variable	Base case estimates
Suspected out-patient case is caused by malaria[1–5]	0.46
Proportion of out-patient cases under 5 years of age[6]	0.4
Drug doses[7]	
Chloroquine	25 mg/kg
SP	25 mg/kg
Amodiaquine	25 mg/kg
Quinine	2100 mg/kg
Average weight assumed for drug cost calculations	
Age <5	10 kg
Age >5	60 kg
Drug stock-out at out-patients	0.15
Drug wastage	10%
Initial total treatment failure in under 5s (from sentinel site data)	
Chloroquine	0.50
SP	0.14
Amodiaquine	0.05
Quinine	0.00
Initial total treatment failure in over 5s (approximated assuming that the TTF in over 5s will be half the TTF in under 5s)	
Chloroquine	0.25
SP	0.07
Amodiaquine	0.02
Quinine	0.00
Compliance (Abdulla unpublished data and Slutsker et al. 1994[8])	
Chloroquine	0.65
SP	0.88
Amodiaquine	0.65
Quinine	0.40
Non-compliers for whom treatment is effective	
Chloroquine	0.2
SP	0
Amodiaquine	0.2
Quinine	0.2
Develop severe malaria if early treatment failure	
Age <5	0.300
Age >5	0.010
Develop severe malaria if late treatment failure	
Age <5	0.043
Age >5	0.010
Proportion of total treatment failure that are early treatment failure	0.43

Table 2.1 (continued)

Model input variable	Base case estimates
Seek out-patient care if treatment failure and uncomplicated[9]	0.48
Proportion of return visits where second-line drug is available[6]	0.06
Seek in-patient care if treatment failure and severe[9]	0.48
Cost per in-patient visit[10]	US$13.38
Percentage of in-patient costs which are variable	22.5%
Case fatality rate if seek formal in-patient care[6]	
Age <5	0.029
Age >5	0.024
Case fatality rate if severe and do not seek formal in-patient care	
Age <5	0.15
Age >5	0.07

[1] Hill et al. 1996; [2] Olivar et al. 1991; [3] Stein et al. 1985; [4] Guiguemde 1997; [5] Brinkman et al. 1991; [6] Ministry of Health 1998; [7] WHO 1995; [8] Slutsker et al. 1994; [9] McCrombie 1996; [10] Health Research for Action 1999.

costs, and cost savings accrue to the Ministry of Health, although there may also be some treatment cost savings for patients as a result of more effective care. Estimates for the model input variables were drawn from published and unpublished literature from Tanzania and other African countries, and consultation with researchers and clinicians. Key decision tree model inputs are documented in Table 2.1. The cost-effectiveness of changing to the SP regimen was assessed by comparing the incremental costs and health benefits of this regimen with the chloroquine regimen, over the chosen timeframe. Two CEA measures were considered: the cost per operational failure averted and the cost per death averted (with the latter being highly tentative due to the problems of estimating the case fatality rate for severe disease without in-patient care).

Results

Costs

Using data from the Tanzanian Health Information System, scaled up to account for under-reporting, it was estimated that 10 millio out-patient diagnoses of malaria are made each year in Tanzania, and that 9 million of these would be initial visits (i.e. first visits for a given episode). Due to the occurrence of stock-outs, not all patients would receive the first-line drug.

Using an estimated stock-out rate of 15%, the number of initial visits where the first-line antimalarial was provided was estimated to be 7.7 million.

The first-line drug costs with the chloroquine regimen were estimated at US$572 000. Assuming that both chloroquine syrup and tablets were replaced with SP tablets, but that chloroquine injections were replaced with injectable quinine and SP tablets, the change in policy was estimated to increase the combined costs of first-line treatment by US$482 000 per year. Non-drug costs of implementation were estimated to total US$424 000 over an 18 month period, equivalent to US$0.01 per capita, or 1% of the total annual Ministry of Health budget for 1998/1999. Subsequent evaluation has shown this to be an underestimate; Mulligan *et al.* (2002) found that the non-drug costs of implementing the switch from chloroquine to SP in Tanzania were over US$800 000.

A conservative estimate of treatment cost savings from the use of a more effective regimen was based on an average cost per admission of US$13.38 [Health Research for Action (HERA) 1999], and the assumption that 22.5% of in-patient costs were variable. (No non-drug cost savings were included at out-patient facilities, as it was unlikely that a significant proportion of these costs would be variable in response to a change in the number of return visits.) The model predicted that in the early years following the switch, substantial in-patient cost savings could be achieved; in year 1, cost savings could recoup 80% of the incremental cost of the new regimen. Over time, potential for cost savings would be reduced as the difference between the efficacy of the two alternatives decreased.

Health outcomes

If the chloroquine regimen were maintained, resistance would continue to grow to chloroquine, leading to an increase in operational failures, severe cases and in-patient admissions (see Fig. 2.4). In the base case, the model predicted that by 2004, 75% of under fives presenting with true uncomplicated malaria would experience operational failure, 21% would become severe and 9% would be admitted. By 2009, 84% of under fives with malaria would experience operational failure, 24% would become severe and 10% would be admitted. If a change were made to the SP regimen in the year 2000, the model predicted an initial substantial improvement in all outcomes, which would then deteriorate over time as resistance to SP increased rapidly. By 2004, 40% of children under five with malaria would experience operational failure, and by 2009 this will rise to 66%. By the end of the 10 year period, health outcomes with the SP regimen would be roughly equal to those with the chloroquine regimen in 2000.

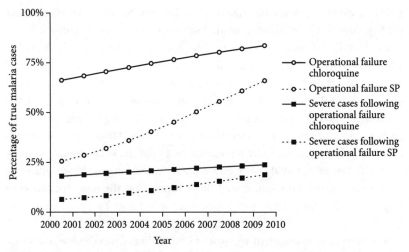

Fig. 2.4 Percentage of out-patients under five with malaria experiencing operational failure after the first visit, and becoming severe after failure with first-line treatment, with either chloroquine maintained as first line, or SP introduced as first line in 2000.

In the base case, the model predicted that average health outcomes across both age groups over the study timeframes would clearly be better using SP as first line. Table 2.2 shows the average probabilities with each regimen for the 5 year period 2000–2004 and the 10 year period 2000–2009. Using the 5 year timeframe, the average operational failure rate would be 57.8% with chloroquine but 26.5% with SP, and the average probability of becoming severe would be 8.3% with chloroquine and 3.6% with SP. Overall, this amounts to an approximately 55% improvement in health outcomes. If a 10 rather than 5 year period is considered, the difference between the two regimens is slightly reduced, as the faster growth of resistance to SP brings the outcomes closer during 2005–2009 than during 2000–2004. However, even over 10 years, the average outcomes are clearly better with SP than with chloroquine, with an improvement in health outcomes of roughly 45%. This translates to approximately 2 million fewer severe cases, 840 000 fewer in-patient admissions and an estimated 160 000 fewer deaths over the whole decade. Incorporating discounting of health benefits would make the SP regimen look relatively more attractive, as it would put more weight on earlier years when the differential in favour of SP is greater. Sensitivity analysis showed that the conclusion that health outcomes would be significantly better using SP was robust to changes in most parameters over reasonable ranges. Varying the relative resistance growth rates, while holding other input values constant, showed that the average effectiveness over the decade would only be greater with the chloroquine regimen if resistance to SP grew more than six times as fast as resistance to chloroquine.

Table 2.2 Average probabilities for health and utilization outcomes over the 5 year period 2000–2004 and the 10 year period 2000–2009 for each regimen (weighted average of patients over and under 5 years of age with true malaria, using base case model assumptions)

	Over a 5 year timeframe		Over a 10 year timeframe	
	Chloroquine	SP	Chloroquine	SP
Operational failure	57.8%	26.5%	61.2%	34.6%
Develop severe malaria	8.3%	3.6%	9.0%	5.1%
In-patient admission	3.5%	1.5%	3.8%	2.2%
Death	0.8%	0.4%	0.9%	0.5%

Table 2.3 Cost-effectiveness of the SP regimen compared with the chloroquine regimen (using base case model assumptions) (US$ in 1999)

	Over a 5 year time period		Over a 10 year time period	
	Cost per operational failure averted	Cost per death averted	Cost per operational failure averted	Cost per death averted
Gross costs (considering outpatient drug costs only)	US$0.44	US$30.49	US$0.46	US$32.85
Net costs (including treatment cost savings)	US$0.15	US$10.47	US$0.20	US$13.82

Cost-effectiveness

Base case cost-effectiveness results are presented in Table 2.3 first considering out-patient drug costs only (gross) and secondly incorporating treatment cost savings (net). Considering gross costs, using the SP regimen rather than the chloroquine regimen over the 10 year period would cost US$0.46 per operational failure averted, or US$32.85 per death averted. According to these results, the change in regimen would represent a highly cost-effective use of resources in comparison with other interventions to improve health. For example, WHO has provided rough guidelines that any intervention with a cost per disability adjusted life year (DALY) averted under US$25 would be considered a highly attractive use of resources (World Health Organization 1996), which would be very roughly equivalent to US$500 per death averted—assuming approximately 20 discounted years of life lost per death averted. If treatment cost savings are included, the switch appears even more cost-effective. For example, considering all drug and non-drug cost savings over the 10 year timeframe, the cost per operational failure averted would be US$0.20, and the cost per death averted US$13.82. If the regimens are compared over the 5 rather than 10 year time-frame, all the cost-effectiveness ratios are slightly improved. Moreover, if the costs of the SP regimen were reduced, for example by reducing the proportion of treatments given as injections, the switch would appear even more cost-effective.

In the base case, a change to the SP regimen therefore appears a highly cost-effective way to improve health outcomes. However, the results have to be interpreted with caution, given the high degree of uncertainty involved.

Sensitivity analysis

As highlighted above, the estimates of the effects and costs of changing regimen are subject to considerable uncertainty. Figure 2.5 shows some examples of the sensitivity analysis conducted to test how the cost per death averted varied when uncertain parameters were changed one by one (using gross costs and a 10 year timeframe). The results were most sensitive to changes in the initial levels of resistance and the relative growth rates of resistance to SP and chloroquine. For example, reducing the initial level of chloroquine TTF in children under five from 50 to 30% (holding other variables constant) increased the cost per death averted from US$33 to US$69. Increasing the assumed ratio of the growth rate of resistance to SP relative to chloroquine from 2 to 4 increased the cost per death averted to US$104. Considering all the variations tested, the cost per operational failure averted ranged between US$0.40 and US$1.05, and the cost per death averted between US$33 and US$104. It was not possible to calculate a cost-effectiveness ratio for the scenario where SP resistance grows six times as fast as chloroquine resistance because the effects are negative, and the chloroquine regimen is therefore dominant.

Contrasting the model results with the ongoing debate

The Tanzanian government formally announced its decision to change to SP as first-line drug in mid-2000, and nationwide implementation began in mid-2001. This CEA study was one of a number of pieces of evidence that contributed to this decision. It indicated that the government could have a high degree of confidence that this change would significantly improve health outcomes over the subsequent 10 years compared with continuing with chloroquine, and that the extra expenditure incurred would be a highly cost-effective use of resources.

However, following the policy decision, considerable debate continued with, on the one hand, some critics arguing that it was unnecessary to abandon

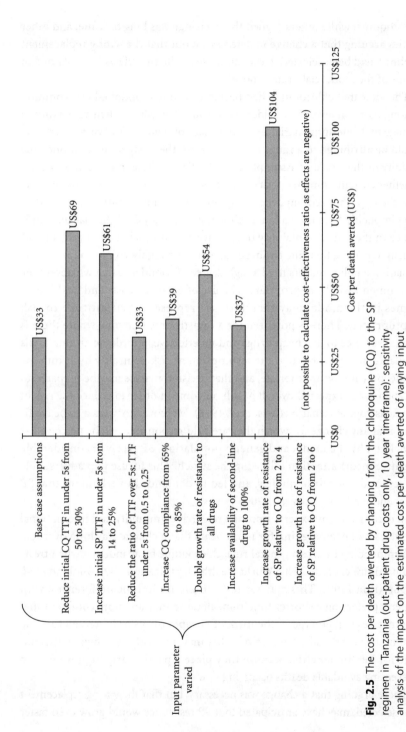

Fig. 2.5 The cost per death averted by changing from the chloroquine (CQ) to the SP regimen in Tanzania (out-patient drug costs only, 10 year timeframe): sensitivity analysis of the impact on the estimated cost per death averted of varying input parameters one by one (US$ in 1999).

chloroquine, while others argued that a change was long overdue, and other critics arguing that a change was necessary, but that the wrong replacement regimen had been selected. How can these conflicting views be explained in terms of the model elaborated above?

The view that chloroquine had been too readily abandoned was common among national level stakeholders (Williams *et al.* 2001). Their reluctance to change first-line antimalarial, even in the face of high levels of drug resistance, could be attributed to a range of factors. First, they may have questioned the validity of the data and assumptions embodied in these models, in particular whether current estimates of drug resistance were accurate and representative, and the hypothesized impact of drug resistance on mortality. Secondly, they may implicitly have used a longer timeframe of analysis, if they lacked confidence in the future availability of effective and affordable alternatives to SP. Finally, changing first-line antimalarial policy is a highly visible policy change, so national policy makers need a high degree of confidence that whatever they recommend will be appropriate. The use of expected costs and health outcomes in the model may therefore not represent their attitude to risk appropriately. There is potential for a catastrophic outcome where there is high resistance to all cheap drugs and no effective, affordable antimalarials available. It is possible that the assumption of risk neutrality built into the model may not be appropriate, and that decision makers may be prepared to accept a lower expected overall health outcome in order to reduce the risk of the catastrophic scenario (Coast *et al.* 1998). Moreover, they need to be confident that any change for which they are held responsible will be perceived as beneficial by the media and general population. SP received considerable negative media attention following the switch. This focused on adverse side effects and poor drug quality, and led to demands in Parliament that SP be abandoned (Williams *et al.* 2003).

In contrast, many experts from the research community and international agencies had been arguing for many years that a change was long overdue, recommending that, as a general rule, chloroquine be abandoned when treatment failure exceeds 25% (World Health Organization 1994; Bloland *et al.* 1998; Kitua 1999). This may reflect a difference in time preferences, with experts preferring a shorter timeframe because they are more confident that alternatives will emerge in the form of cheaper drugs or increased funding within the next decade. Alternatively, they may implicitly use a higher discount rate for health benefits, because they place a particularly high weight on preventing avoidable deaths occurring now.

Those arguing that a change was necessary, but that the wrong replacement was selected, may have anticipated that SP resistance would grow even faster than postulated in the base case. They may also have been concerned with implications beyond the scope of the model described. Some analysts were worried that introducing SP as first line, and as a result increasing the growth rate of SP resistance, could compromise the efficacy of potential future first-line regimens, such as chloroproguanil-dapsone (Lapdap), or a combination therapy of SP or Lapdap with an artemisinin derivative, such as artesunate. It was anticipated that there would be cross-resistance between SP and Lapdap (Winstanley 2000), and experience in Southeast Asia suggested that combination therapies may be more effective at slowing the development of resistance when initial resistance levels to both drugs are relatively low (White 1999). Many national and international experts now favour an immediate switch to combination therapy using artemisinin derivatives combined with another drug with limited current resistance such as amodiaquine or lumefantrine. In terms of the model, these views imply that the choice of alternative regimens compared in the CEA was inappropriate, and the timeframe too short.

The way forward

To evaluate accurately the cost-effectiveness of drug policy change in a setting of growing drug resistance, policy makers ideally need information on the health outcomes and costs over time of a range of alternative drug regimens. However, the information they have at their disposal is generally restricted to current drug prices and limited data on current resistance levels from controlled trial settings. CEA models provide a useful framework to synthesize information on epidemiological, cost and behavioural factors over time; to estimate outcomes relevant to policy makers from the highly intermediate measures of efficacy available; and to put ranges on the likely cost-effectiveness of different regimens. However, their users should be aware that the models cannot provide definitive answers to highly complex drug policy questions. It would be more appropriate to view them as an analytical tool to help researchers and policy makers think through the issues in detail. This allows them to structure the problem, explicitly explore the trade-offs involved and pinpoint data gaps. Concern will remain about the use of such models for policy making because the degree of analyst discretion is high, and there is potential for both inaccuracies in the parameter estimates used and bias in the way the model is structured (Sheldon 1996; Buxton et al. 1997). However, where urgent policy decisions are required, but the magnitude of key variables is not known and experimental observation is not possible, modelling will remain an essential feature of such work (Buxton et al. 1997; Halpern et al. 1998).

Where analysts find they disagree with the policy recommendations from CEA results, the model provides a framework to think through exactly why this is, for example whether due to the reliability of the data or assumptions, the choice of comparators, timeframe or discount rate, or the assumed attitude to risk. Exploring the contrasting views on the Tanzanian policy change discussed above highlights that some of the areas of disagreement could be resolved by further data collection. CEA is often seen as the realm of economists, but it is clear that the most significant barrier to the production of accurate cost-effectiveness estimates is the lack of information on the health impact of given levels of resistance, and the growth rates of resistance over time and the factors that influence these rates. However, the growth rate of resistance to SP following its adoption in Tanzania in 2001 has to date been in line with that assumed in this model. The model predicted that 2.5 years after SP implementation its TTF (14 day clinical failure) would be 24.6%, which compares with an average recorded across sentinel sites of 23.1% in the first half of 2004 (R Mandike, NMCP, personal communication). Estimations of the impact of drug resistance on final health outcomes could be improved with better data on compliance with different drugs, and on treatment-seeking behaviour following treatment failure. Comprehensive evaluations of the implementation of drug policy changes would help to test the accuracy of the models in predicting both the cost and health outcomes, and improve future modelling studies.

Other contrasting views could be incorporated by extending the model to incorporate a wider range of alternative drug regimens. The debate surrounding drug policy change in Africa has been evolving rapidly. For many countries, the policy options used in the Tanzanian analysis are already out of date, where a switch to SP has already been made, or inappropriate if the simple two-way comparison does not reflect the full range of alternative regimens under consideration. The model has subsequently been extended to consider ACT, demonstrating that such combinations are likely to be cost-effective under most scenarios explored (Coleman *et al.* 2004). The model could also be extended to incorporate fully treatment seeking outside facilities; or to integrate a full model of the growth of drug resistance (Yeung *et al.* 2004). A key challenge in improving the model structure is the clear trade-off between the need for greater realism and the greater complexity that realism brings. When such analyses are presented to policy makers and experts, the number of requests for the model to be extended to be more comprehensive and realistic is usually balanced by the number of pleas for the model to be simplified, to aid transparency and comprehension by a wider audience.

Other sources of disagreement are inherently more intractable. Some relate to the accuracy of model variables for which it is not possible to collect better data. This may be due to the ethical constraints on research (e.g. measuring case fatality rates in the absence of in-patient care), or the problems of predicting the future (e.g. the future price and availability of antimalarials, or the growth rates of drug resistance in specific settings). For example, predictions that ACT costs would fall dramatically (Kindermans *et al.* 2002) have proved optimistic. Finally, but perhaps most importantly, many other sources of disagreement relate to the framing of the analysis, such as the specification of the alternatives or the timeframe considered. These choices reflect the subjective views of the analysts concerned, and cannot be addressed simply by better data or model extensions. However, they are central to an understanding of the evaluation of drug policy change. While they cannot be easily resolved, CEA models can play a crucial role in making them explicit.

Acknowledgements

We would like to thank the following organizations for their advice and support with the Tanzanian case study: the staff of the Planning & Policy Unit and the National Malaria Control Programme of the Ministry of Health, the Pharmacy Board, Mlimba Health Centre, Kilombero District Health Management Team, the Ifakara Health Research and Development Centre (IHRDC), Tanzanian Essential Health Interventions Project (TEHIP), Adult Morbidity and Mortality Project (AMMP), Medical Stores Department (MSD), Muhimbili Medical Centre, WHO Tanzania Office, WHO Regional Office for Africa, The Malaria Consortium, Centres for Disease Control and Prevention, Atlanta (CDC) and the UK Department for International Development-Eastern Africa. Funding for the Tanzanian case study was provided by the WHO Regional Office for Africa, through the Ministry of Health, Tanzania. S.A. was supported by the Swiss Agency for Development and Cooperation. C.G. and A.M. are members of the LSHTM Health Economics and Financing Programme, which receives support from the UK Department for International Development

References

Abdulla, S., Goodman, C., Coleman, P., Mubyazi, G., Kikumbih, N. and Okorosobo, T. (2000) The costs, effects and cost-effectiveness of changing the first line drug for the treatment of malaria in Tanzania: HEFP working paper 01/00, LSHTM, http://www.hefp.lshtm.ac.uk/publications/working_papers.php.

Attaran, A., Barnes, K.I., Curtis, C., d'Alessandro, U., Fanello, C.I., Galinski, M.R., Kokwaro, G., Looareesuwan, S., Makanga, M., Mutabingwa, T.K., Talisuna, A., Trape, J.F. and Watkins, W.M. (2004) WHO, the Global Fund, and medical malpractice in malaria treatment. *Lancet* **363**, 237–240.

Barat, L.M., Himonga, B., Nkunika, S., Ettling, M., Ruebush, T.K., Kapelwa, W. and Bloland, P.B. (1998) A systematic approach to the development of a rational malaria treatment policy in Zambia. *Tropical Medicine and International Health* **3**, 535–542.

Baume, C. and Macwan'gi, M. (1998) *Care-seeking for Illnesses with Fever or Convulsions in Zambia, Final Report: The BASICS Project.* USAID.

Bloland, P.B., Kazembe, P.N., Oloo, A.J., Himonga, B., Barat, L.M. and Ruebush, T.K. (1998) Chloroquine in Africa: critical assessment and recommendations for monitoring and evaluating chloroquine therapy efficacy in sub-Saharan Africa. *Tropical Medicine and International Health* 3, 543–552.

Brinkman, U., and Brinkman, A. (1991) Malaria and health in Africa: the present situation and epidemiological trends. *Tropical Medicine and Parasitology* 42 (3), 204–13.

Buxton, M.J., Drummond, M.F., Van Hout, B.A., Prince, R.L., Sheldon, T.A., Szucs, T. and Vray, M. (1997) Modelling in economic evaluation: an unavoidable fact of life [editorial]. *Health Economics* 6, 217–227.

Cairns, J. (2001) Discounting in economic evaluation. In Drummond, M.F. and McGuire, A. (eds), *Economic Evaluation in Health Care—Merging Theory with Practice.* Oxford University Press, Oxford, pp. 236–255.

Coast, J., Smith, R.D. and Millar, M.R. (1998) An economic perspective on policy to reduce antimicrobial resistance. *Social Science and Medicine* 46, 29–39.

Coleman, P.G., Morel, C., Shillcutt, S., Goodman, C. and Mills, A.J. (2004) A threshold analysis of the cost-effectiveness of artemisinin-based combination therapies in sub-Saharan Africa. *American Journal of Tropical Medicine and Hygiene* 71, 196–204.

EANMAT (2003) The efficacy of antimalarial monotherapies, sulphadoxine-pyrimethamine and amodiaquine in East Africa: implications for sub-regional policy. *Tropical Medicine and International Health* 8, 860–867.

Foster, S.D. (1991) Pricing, distribution, and use of antimalarial drugs. *Bulletin of the World Health Organization* 69, 349–363.

Gold, M.R., Siegel, J.E., Russell, L.B. and Weinstein M.C. (1996) *Cost Effectiveness in Health and Medicine.* Oxford University Press, New York.

Goodman, C.A., Coleman, P.G. and Mills, A.J. (2001) Changing the first line drug for malaria treatment—cost-effectiveness analysis with highly uncertain inter-temporal trade-offs. *Health Economics* 10, 731–749.

Guiguemde, T.R., Ouedraogo, I., Ouedraogo, J.B., Coulibaly, S.O., and Gbary, A.R. (1997) Malaria morbidity in adults living in urban Burkina Faso. *Medicine Tropicale Marseilles* 57 (2): 165–8.

Halpern, M.T., McKenna, M. and Hutton, J. (1998) Letter to the editors. *Health Economics* 7, 741–742.

Health Research for Action (HERA) (1999) *Health Care Financing in Tanzania: Costing Study of Health Services.* Final Report, Volume I, October 1999. Laarstraat, Belgium.

Hill, J.A., Lake, S., Meek, S.R., Mehra, S., and Standing, H. (1996) *Approaches to malaria control in Africa, Part I: analysis and opportunities for malaria control support in selected countries in Africa.* London/Liverpool Consortium.

Institute of Medicine (2004) *Saving Lives, Buying Time: Economics of Malaria Drugs in an Age of Resistance.* National Academies Press, Washington, DC.

Kindermans, J., Pecoul, B., Perez-Casas, C., Den Boer, M., Berman, D. and Cox, I. (2002) *Changing National Malaria Treatment Protocols in Africa: What is the Cost and Who Will Pay?* Campaign for Access to Essential Medicines, MSF.

Kitua, A.Y. (1999) Antimalarial drug policy: making systematic change. *Lancet* 354 Supplement, Siv32.

McCrombie, S.C. (1996) Treatment seeking for malaria – a review of recent research. *Social Science and Medicine* **43**(6), 933–945.

Management Sciences for Health (1999) *International Drug Price Indicator Guide.* Management Sciences for Health, Boston.

Ministry of Health (1998) *Health Statistics Abstract, Vol. 1 Morbidity and Mortality Data.* Health Information and Research Section, Planning and Policy Department, Ministry of Health, Dar es Salaam, United Republic of Tanzania.

Ministry of Health (1999) *Summary Report of the Task Force on Antimalarial Drug Policy*, July 23, 1999. Ministry of Health, Dar es Salaam, United Republic of Tanzania.

Mulligan, J., Mandike, R., Palmer, N., Williams, H.A., Abdulla, S., Mills, A. and Bloland, P. (2002) *Costs of implementing the policy change of first line drug for malaria in Tanzania.* Paper presented at the 3rd Pan-African Conference on Malaria, Arusha, Tanzania, November 2002.

Murray, C.J., Evans, D.B., Acharya, A. and Baltussen, R.M. (2000) Development of WHO guidelines on generalized cost-effectiveness analysis. *Health Economics* **9**, 235–251.

Olivar, M., Develoux, M., Chegou Abari, A., and Loutan, L. (1991) Presumptive diagnosis of malaria results in a significant risk of mistreatment of children in urban Sahel. *Transactions of the Royal Society of Tropical Medicine and Hygiene*, **85**(6), 729–30.

Sheldon, T.A. (1996) Problems of using modelling in the economic evaluation of health care. *Health Economics* **5**, 1–11.

Shretta, R., Walt, G., Brugha, R. and Snow, R.W. (2001) A political analysis of corporate drug donations: the example of Malarone® in Kenya. *Health Policy and Planning* **16**, 161–170.

Slutsker, L., Chitsulo, L., Macheso, A. and Steketee, R.W. (1994) Treatment of malaria fever episodes among children in Malawi: results of a KAP survey. *Tropical Medicine and Parasitology* **45**, 61–64.

Stein, C.M., and Gelfand, M. (1985) The clinical features and laboratory findings in acute *plasmodium falciparum* malaria in Harare, Zimbabwe. *Central African Journal of Medicine* **31**(9), 166–70.

Trape, J.F., Pison, G., Preziosi, M.P., Enel, C., Desgrees du Lou, A., Delaunay, V., Samb, B., Lagarde, E., Molez, J.F., and Simondon, F. (1998) Impact of chloroquine resistance on malaria mortality. *Compte Rendu de l'Academie des Sciences Paris, Sciences de la Vie* **321**, 689–697.

White, N. (1999) Antimalarial drug resistance and combination chemotherapy. *Philosophical Transactions of the Royal Society of London Series B*, 739–749.

White, N.J. and Olliaro, P.L. (1996) Strategies for the prevention of antimalarial drug resistance: rationale for combination chemotherapy for malaria. *Parasitology Today* **12**, 399–401.

Williams, H.A., Trupin, C. and Mwisongo, A. (2001) *A case study of the change in national malaria treatment guidelines in Tanzania: Preliminary findings.*: Paper presented at the annual meetings of the American Society for Tropical Medicine and Hygiene, Atalanta, GA, 13 November.

Williams, H.A., Masanja, I., Metta, E., Msechu, J. and Khatibu, R. (2003) *Sulfadoxine-Pyrimethamine (SP) Implementation in Tanzania: Two Year Evaluation.* IMPACT-Tz Debriefing for Stakeholders, 14 November 2003. Dar es Salaam, Tanzania.

Winstanley, P.A. (2000) Chemotherapy for falciparum malaria: the armoury, the problems and the prospects. *Parasitology Today* 16, 146–153.

World Health Organization (1994) *Antimalarial Drug Policies: Data Requirements, Treatment of Uncomplicated Malaria and Management of Malaria in Pregnancy*. World Health Organization-Division of Control of Tropical Diseases, Geneva, WHO/MAL/94.1070.

World Health Organization (1995) *Model Prescribing Information: Drugs used in Parasitic Diseases*. Geneva: WHO.

World Health Organization (1996) *Investing in Health Research and Development: Report of the Ad Hoc Committee on Health Research Relating to Future Intervention Options*. World Health Organization, Geneva. TDR/Gen/96.1.

World Health Organization/CTD (1996) *Assessment of Therapeutic Efficacy of Antimalarial Drugs for Uncomplicated Falciparum Malaria in Areas with Intense Transmission*. World Health Organization, Geneva. WHO/MAL/96.1077.

World Health Organization RMB (2003) *Improving Access to Antimalarial Medicines: Report of the RBM Partnership Meeting*. WHO/CDS/RBM/2003.44.

World Health Organization RMB (2004) Global antimalarial drug policy database—AFRO. http://mosquito.who.int/amdp/amdp_afro.htm.

World Health Organization/RBM, UNICEF, PSI and MSH (2004) *Sources and Prices of Selected Products for the Prevention, Diagnosis and Treatment of Malaria*. World Health Organization, Geneva.

Yeung, S., Pongtavornpinyo, W., Hastings, I.M., Mills, A.J. and White, N.J. (2004) Antimalarial drug resistance, artemisinin-based combination therapy, and the contribution of modeling to elucidating policy choices. *American Journal of Tropical Medicine and Hygiene* 71, 179–186.

Zucker, J.R., Lackritz, E.M., Ruebush, T.K. 2nd, Hightower, A.W., Adungosi, J.E., Were, J.B., Metchock, B., Patrick, E. and Campbell, C.C. (1996) Childhood mortality during and after hospitalization in western Kenya: effect of malaria treatment regimens. *American Journal of Tropical Medicine and Hygiene* 55, 655–660.

Chapter 3

Economic issues related to antimicrobial resistance

Ramanan Laxminarayan*

Introduction

The rise of antimicrobial resistance in recent times poses a serious threat to our ability to treat infectious diseases successfully (Cohen 1992; Levy 1992; Office of Technology Assessment 1995). Selection pressure resulting from increasing antimicrobial use has been identified as a primary causal factor, and is strongly influenced by the behaviour of individuals and institutions. More specifically, this increase is blamed on the overuse and misuse of anti-microbials by patients, physicians and the farm animal industry. From an economic perspective, antimicrobial resistance is a result of the absence of sufficiently strong incentives for individuals, physicians and drug manufacturers to consider the cost of resistance associated with antimicrobial use (Laxminarayan 2003). In this chapter, an economic perspective is used to characterize the resistance problem in both hospital and community settings, and to describe policy responses to encourage judicious use of antimicrobials. Incentives faced by patients, physicians, hospital administrators and the pharmaceutical industry with respect to antimicrobials are discussed.

Antimicrobial effectiveness as a resource

From an economic perspective, antimicrobial effectiveness (or susceptibility), the converse of antimicrobial resistance, can be thought of as a natural resource (Brown and Layton 1996) where current antimicrobial use lowers future effectiveness (McGowan 1983). This resource enables doctors to both prevent and treat infections and is therefore valuable to society. The current debate surrounding antimicrobial resistance is about whether the current rate of depletion of this resource, i.e. antimicrobial effectiveness, is greater than is optimal from society's standpoint.

When a doctor prescribes an antimicrobial, he/she evaluates the benefit and cost to the patient (and themselves) of using the antimicrobial. These benefits

* Contribution originally submitted in 2001.

(and costs) include factors such as convenience of dosing, risk of adverse events and speed of patient recovery. Admittedly, this characterization conflates the multiple criteria that a physician must evaluate when prescribing antimicrobials to a single metric, but succinctly describes the underlying decision-making process. The key issue here is that this decision may implicitly ignore the impact that antimicrobial use may have on resistance in the future when such considerations are in conflict with the perceived current benefits of antimicrobial use. In these situations, physicians may prefer to prescribe antimicrobials even when there is little or no benefit of doing so, because they may have no incentive to consider the cost to society associated with a potential increase in drug resistance. In the language of economics, antimicrobial effectiveness is an open access resource, in the same way that fish stocks or village commons are resources that are accessible to many users. Since no single fisherman or herdsman has an incentive to care about the depletion of fisheries or the commons, there is a tendency to overuse them. In the case of overfishing, the situation can be dealt with through regulations such as taxes, quotas or gear restrictions to force fishermen to take the effect of their behaviour on society into account when determining how much and when to fish. Similar mechanisms would be needed to force users of antimicrobials to take the cost of resistance into consideration.

Optimal policy for antimicrobial use, from the 'natural resource' perspective, depends to some extent on whether its effectiveness is a renewable resource (like a stock of fish) or a non-renewable resource (like petroleum). This distinction is facilitated by the biological concept of fitness cost of resistance. Fitness cost is the evolutionary disadvantage placed on resistant strains in an environment where antimicrobial selection pressure has been removed. If the fitness costs associated with resistance were large, resistant bacteria would be less likely than susceptible bacteria to survive in the absence of antimicrobials. One can then potentially remove an antimicrobial from active use to enable it to recover its effectiveness, before bringing it back into active use. Antimicrobial effectiveness would be considered a renewable resource, in much the same way as a stock of fish that is harvested periodically, but regenerates between harvest seasons. If, however, the fitness cost of resistance is zero or small, then antimicrobial effectiveness does not increase even if antimicrobial use is terminated. Antimicrobial effectiveness can be thought of as a non-renewable or exhaustible resource, similar to a mineral deposit. The magnitude of the fitness cost of resistance is still under debate, and may be context specific. While some studies have shown that fitness cost can be significant (Musher and Baughn 1977; Bennett and Linton 1986; Bouma and Lenski 1988; Seppala *et al.* 1997; Laufer and Plowe 2004), other studies have

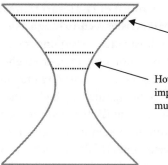

At this level of effectiveness, treating one more patient has a relatively small impact on bacterial susceptibility to the antimicrobial.

However, as susceptibility (effectiveness) declines, the impact on susceptibility of treating an additional patient is much greater.

Fig. 3.1 Logistic extraction of antimicrobial effectiveness: the hourglass analogy.

questioned if less antimicrobial use would be accompanied by a decrease in the incidence of drug resistance (Schrag *et al.* 1997; Bjorkman *et al.* 1998).

A feature of antimicrobial resistance is that the increase in resistance in response to constant use over time follows a logistic, or S-shaped path (Anderson and May 1991). Initially, the increase in resistance is gradual, but, as resistance increases, the rate of increase becomes more rapid. Translating this functional form to the natural resource metaphor, the stock of effectiveness of an antimicrobial may be modelled as an hourglass-shaped oil well, where the level of oil in the well is indicative of the effectiveness of the antimicrobial (see Fig. 3.1). The volume of oil extracted each month represents the number of patients treated each month. The oil well representation reflects an observation from the population genetics of resistance that the decrease in antimicrobial effectiveness with antimicrobial use follows a logistic path (Anderson and May 1991). Initially, the use of an antimicrobial has a fairly small effect on resistance. However, after a long period of fairly low levels of resistance, resistance is observed to increase dramatically in a fairly short span of time. These parallels are useful in the formal economic analysis of antimicrobial effectiveness as a natural resource.

Economic costs

There are at least two sources of economic costs arising from antimicrobial resistance. First, resistant infections are more expensive to treat. Studies have shown that patients infected with resistant strains of bacteria are more likely to require longer hospitalization and face higher treatment costs than patients infected with drug-susceptible strains (Holmberg *et al.* 1987; Genesis Report 1994). In fact, some large hospitals in the USA spend as much as 15% of their pharmacy budget on vancomycin, the antimicrobial of last resort to treat methicillin-resistant *Staphylococcus aureus* (MRSA). Between 1997 and 1998, empiric use of vancomycin increased 18%, at least partly in response to the increase in the prevalence of MRSA (Lavin 2000). Moreover, there is a higher risk of mortality in resistant infections. For instance, the mortality rate for patients infected with MRSA has been found to be significantly higher than for patients infected with a methicillin-sensitive strain (Rubin *et al.* 1999). A second cost of resistance is that associated with the cost of introducing new, expensive, antimicrobials to replace old ineffective ones (Office of Technology Assessment 1995). This represents forgone resources that society could deploy elsewhere (Reed *et al.* 2001). According to one estimate, between 1997 and 1998, increases in drug resistance have raised the cost of treating ear infections by about 20% (US$216 million) (Howard and Rask 2002).

The annual figure quoted most often for the economic impact of resistance in the USA ranges from US$350 million to US$35 billion (in 1989 dollars). These estimates assume 150 million prescriptions are generated each year and vary depending on, among other factors, the rate at which resistance grows with respect to increasing antimicrobial use, and the probability that a patient will die following infection with a resistant pathogen (Phelps 1989). A more recent study measured the deadweight loss associated with the loss of anti-microbial effectiveness associated with out-patient prescriptions in the USA to be US$378 million and as high as US$18.6 billion (Elbasha 1999). A report by the Office of Technology Assessment to the US Congress estimated the annual cost associated with antimicrobial resistance in hospitals, attributable to five classes of hospital-acquired infections from six different antimicrobial-resistant bacteria, to be at least US$1.3 billion (in 1992 dollars) (Office of Technology Assessment 1995). The US Centers for Disease Control and Prevention estimated that the cost of all hospital-acquired infections, including both antimicrobial-resistant and antimicrobial-susceptible strains in their figures, was $4.5 billion (for the UK, see Plowman Chapter 8). The lack of time series data on both antimicrobial use and bacterial resistance has made it difficult to estimate the dose-response relationship between antimi-crobial use and resistance, further complicating an assessment of the economic costs of resistance.

Measuring the economic burden of resistance shows only one side of the story, however, since antimicrobial use implies both costs and benefits. Effective antimicrobial treatment cures, and benefits the patient, because he/she recovers more rapidly than in the absence of treatment; as well as benefit-ing society because of the potential of successful treatment (or prophylaxis) to reduce transmission of the infection to other healthy individuals. On the cost side, antimicrobial use increases selection pressure on bacteria and decreases the effectiveness of future antimicrobial treatment. Therefore, policy makers must examine the trade-offs between the benefits and the costs of antimicrobial use when designing policies to influence their use. Currently, however, resistance costs are rarely considered even in economic evaluations of antimicrobial treatment alternatives (Coast *et al.* 1996).

The role of economics in finding solutions

The following sections describe the central economic issues that influence antimicrobial use policy in hospital and community settings. Institutional responses to the antimicrobial resistance problem, such as through the design of formulary management strategies and optimal patent rules in order to influence the behaviour of key players such as patients, physicians, hospital infection control committees and pharmaceutical firms in favour of judicious antimicrobial use, are discussed.

Managing resistance in a hospital setting

The upward trend in resistant nosocomial infections in the USA has been cause for much concern and has been attributed to growing antimicrobial use in many hospitals(McGowan 1983). Antimicrobial-resistant bacteria such as vancomycin-resistant enterococci (VRE) and MRSA are leading causes of hospital-acquired infections, and they have proved difficult to eradicate and control. One strategy used by hospitals to control antimicrobial use is to use drug formularies that limit the menu of antimicrobials available to physicians (Klem and Dasta 1996). These were originally introduced to hold down prescription drug costs, but in recent years, have assumed the added role of discouraging antimicrobial use.

In a hospital setting, there is often a choice made between two or more available antimicrobials, giving rise to the question of whether to use only one antimicrobial, both or alternate between the two in sequence (cycling) in order to minimize resistance. Using mathematical models, it is possible to show that if one were faced with choosing between two antimicrobials with independent modes of antibacterial activity, that were identical in all other respects, then the optimal strategy would be to use both antimicrobials on all patients simultaneously (Bonhoeffer *et al.* 1997). In other words, it may be short-sighted to use a single antimicrobial on all patients just because that antimicrobial appears to be the most cost-effective option. Indeed, it may be optimal, from society's point of view, to use different drugs on different, but observationally identical, patients and include among this menu of drugs some that may not be cost-effective from the individual patient's perspective (Laxminarayan and Weitzman 2002). Cycling between antimicrobials is analytically similar to long-studied questions in natural resource economics, such as those of crop rotation and cycling between two or more stocks of fish for harvesting (Niederman 1997; Laxminarayan 2000). Under this analogy, cycling may be feasible under two conditions (Laxminarayan 2000). First, there must be a fixed cost associated with maintaining an antimicrobial on the hospital formulary. If there is no fixed cost of storing, i.e. keeping an anti-microbial on the formulary, then it makes sense to maintain the greatest diversity of antimicrobials on the formulary. This minimizes the likelihood that selec-tive pressure to any single drug or class of drugs would be great enough to lead to bacterial resistance to that drug. The second condition for cycling is that there should be a cost of switching from one antimicrobial to another. If this second condition is not satisfied, then the optimal switching strategy may instantaneously switch back and forth between the two or more antimicro-bials. In the absence of these two conditions, cycling may be an inefficient strategy compared with simultaneously treating equal proportions of the population with two different drugs, even if the fitness cost of resistance is large (Bonhoeffer *et al.* 1997; Laxminarayan 2000).

If the economic conditions for cycling are met, a critical question in imple-menting this strategy relates to optimal rotation time (period of using one antimicrobial before switching to the other). The optimal rotation time would be such that at the switching point the marginal benefit associated with the difference in effectiveness between the antimicrobial that is being used and the one that is being held in reserve is equal to the marginal cost of switching between the two antimicrobials. The optimal rotation time is a function of biological parameters such as pathogen virulence and the fitness cost of resistance.

While optimal antimicrobial use is one way in which hospitals can respond to nosocomial resistance, another involves strengthening infection control measures that are already in place. For instance, infection control measures such as sequestering nursing staff to a limited number of patients and enforc-ing hand washing rules are effective methods to reduce the transmission of resistant (and sensitive) infections in hospitals, and to lower their prevalence (Austin *et al.* 1999). These policies have been shown to be capable of reducing the prevalence of resistance in hospital settings (Austin *et al.* 1999). However, stronger infection control measures may require greater commitment of resources by the hospital, and policy makers may have to make trade-offs between the cost of boosting infection control measures and the cost of reducing antimicrobial use. Further studies are required to determine the relative costs of these different policy options and their impact on reducing resistant infections in order to develop the optimal mix of strategies to reduce resistance cost-effectively.

Managing resistance in a community setting

Of the 335 million daily defined doses of antimicrobials prescribed each year in the USA, nearly 110 million are used in out-patient settings (Harrison and Lederberg 1992; Hanberger et al. 1997). Designing economic incentives to reduce antimicrobial use and resistance in the community is challenging primarily because there is no single central agent (similar to a hospital administrator or infection control committee) that is able to set and effectively enforce judicious use policy. Consequently, efforts to restrict antimicrobial use in out-patient settings have been less successful than in hospitals. The opposite appears to be the case in the UK (see House of Lords 2001).

While there are good reasons for patients both to decrease antimicrobial use and to complete a full dose of therapy, even if they were to ignore the impact of their antimicrobial use on future resistance, they may lack information to make an informed decision. From a patient's perspective, the decision to request an antimicrobial is based on two factors: the perceived benefit associated with each day of expedited recovery from infection, and the cost of the antimicrobial. With insurance coverage, and public provision, the patient is often shielded from being directly responsible for the cost of the antimicrobial. Studies have demonstrated conclusively that prior antimicrobial use is an important risk factor for acquiring a resistant infection (Hanberger et al. 1997; Castillo et al. 1998). Educating patients about the risks associated with misuse of antimicrobials could motivate rational behaviour and is therefore an important agenda to pursue. A patient who is aware of the cost of current antimicrobial use in terms of future risk of resistant infection may be more careful about demanding antimicrobials from the doctor.

A number of studies and reports have advocated clinical practice guidelines for judicious antimicrobial use in the era of resistance (Marr et al. 1988; Goldmann et al. 1996; Dowell et al. 1998, 1999). However, past experience with efforts to encourage judicious use through educational efforts or through a combination of education and clinical guidelines has been mixed (McGowan and Gerding 1996). One reason for the limited impact of guidelines is that they tend to be of an advisory nature, and may therefore be ineffective when they run counter to incentives faced by physicians in their practice of medicine. For instance, physicians may be reimbursed based on the number of patients they see and not necessarily the number of office visits that each patient makes. This encourages physicians to prescribe an antimicrobial to reduce the likelihood of a repeat office visit. Short of directly monitoring clinical practice, there are few mechanisms that the public health policy makers can use to enforce restrictions on antimicrobial use directly. Attempts to discourage antimicrobial use by admonishing physicians for overusing them are likely to face strong opposition from the medical community (Stephenson 1996; Schrader 1997). Moreover, monitoring antimicrobial prescriptions written by each physician is likely to be both expensive and unenforceable, although there have been a few exceptions.

Physicians face few incentives to withhold antimicrobials from patients. The high cost of liability in the case of treatment failure may induce physicians to err on the side of using stronger and broader spectrum antimicrobials than may be called for. This has the effect of increasing the overall community level of resistance, but the impact of each individual prescription on this level is so small that the benefit perceived by the physician of prescribing antimicrobials often outweighs the small uncertain costs associated with resistance. One solution is to design antimicrobial use guidelines that use community-specific surveillance data to minimize the overall total cost of treatment and future resistance (Laxminarayan *et al.* 1998).

Incentives faced by industry

The incentives faced by firms that manufacture antimicrobials with respect to resistance are complex. On the one hand, these firms are concerned about increasing bacterial resistance to their products and the resulting decrease in the market demand for their products. On the other hand, increasing resistance increases their financial returns from investing in new antimicrobials.

The cost of bringing a new antimicrobial agent to market is estimated to be of the order of US$300 miilon–US$450 million (Harrison and Lederberg 1992; Murray 1994). However, increasing antimicrobial resistance could increase the returns to R&D spending on new antimicrobials. In the 1980s, with many effective antimicrobials available to physicians on the market, many drug manufacturers abandoned efforts to find new antimicrobials and turned their research funding towards 'more profitable' diseases such as cancer, diabetes, arthritis and cardiovascular diseases (Stinson 1996). In fact, the last major antimicrobial class to be discovered, carbapenems, was first identified nearly two decades ago (Chopra *et al.* 1996). However, with increasing resistance, the returns to producing new antimicrobials have increased dramatically. In the early 1990s, drug firms turned their attention back to anti-infectives, and the new antimicrobials such as oxazolidinones (Zyvox) that are a result of this research activity are beginning to enter the market.

These new discoveries notwithstanding, it is apparent that the pool of potential antimicrobials is shrinking and the cost of discovering and introducing new antimicrobial classes is high and increasing (Bax 1997). Fewer than six new antimicrobials have been introduced during the past decade, and most of these are variations of the same 16 compounds that most antimicrobials are derived from. New approaches to countering resistance such as developing antimicrobials that are stable to enzymatic inactivation are likely to be prohibitively expensive (Chopra *et al.* 1996).

Patents may be the single most influential factor in production decisions made by pharmaceutical firms (Grabowski and Vernon 1992). Firms are driven to maximize profits during the course of the antimicrobial's effective patent life, i.e. the period of time between obtaining regulatory approval for the antimicrobial and the expiration of product and process patents to manufacture the drug. Given the paucity of tools at the policy maker's disposal, the use of optimal patent length and breadth to influence antimicrobial use has direct and valuable practical applicability in achieving optimal and judicious antimicrobial use. A longer effective patent life may increase incentives for a patentee to conserve resistance for the future, since the patentee enjoys a longer period of monopoly benefits from antimicrobial effectiveness. One reason why firms aggressively market antimicrobials without any apparent concern for resistance may be linked to the relatively short effective patent lives of antimicrobials.

The Kefauver-Harris Drug Amendments enacted by the US Congress in 1962 had the effect of reducing the effective patent life on antimicrobials. While they required drug firms to conduct clinical trials to demonstrate drug efficacy and safety prior to obtaining regulatory approval from the Food and Drug Administration (FDA), they exempted the manufacturers of generic antimicrobials alone from repeating these trials at the expiration of patent life (Temin 1980). Consequently, generic substitutes for patented antimicrobials have been particularly fast in entering the market, resulting in strong price competition that may have undesirable consequences in the case of antimicrobials (Grabowski and Vernon 1992). Although additional testing may be a waste of economic resources, one solution to the issue of extremely short effective patent lengths would be to increase them under the provisions of existing law. For instance, the Drug Price Competition and Patent Term Restoration Act of 1984 extends the patent life on antimicrobials (and other drugs) by 5 years. However, this extension is not permitted to exceed 14 years of effective patent life. In a parallel development, the General Agreement on Trade and Tariffs (GATT) extended 20 year patent protection to new drugs (Office of Technology Assessment 1995).

Patent scope is a critical parameter that influences the extent of monopoly power assigned to a patentee. When resistance is a significant problem, other things being equal, it may be optimal to assign broader patents to antimicrobials that cover an entire class of antimicrobials. Society's benefit from preserving effectiveness may outweigh the societal cost of greater monopoly power associated with broader patents by preventing many firms from competing (inefficiently) for the same stock of effectiveness (Laxminarayan 1999). Moreover, broader patents could increase the return to finding new classes of antimicrobials and encourage investment in research and development. A 1995 report to the US Congress warned of the growing costs of antimicrobial resistance and suggested that changes in the patent laws governing antimicrobials might be an effective way to increase the stake of pharmaceutical manufacturers in antimicrobial resistance, but did not address the issue of patent scope (Office of Technology Assessment 1995).

Subtherapeutic antimicrobial use in farm animal feed

Antimicrobials are used in the animal industry for improving feed efficiency and rate of weight gain, and for disease prevention and treatment. There is growing evidence that antimicrobial use for growth promotion in animals also contributes to the pool of resistant pathogens that put humans at risk (Bates *et al.* 1994; Gordts *et al.* 1995; National Research Council 1999; Wegener *et al.* 1999). For instance, there has been a sharp increase in the prevalence of fluoroquinolone-resistant *Campylobacter jejuni* in both poultry meat and infected humans since flouroquinolones were approved for use in poultry (World Health Organization 1997).

However, there is some uncertainty about the magnitude of the effect that antimicrobial use in animals has on selecting for resistant organisms that infect humans and the size of this effect relative to that caused by antimicrobial use in humans. A recent report by the World Health Organization (WHO) calls for the termination of the subtherapeutic use in animals of any antimicrobial agent that is either itself used in humans or known to select for cross-resistance to antimicrobials used in humans (World Health Organization 1997). Many countries in Europe have either banned or restricted the use of antimicrobials for this purpose, and there is pending legislation in the US Congress with this objective. While the use of antimicrobials as growth promoters in farm animals increases the likelihood that resistance will arise in infections in humans, a secondary effect is that the depletion of effectiveness by antimicrobial use in animals may encourage greater antimicrobial use in humans, because use in animals diminishes the value of preserving effectiveness for the future. Therefore, the threat of depletion of effectiveness caused by antimicrobial use in animals reduces incentives for pharmaceutical firms that manufacture antimicrobials for use in humans to conserve the effectiveness of their product.

Subtherapeutic antimicrobial use reduces the cost of raising cattle or poultry, and thereby benefits both producers and consumers. The benefit of antimicrobial use in animals is diminished to the extent by which there are substitutes for antimicrobials in raising animals, such as better hygiene. The resistance-related costs of subtherapeutic antimicrobial use in farm animals must be balanced against the benefit to society of such use. Even if the gains of antimicrobial use in animals outweigh the losses (and there is no evidence to support this), it is possible that the 'gainers' from permitting such use (producers and consumers of meat and poultry) may be quite different from the 'losers' (sick patients).

Costs of resistance in the developing world

Bacterial resistance to inexpensive, broad-spectrum antimicrobials is increasing in developing countries and is cause for particularly serious concern (Okeke *et al.* 1999). Although selection pressure of antimicrobials is currently low in developing countries, this is expected to rise with rising incomes. For instance, macrolide use in children in China may be preferred to the use of β-lactams, and in the large cities of Beijing and Shanghai, the highest global rates of macrolide resistance are encountered in nasopharyngeal isolates from children. Tetracycline use remains widespread in developing countries, and even in isolates from children, relatively higher rates of tetracycline resistance than of β-lactam or macrolide resistance may be encountered in poor African countries, such as the Central African Republic.

The health consequences of resistance may be greater in developing countries because of the unaffordable costs of new antimicrobials necessitated by growing resistance to older drugs. Unlike in developed countries, where a large section of the population can afford more effective and expensive alternatives, drug resistance in developing countries could significantly increase mortality from common infectious diseases. A comparable situation has already developed with respect to malarial resistance, where most strains of the malarial parasite in Africa and Southeast Asia are highly resistant to most affordable and commonly available antimalarials (Bjorkman and Philipps-Howard 1990; Brinkmann and Brinkmann 1991; Wernsdorfer 1991; see Goodman *et al.* Chapter 2). Finally, exacerbating factors such as poor hygiene, lack of reliable water supply and an increase in the number of immunocompromised patients attributable to the ongoing human immunodeficiency virus (HIV) epidemic are likely to increase the cost of antimicrobial resistance further still (Bax 1997).

Directions for future research

Since resistance is primarily caused by selective pressure on sensitive strains of bacteria, it is likely to remain an issue as long as we use antimicrobials. The importance of scientific research in providing a reliable foundation, on the basis of which sound economic policies may be formulated, cannot be understated. With an increasing number of surveillance programmes at work, more complete data on the impact of antimicrobial use on resistance as well on the socio-economic factors that mediate this relationship are becoming available. These data will be useful in accurately estimating the relationships between antimicrobial use and resistance, which in turn will help quantify the social costs of resistance. Also, quantifying the relationship between subtherapeutic use of antimicrobials in animals and resistance in humans could further clarify the economic trade-offs associated with the use of antimicrobials as growth promoters in farm animal feed.

A number of policy questions that remain unanswered are open to economic analysis, and could benefit from further research. These fall into four broad categories. The first deals with the issue of optimal antimicrobial use when antimicrobial effectiveness is treated as a societal resource. For instance, the problem of optimal use of antimicrobials in a community setting remains to be addressed. Ideally such an analysis would require taking into consideration both patient and physician behaviour in an out-patient setting to determine optimal antimicrobial therapy. From the practitioner's perspective, it may be useful to determine separate cost-effective empiric antimicrobial treatment strategies by geographical region using local surveillance data for resistance (Dowell *et al.* 1998).

Secondly, economic analysis can help in the design of incentives for antimicrobial users to encourage judicious use of antimicrobials. Implementing judicious antimicrobial use guidelines developed by federal and state agencies is difficult by mandatory rule because of practical problems in monitoring individual physicians or patients to ensure compliance. In this situation, economic instruments such as taxes, subsidies and optimally designed prescription drug insurance programmes may ensure that incentives faced by individual physicians and patients are aligned with the interests of society.

Thirdly, economic analysis may be useful in analysing the behaviour of pharmaceutical firms in investing in the development of new antimicrobials and the impact of patent and drug approval rules on their incentives to do so. While extending patent length and scope may give firms a greater incentive to consider resistance, the benefits to society from doing so must be weighed against the social cost associated with monopoly distortions and altered incentives to innovate.

Finally, there is an unfilled gap in quantifying the net social costs of resistance in a manner that takes into account the important benefits of antimicrobial use and the complex biological dynamics of drug resistance.

References

Anderson, R.M. and May, R.M. (1991) *Infectious Diseases of Humans: Dynamics and Control.* Oxford University Press, New York.

Austin, D.J., Bonten, M.J.M. *et al.* (1999) Vancomycin-resistant enterococci in intensive-care hospital settings: transmission dynamics, persistence, and the impact of infection control programs. *Proceedings of the National Academy of Sciences of the USA* **96**, 6908–6913.

Bates, J., Jordens, J. *et al.* (1994) Farm animals as putative reservoir for vancomycin resistant enterococcal infections in man. *Journal of Antimicrobial Chemotherapy* **34**, 507–516.

Bax, R.P. (1997) Antibiotic resistance: a view from the pharmaceutical industry. *Clinical Infectious Diseases* 24 (Supplement 1), S151–S153.

Bennett, P.M. and Linton, A.H. (1986) Do plasmids influence the survival of bacteria? *Journal of Antimicrobial Chemotherapy* 18 (Supplement C), 123–126.

Bjorkman, A. and Philipps-Howard, P.A. (1990) The epidemiology of drug-resistant malaria. *Transactions of the Royal Society for Tropical Medicine and Hygiene* **84**, 177–180.

Bjorkman, J., Hughes, D. *et al.* (1998) Virulence of antibiotic-resistant *Salmonella typhimurium. Proceedings of the National Academy of Sciences of the USA* **95**, 3949–3953.

Bonhoeffer, S., Lipsitch, M. *et al.* (1997) Evaluating treatment protocols to prevent antibiotic resistance. *Proceedings of the National Academy of Sciences of the USA* **94**, 12106–12111.

Bouma, J.E. and Lenski, R.E. (1988) Evolution of a bacteria/plasmid association. *Nature* **335**, 351–352.

Brinkmann, U. and Brinkmann, A. (1991) Malaria and health in Africa: the present situation and epidemiological trends. *Tropical Medicine and Parasitology* **42**, 204–213.

Castillo, F.D., Bacquero-Artigao, F. *et al.* (1998) Influence of recent antibiotic therapy on antimicrobial resistance of *Streptococcus pneumoniae* in children with acute otitis media in Spain. *Pediatric Infectious Disease Journal* **17**, 94–97.

Chopra, I., Hodgson, J. *et al.* (1996) New approaches to the control of infections caused by antibiotic resistant bacteria—an industry perspective. *Journal of the American Medical Association* **275**, 401–403.

Coast, J., Smith, R.D. *et al.* (1996) Superbugs: should antimicrobial resistance be included as a cost in economic valuation? *Health Economics* **5**, 217–226.

Cohen, M.L. (1992) Epidemiology of drug resistance: implications for a post-antimicrobial era. *Science* **257**, 1050–1055.

Dowell, S.F., Butler, J.C. *et al.* (1998) Otitis media—management and surveillance in an era of pnemococcal resistance: a report from the Drug-resistant *S. pneumoniae* Therapeutic Working Group (DRSPTWG). *Pediatric Infectious Disease Journal* **18**, 1–9.

Dowell, S.F., Butler, J.C. *et al.* (1999) Acute otitis media: management and surveillance in an era of pneumococcal resistance—a report from the Drug-resistant *Streptococcus pneumoniae* Therapeutic Working Group. *Pediatric Infectious Disease Journal* **18**, 1.

Elbasha, E. (1999) *Deadweight Loss of Bacterial Resistance Due to Overtreatment.* Mimeo, Atlanta, pp. 1–53.

Genesis Report (1994) *The Real War on Drugs: Bacteria are Winning*. New Jersey.

Goldmann, D.A., Weinstein, R.A. *et al*. (1996) Strategies to prevent and control the emergence and spread of antimicrobial resistant microorganisms in hospitals—a challenge to hospital leadership. *Journal of the American Medical Association* 275, 234–40.

Gordts, B., Landuyt, H.V. *et al*. (1995) Vancomycin-resistant enterococci colonizing the intestinal tract of hospitalized patients. *Journal of Clinical Microbiology* 33, 2842–2846.

Grabowski, H.G. and Vernon, J.M. (1992) Brand loyalty, entry and price competition in pharmaceuticals after the 1984 drug act. *Law and Economics* 35, 331–350.

Hanberger, H., Hoffmann, M. *et al*. (1997) High incidence of antibiotic resistance among bacteria in four intensive care units at a university hospital in Sweden. *Scandinavian Journal of Infectious Diseases* 29, 607–614.

Harrison, P.F. and Lederberg, J. (eds) (1992) *Antimicrobial Resistance: Issues and Options, Workshop Report*. Forum on Emerging Infections. Institute of Medicine, Washington, DC.

Holmberg, S.D., Solomon, S.L. *et al*. (1987) Health and economic impacts of antimicrobial resistance. *Review of Infectious Diseases* 9, 1065–1078.

Howard, D. and Rask, K. (2002) The impact of resistance on antibiotic demand in patients with ear infections. In: Laxminarayan, R. (ed.), *Battling Resistance to Antibiotics and Pesticides: An Economic Approach*. RFF Press, Washington, DC, pp. 119–133.

Klem, C. and Dasta, J.F. (1996) Efforts of pharmacy to reduce antibiotic resistance. *New Horizons* 4, 377–384.

Laufer, M.K. and Plowe, C.V. (2004) Withdrawing antimalarial drugs: impact on parasite resistance and implications for malaria treatment policies. *Drug Resistance Update* 7, 279–288.

Lavin, B.S. (2000) Antibiotic cycling and marketing into the 21st century: a perspective from the pharmaceutical industry. *Infection Control and Hospital Epidemiology* 21 (Supplement), S32–S35.

Laxminarayan, R. (1999) Optimal breadth for antibiotic patents. *Economics*. University of Washington, Seattle, p. 38.

Laxminarayan, R. (2000) *Economics of antibiotic resistance: on cycling*. Presented at a conference on antibiotic resistance: Global Policies and Options. Harvard University, Cambridge MA.

Laxminarayan, R. (2003) *Battling Resistance to Antibiotics and Pesticides: An Economic Approach*. Resources for the Future, Washington, DC.

Laxminarayan, R. and Weitzman M.L. (2002) On the implications of endogenous resistance to medications. *Journal of Health Economics* 21, 709–718.

Laxminarayan, R., Jernigan, D.B. *et al*. (1998) *Using antibiotic resistance surveillance data in the optimal treatment of acute otitis media*. Presented at the Infectious Diseases Society of America 36th Annual Meeting, Denver, CO.

Levy, S.B. (1992) *The Antibiotic Paradox: How Miracle Drugs are Destroying the Miracle*. Plenum Press, New York.

Marr, J.J., Moffitt, H.L. *et al*. (1988) Guidelines for improving the use of antimicrobial agents in hospitals: a statement by the Infectious Diseases Society of America. *Journal of Infectious Diseases* 157, 869–876.

McGowan, J.E. (1983) Antimicrobial resistance in hospital organisms and its relation to antibiotic use. *Review of Infectious Diseases* 5, 1033–1048.

McGowan, J.E. and Gerding, D.N. (1996) Does antibiotic restriction prevent resistance. *New Horizons* **4**, 370–376.

Murray, B. (1994) Can antibiotic resistance be controlled? *New England Journal of Medicine* **330**, 1229–1230.

Musher, D.M., Baughn, R.E. *et al.* (1977) Emergence of variant forms of *Staphylococcus aureus* after exposure to gentamicin and infectivity of the variants in experimental animals. *Journal of Infectious Diseases* **136**, 360–369.

National Research Council (1999) *The Use of Drugs in Food Animals: Benefits and Risks.* National Academic Press, Washington, DC.

Niederman, M.S. (1997) Is 'crop rotation' of antibiotics the solution to a 'resistant' problem in the ICU? *American Journal of Respiratory and Critical Care Medicine* **156**, 1029–1031.

Office of Technology Assessment (1995) *Impact of Antibiotic-resistant Bacteria: A Report to the U.S. Congress.* Government Printing Office.

Okeke, I.N., Lamikanra, A. *et al.* (1999) Socioeconomic and behavioral factors leading to acquired bacterial resistance to antibiotics in developing countries. *Emerging Infectious Diseases* **5**, 18–27.

Phelps, C.E. (1989) Bug/drug resistance: sometimes less is more. *Medical Care* **27**, 194–203.

Reed, S., Sullivan, S. *et al.* (2001) Socioeconomic issues related to antibiotic use. In: Low, D.E. (ed.), *Appropriate Antibiotic Use.* The Royal Society of Medicine Press, London, pp. 41–46.

Rubin, R.J., Harrington, C.A. *et al.* (1999). The economic impact of *Staphylococcus aureus* in New York city hospitals. *Emerging Infectious Diseases* **5**(1).

Schrader, A. (1997) Bill would punish overprescription of antibiotics. *Denver Post* Denver, B-06.

Schrag, S.J., Perrot, V. *et al.* (1997) Adaptation to the fitness costs of antibiotic resistance in *Escherichia coli. Proceedings of the Royal Society of London, Series B* **264**, 1287–1291.

Seppala, H., Klaukka, T. *et al.* (1997) The effect of changes in the consumption of macrolide antibiotics on erythromycin resistance in group A streptococci in Finland. Finnish Study Group for Antimicrobial Resistance. *New England Journal of Medicine* **337**, 441–446.

Stephenson, J. (1996) Fighting infectious diseases threats via research: a talk with Anthony Fauci. *Journal of the American Medical Association* **275**, 173–174.

Stinson, S.C. (1996) Drug firms restock antibacterial arsenal. *Chemical and Engineering News* 75–100.

Temin, P. (1980) *Taking your Medicine: Drug Regulation in the United States.* Harvard University Press, Cambridge, MA.

Wegener, H.C., Aarestrup, F.M. *et al.* (1999) Use of antimicrobial growth promoters in food animals and *Enteroccus faecium* resistance to therapeutic antimicrobial drugs in Europe. *Emerging Infectious Diseases* **5** (3).

Wernsdorfer, W.H. (1991) The development and spread of drug-resistant malaria. *Parasitology Today* **7**, 297–303.

World Health Organization (1997) *The Medical Impact of Antimicrobial Use in Food Animals.* Report of a WHO meeting. World Health Organization, Berlin, Germany.

Chapter 4

Economic evaluation of HIV prevention activities: dynamic challenges for cost-effectiveness analysis

Lilani Kumaranayake, Charlotte Watts, Peter Vickerman and Fern Terris-Prestholt

Introduction

The culture of international public health discourse and infectious disease can be characterised in part by the reigning logic of cost-effectiveness

(Henry and Farmer 1999).

Current estimates suggest that globally there about 40 million people living with human immunodeficiency virus (HIV)/acquired immune deficiency syndrome (AIDS), and 3 million people died of AIDs in 2004. Of the nearly 5 million new infections in 2004, 2.7–3.8 million occurred in sub-Saharan Africa, where across the region the adult prevalence rates are between 6.9 and 8.3%. In a belt across Southern Africa, the epidemic is rampant, and population levels of HIV infection are high—antenatal HIV prevalence is levelling off at 40% in Gaberone, Botswana and Manzini, Swaziland, at 16% in Blantyre, Malawi, 18% in Maputo, Mozambique, 20% in Lusaka, Zambia and over 25% in Kinshasa, Zaire. Antenatal HIV prevalence is above 25% in South African 20–34 year olds, and in Windhoek, Namibia (UNAIDS 2004). However, there is also evidence of declining incidence—with declining HIV prevalence among 15–19 year olds attending antenatal services in Addis Abbaba, Kigali and Kampala. In other regions in sub-Saharan Africa, levels of infection are lower, but do not show signs of abating (UNAIDS 2004).

Driven by risky sex and widespread injecting drug use, the HIV epidemics continue to grow in Eastern Europe and Central Asia, and are spreading into populous countries such as China, Indonesia and Vietnam. In Thailand and Cambodia, who responded decisively to the epidemic in the 1990s, the antenatal HIV prevalence is now between 2 and 3%. However, even though much transmission via commercial sex has been averted, HIV infection between long-term partners has become a more prominent mode of transmission. The epidemic is South Asia is dominated by India, where nationally about 5.1 million people were infected with HIV in 2003 alone (UNAIDS 2004).

The scale of the global response to the HIV epidemic has increased rapidly in the past few years, but is still not on the scale needed to address the HIV epidemic (Schwartlander *et al.* 2001). Targets to increase access to antiretroviral treatment (ART) have also been set—with the World Health Oragnization (WHO) '3 by 5' initiative aiming to provide 3 million people with ART by 2005. Alongside this is the challenge to expand the coverage and scope of HIV prevention programmes. Given these different demands on resources, it is important that all investment in prevention achieves the maximum possible impact. Economic evaluation can be used to help inform how best to make use of limited resources. Derived from the principles of welfare economics, cost-effectiveness analysis (CEA) attempts to compare the resources ('costs') required to implement different interventions with the epidemiological impact ('effectiveness') of different options. For more than 30 years, CEA has helped determine how economic resources should be combined and allocated, and to evaluate and compare different interventions within the health sector.

Economic evaluations use economic theory to develop a systematic framework by which to assess the relative costs and consequences of different interventions. In practice, this framework can be applied to a whole range of questions such as: whether a new drug should be used for a particular treatment, whether free-standing or mobile clinics are the best way to deliver a particular service or whether priority should be placed on some types of preventive activities relative to others. The advantage of such a framework is that it allows clear identification of the relevant alternatives and makes the viewpoint (e.g. whose perspective—the provider? the consumer? society as a whole?) more explicit. The basic task of any economic evaluation is to identify, measure, value and compare the costs and consequences of alternatives being considered (Drummond *et al.* 1997). The result of an economic evaluation is a ratio of numbers representing the cost per outcome of a particular alternative. More importantly, it gives an idea of the relative magnitude of cost per outcome of the alternatives (e.g. is the difference really hundreds of dollars or a few cents?). Economic evaluation makes the comparison between alternatives explicit and transparent, and, as such, facilitates priority setting and hence resource allocation.

CEA was spearheaded onto the international public health agenda by the publication of the World Bank's 1993 World Development Report (WDR), and its background studies (Jamison *et al.* 1993; World Bank 1993). This was the first attempt to make comparisons both internationally (involving two or more countries) and globally (broader worldwide comparisons, by low- and middle-income country categorization). The influence of CEA in health policy debates has arisen for a number of reasons. While priority setting and planning have been emphasized in the health sectors since the 1960s, the greater prominence of CEA reflects the broader trend of evidence-based planning and priority setting in the context of health sector reform. Secondly, the emergence of the World Bank, an institution dominated by economists, as the largest external donor to the health sector has led to a greater emphasis on economic approaches to priority setting in low- and middle-income countries.

Despite the high demand for evidence of CEA, it is in the face of limited availability of data from low- and middle-income countries. Accordingly, there have been attempts to generalize the results of specific studies to other settings (Kumaranayake and Walker 2002). Following the re-organization of the WHO in 1998, a new programme 'Choosing Interventions: Costs, Effectiveness, Quality and Ethics' (EQC) was established as part of the Global Programme on Evidence for Health Policy. EQC aims to collaborate with international organizations to provide international guidelines for CEA intended to provide a more standardized evidence base, and addressing some of the concerns surrounding the WDR methodology (Murray *et al.* 2000). There is also ongoing work by the WHO to collect CEA data for over 100 interventions, including those related to HIV/AIDS. Comparisons of interventions between disease groups were facilitated by the development of a generic indicator—the disability adjusted life years (DALYs) saved by an intervention (World Bank 1993; Murray and Acharya 1997).

Cost-effectiveness of HIV interventions

The rapid spread of the disease both within sub-Saharan Africa and now South and East Asia has placed HIV/AIDS at the forefront of international public health resource mobilizations [e.g. The Global Fund Against AIDS, Malaria and Tuberculosis, the United Nations Special Session on HIV/AIDS (UNGASS) in 2000]. Central to the debate around how new resources should be used has been an ongoing discussion about the cost-effectiveness of alternative strategies for HIV prevention, the role of different forms of prevention intervention in countries with different levels of HIV infection, and the need to increase the provision of resources for care and treatment (Jha *et al.* 2001; Moatti *et al.* 2003). In this chapter, we review the evidence on the cost-effectiveness of different HIV prevention interventions, highlighting the particular methodological issues related to linking costs and effects, and the generalizability of cost-effectiveness findings from one setting to another.

The range of HIV/AIDS prevention interventions

A wide range of HIV prevention interventions are being used to reduce the rate of new infections (incidence) of HIV/AIDS. Prevention strategies include different methods to promote abstinence, behavioural change and condom use (such as peer education activities with different subgroups, mass media campaigns and in-school and workplace-specific education); the distribution of male and female condoms (including through social marketing, public sector distribution and community-based distribution); and initiatives to ensure a safe blood supply.

As infection with another sexually transmitted infection (STI) can facilitate HIV transmission, there are a range of interventions that aim to reduce the incidence, duration and prevalence of STI. These include the targeted treatment of groups such as sex workers and their clients—who often have high levels of STI infection, and the strengthening of public and private sector STI treatment services.

Voluntary counselling and testing (VCT) has received increased prominence due to the increasing profile of interventions to prevent mother-to-child transmission (MTCT) and options for care and management of opportunistic infections related to HIV status [e.g. preventative therapy for tuberculosis (Aisu *et al.* 1995) and treatment of the virus itself (ART)]. As part of the counselling process, VCT can help inform uninfected clients of the risks of HIV and educate HIV-positive people about preventing further transmission and how to live positively.

Pregnant HIV-infected women are at risk of transmitting HIV infection to their child either *in utero*, during delivery or whilst breastfeeding. MTCT interventions entail the routine counselling and HIV testing of pregnant women, and the delivery of antiretroviral drugs to women testing HIV positive and requesting their test results. This is generally done in facilities where women deliver and are attended by trained birth attendants. Interventions may also offer formula milk or replacement feeding strategies for HIV-positive mothers, and there are currently MTCT initiatives to enable women to access ART (Stringer *et al.* 2003).

Blood safety strategies aim to reduce the estimated 5–10% of HIV infections in developing countries that occur through the transfusion of HIV-infected blood. Strategies to ensure a safe blood supply include the selective recruitment of blood donors from low-risk populations (such as male adolescents), a reduction in the levels of unnecessary transfusion, and the testing of all blood donations for HIV antibodies before transfusion (Watts *et al.* 2000a).

The transmission of HIV through needle sharing has led to explosive HIV epidemics amongst numerous injecting drug user (IDU) populations (Rhodes *et al.* 1999). Harm reduction interventions for IDUs attempt to reduce the transmission of HIV amongst IDUs through reducing the frequency with which they share syringes or increasing the regularity with which they sterilize their syringes and needles before re-use. The interventions try to do this mainly through education and the distribution of new syringes, needles and bleach through distribution points and peer educators. Many of these interventions have been initiated over the last 10 years (Gibson *et al.* 2001) and, although no randomized controlled trials (RCTs) have been undertaken to estimate their effectiveness, there is still substantial evidence that they reduce the transmission of HIV (Gibson *et al.* 2001; MacDonald *et al.* 2003).

In general, some forms of prevention activity are tailored towards the needs of different groups. Targeted interventions generally focus on the groups most vulnerable to HIV infection and transmission (sometimes called 'core groups'), including sex workers and their clients, other high-risk occupation groups such as miners, truck-drivers and the military, and IDUs. These interventions aim to reduce rates of infection among these groups, and through this activity limit the extent to which this group contributes to more widespread levels of infection. Population-based strategies include mass media educational campaigns and the integration of HIV activities into workplace and schools.

Evidence base on the cost-effectiveness of HIV/AIDs prevention interventions

What is the evidence base about the cost-effectiveness of HIV/AIDs interventions in low- and middle-income countries? Two reviews summarize existing studies of the cost-effectiveness of different forms of HIV/AIDS interventions. Creese *et al.* (2002) reviewed more than 60 studies of prevention, care and treatment in sub-Saharan Africa. Inclusion criteria included:

+ containing data for Africa
+ measuring both cost and effectiveness
+ appearing to use standard practice methods for estimating costs and outcomes
+ appearing to include all major cost items
+ allowing a generic measure of outcome (either HIV infections prevented or DALYs gained) to be calculated.

Of the studies reviewed, only 24 qualified for inclusion in the comparative analysis.

Table 4.1 summarizes the CEA findings from their analysis. The results illustrate how the cost per HIV infection averted and cost per DALY gained

Table 4.1 HIV/AIDS intervention groups, individual interventions and standardized cost-effectiveness results, 2000 US$

Intervention groups (numbered) and individual interventions	Place and year of publication (reference)	Cost per HIV infection prevented	Cost per DALY gained*
1. Condom distribution			
Condom distribution plus STI treatment for commercial sex workers[1]	Kenya (Moses et al. 1991)	11–17	1
Female condoms:	Kenya (Homan et al. 1999)		
targeted to commercial sex workers		275	12
targeted to high-risk women		1066	48
targeted to medium-risk women		2188	99
2. Blood safety			
Hospital-based screening	Tanzania (Jacobs and Mercer 1999)	18	1
	Zambia (Foster and Buve 1995)	107	5
Strengthening blood transfusion services through:			
Defer high risk donors	Zimbabwe (McFarland et al. 1995)	18–107	1–5
Test and defer high-risk donors[2]	Zimbabwe, 1995	48–74	2–3
Rapid test	Zimbabwe, 1995	62	3
Improved transfusion practice, routine blood screening, with outreach for blood donors[3]	Lusaka, Zambia (Watts et al. 2000a)	208–256	10–12
Improved blood collection and transfusion	Tanzania (Jacobs and Mercer, 1999)	950	43
3. Peer education for commercial sex workers[4]	Cameroon (Kumaranayake et al. 1998)	79–160	4–7
4. Prevention of mother-to-child-transmission			
Single dose nevirapine—targeted	Sub-Saharan Africa (Stringer et al. 2000)	20–341	1–1210
Single-dose nevirapine[5]—universal	Uganda (Marseille et al. 1999)	308	5
ZDV Petra regimen	Uganda (Marseille et al. 1999)	143	9

ZDV CDC regimen[6]	Sub-Saharan Africa (Stringer et al. 2000)	268	9
Formula recommendation	South Africa (Soderlund et al. 1999)	268	33–75
Breastfeeding 3 months	South Africa (Wilkinson et al. 2000)	949–2198	81
Formula provision	South Africa (Soderlund et al. 1999)	2356	131
Breastfeeding 6 months	South Africa (Soderlund et al. 1999)	3834	171
		5006	218
		6355	
		21 355	731
5. Diagnosis and treatment of STIs	Tanzania (Gilson et al. 1997)	271	12
6. Voluntary counselling and testing[7]	Kenya and Tanzania (Sweat et al. 2000)	393–482	18–22

Ranges reflect:

1 Sensitivity analysis for variation in condom use, HIV transmission and efficacy.

2 Sensitivity analysis undertaken within the study to explore the changes in HIV prevalence, STI incidence and prevalence of STI history.

3 Sensitivity analysis carried out to explore the changes of adding outreach services to identify donors and varying HIV prevalence in the donor and recipient populations.

4 Sensitivity analysis undertaken within the study to explore the changes in coverage, HIV prevalence, condom use and transmission probabilities.

5 Ranges show results of an analysis undertaken to explore all plausible scenarios of costs and effects including targeted versus universal coverage.

6 Analysis was undertaken for each province, and cost-effectiveness varied among provinces, principally due to variation in HIV prevalence (which affects the costs per pregnant women identified to be eligible for the intervention). The difference in the cost-effectiveness ratios for universal and targeted coverage were also explored.

7 Study undertaken in two countries.

Source: Adapated from Creese et al. (2002).

varies widely. Costs for condom distribution ranged from US$11 to more than US$2000, while the cost per HIV infection averted for blood safety measures ranged from under US$20 to about US$1000. The cost per HIV infection prevented by diagnosing and treating other STIs averaged little more than US$270, and the cost of VTC averaged between US$400 and US$500. The costs of interventions to prevent MTCT varied the most, with prices for the cheapest, single dose drug (nevirapine) ranging from US$20 to US$341, whilst the cost-effectiveness of breastfeeding and formula interventions ranged in cost from US$4000 to more than US$20 000 per HIV infection prevented. The cost per DALY gained by interventions also varied accordingly. The cost for combined STI treatment and condom distribution was about US$1 per DALY gained.

A key limitation identified from the review of Creese et al. was the lack of studies for comparison, and the diversity of settings in which the interventions were being implemented. Although results were taken from 11 countries, for 4 forms of intervention only one study was found. No intervention was analysed in more than 4 studies and in no one country were all the interventions studied. In particular, a number of HIV prevention strategies that are being widely implemented do not have cost-effectiveness data published—most noteworthy being youth- and media-based strategies. These studies were not classified by timeframe of analysis, HIV prevalence or the method of estimating impact.

Walker (2003) reviewed the published literature on the cost and cost-effectiveness of prevention activities in all developing countries. He found 38 studies, of which 23 were from sub-Saharan African countries, five from Asian countries, three from Eastern European countries and seven studies presenting results for developing countries as a whole. No studies were found for Latin America. The review also considered a broader range of interventions relative to Creese et al. including mass media, interventions related to schools and youth, interventions working with IDUs, vaccines and hypothetical analyses to consider the potential cost-effectiveness of alternative female controlled methods of HIV prevention (microbicides). Similar to Creese et al. (2002), the majority of studies provided evidence of the costs and cost-effectiveness of preventing MTCT (10 studies), eight studies focused on VTC, eight studies focused on strengthening blood safety systems, and five studies examined the cost-effectiveness of treating symptomatic STIs. There was limited or no evidence for other prevention strategies such as mass media, working with schools and youth, working with IDUs, and interventions working with men who have sex with men. However, since this review, the results of an RCT of a youth-based intervention in Tanzania has been released (no impact on HIV was documented) (Changalucha *et al.* 2003; Ross *et al.* 2003), and analyses of the cost-effectiveness of IDU interventions have been conducted (Jacobs *et al.* 1999; Laufer 2001; Kumaranayake *et al.* 2004).

Why the limited evidence base?

This limited evidence base reflects in part the complexity of trying to estimate how specific forms of prevention activity may impact on patterns of HIV transmission. For HIV prevention, the primary impact measure for use in comparison is the number of HIV infections averted. The 'gold standard' method for quantifying the impact of an intervention is an RCT. For a community level intervention, impact is measured by randomly allocating an intervention to specific communities, and comparing patterns of HIV incidence in these settings with comparable communities that have not received the intervention. However, community RCTs for HIV prevention are time-consuming, expensive and difficult to implement, and so far have only been conducted in a limited number of settings (e.g. Grosskurth *et al.* 1995; Gilson *et al.* 1997; Wawer *et al.* 1998, 1999; Voluntary HIV-1 Counselling and Testing Efficacy Study Group 2000; Changalucha *et al.* 2003; Ross *et al.* 2003).

An alternative is to use mathematical modelling, in combination with epidemiological intervention-specific and behavioural data, to estimate how specific changes in reported behaviour or improvements in STI treatment may translate into averting HIV infection. For blood safety or MTCT interventions, it is relatively straightforward to estimate the extent of HIV transmission averted through the effective screening or blood, or the delivery of nevirapine to an HIV-infected pregnant women.

However, because of the ongoing nature of sex and the dynamic nature of infectious disease transmission, calculating the full impact of other forms of HIV prevention interventions requires that both the infections averted among people having direct contact with the intervention and the secondary infections averted because the chain of transmission has been broken must be estimated. The mathematical models used to do this use behavioural, epidemiological and intervention-specific data to make projections about the patterns of HIV transmission with and without the intervention. Comparisons are used to obtain estimates of HIV impact. This is a more complex calculation, but is necessary, as if one only considers the direct benefits to groups in contact with an intervention, the overall impact on HIV prevention may be greatly under- or overestimated (Watts *et al.* 2001).

Challenges to linking costs and effects for HIV/AIDS prevention interventions

The dynamic nature of HIV transmission raises several methodological questions associated with what are the appropriate methods to link cost and effectiveness data. At present, there is a limited body of evidence which combines this technical level of modelling analysis with intervention- and country-specific intervention cost and output data, or uses these data to explore methodological aspects of CEA. Drawing upon existing research conducted by the *HIV Tools* Research Group at the London School of Hygiene and Tropical Medicine and the published literature, we discuss below several methodological issues. The *HIV Tools* Research Group uses economic analysis, mathematical modelling and behavioural research to explore applied issues in HIV/AIDS planning and intervention evaluation in low- and middle-income countries. As part of this work, guidelines on costing different HIV prevention activities have been developed (Kumaranayake *et al.* 2000), data on the costs of a range of prevention interventions have been compiled and several mathematical epidemiological models have been developed to estimate the effectiveness of specific interventions (Vickerman and Watts 2002, www.hivtools.lshtm.ac.uk/models.htm).

Measuring cost-effectiveness: static or dynamic perspective?

Many existing CEAs use static models to estimate how an intervention impacts on HIV transmission. These include the only existing study on the cost-effectiveness of VCT (Sweat *et al.* 2000), a study of a sex worker intervention in Kenya (Moses *et al.* 1991) and studies of IDUs (Jacobs *et al.* 1999; Laufer 2001). To illustrate the extent to which such static estimates of impact

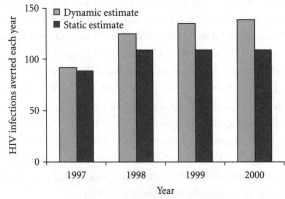

Fig. 4.1 Project effectiveness in Belarus over a 4 year period.

Source: Re-analysis of data from Vickerman and Watts (2002).

may influence cost-effectiveness, Table 4.2 shows the impact and cost-effectiveness estimates of three targeted strategies (targeting commercial sex workers and IDUs) implemented in different settings. Both static and dynamic estimates of HIV infections averted are presented. For both the static and dynamic examples, the costs associated with the intervention are identical, regardless of whether a static or dynamic perspective is adopted. The findings illustrate how, for these examples of targeted interventions that focus on vulnerable groups, failing to take account of secondary infections results in a 10–140% underestimate of cost-effectiveness. More generally, the direction of the bias associated with using a static estimate of impact will differ between settings, and between different forms of intervention. Where there is little competing source of HIV risk among the sexual partners of the groups targeted by an intervention, a static estimate is likely to underestimate intervention impact. Where there are large, competing potential sources of HIV risk that are not adequately incorporated into a static analysis, impact may be overestimated.

Time horizon: measuring duration of impact relative to investment of resources

A related issue associated with using a dynamic perspective to estimate how an intervention may impact on a chain of HIV transmission is the timeframe that is used to measure effectiveness relative to the timing of the investment of resources. If we measure the cost-effectiveness of a project simply by using one year of costs and one year effectiveness, this allows a very short timeframe for the dynamic effect of averting secondary infections to occur. However, if we consider longer timeframes for effects, we must also take into account the resources required to sustain a project's impact in subsequent years (such as the ongoing provision of information and condoms). In Table 4.3, we illustrate how the projected cost-effectiveness of the Cameroon sex worker intervention shown in Table 4.2 varies depending upon the underlying assumptions used in the analysis.

In scenario A, we present the static and dynamic cost-effectiveness estimates, allowing for a 1, 2 and 3 year time horizon for effects, but only a 1 year timeframe for costs. As would be expected, including a longer timeframe of effect substantially improves the cost-effectiveness estimates—with the dynamic cost-effectiveness measure improving by 75% by the third year.

However, for this example, it is not realistic to assume that programme impact can be sustained without any additional investment in resources after the first year. As the condom use achieved by the intervention relies on the continued supply of condoms, the costing needs to reflect that, at a minimum, these supplies continue to be available. In scenario B of Table 4.3, the required

Table 4.2 Differential estimates of cost-effectiveness of HIV/AIDS interventions by static and dynamic measures of effectiveness

Intervention	Initial HIV prevalence	Timeframe for analysis	Costs (US$)	Static estimate of HIV infections averted	Dynamic estimate of HIV infections averted	Cost-effectiveness: cost (US$) per HIV infection averted (static measure of impact)	Cost-effectiveness: cost (US$) per HIV infection averted (dynamic measure of impact)
Intervention targeting CSWs, Yaounde, Cameroon[1]	CSW	1 year	50 000	182	443	275	113
Intervention targeting IDUs, Svetlogorsk, Belarus[2]	IDU	2 years	40 473	198	217	204	183
Intervention providing STI treatment for sex workers in Johannesburg, South Africa[3]	CSW	1 year	110 301	37	90	2981	1226

[1] Intervention in Cameroon targeting 9000 commercial sex workers (CSWs) (Kumaranayake et al. 2000).

[2] Intervention in Belarus targeting injecting drug users (IDUs). Estimate of cost and impact assumes no gap in service delivery (Vickerman and Watts 2002; Walker et al. 2001; Kumaranayake et al. 2003). Costs have been purchasing-power parity adjusted to reflect cost structures in Sub-Saharan Africa.

[3] The static estimate is only infections averted in sex workers and clients. The dynamic estimate includes infections averted in the whole population (Terris-Prestholt et al. 2003).

Table 4.3 Effect of duration on impact and cost-effectiveness estimates: case study of the Cameroon sex worker intervention

	Total costs (US$)	Cumulative HIV infections averted		Cost-effectiveness [cost (US$) per HIV infection averted)	
		Static	Dynamic	Static	Dynamic
Scenario A					
Year 1	50 000	182	443	275	113
Year 2	50 000	365	1116	137	45
Year 3	50 000	548	1765	91	28
Scenario B					
Year 1	50 000	182	443	275	113
Year 2	56 000	365	1116	153	50
Year 3	62 720	548	1765	114	36
Scenario C					
Year 1	50 000	182	443	275	113
Year 2	100 000	365	1116	274	90
Year 3	150 000	548	1765	274	85

Scenario A was a 1 year investment in resources and differential measures of effectiveness. Scenario B includes costs of condoms. Scenario C assumes that programme investment is the same in each of 3 years. Adapted from Kumaranayake *et al.* (2000).

costs of ensuring adequate condom supplies to the target population for each of the three years is included. In this case, we still see that the cost-effectiveness measures continue to improve with longer timeframes. However, if as research suggests, that behaviour change needs to be supported by ongoing intervention activity and outreach, the actual degree of resources that are required to sustain an impact in subsequent years may be greater. For this reason, in the most conservative case (scenario C), we estimate cost-effectiveness assuming full resources continue to be invested in each year to reach the targeted group of commercial sex workers. In this case, the static cost-effectiveness ratio remains constant but the dynamic cost-effectiveness estimate continues to improve—with the dynamic cost-effectiveness measure improving by 25% by the third year. These examples illustrate how a simple difference in the way in which costs and effects are calculated can lead to striking differences in assessments of cost-effectiveness, with, for these targeted interventions, impact and cost-effectiveness increasing over longer time periods.

Consequently, an assessment of the relative cost-effectiveness of different interventions may vary, depending upon the timeframes used for the analysis, and the extent to which the dynamic effects of an intervention are incorporated. Traditionally, RCTs are implemented over a 2–3 year timeframe. In reality, the impact and cost-effectiveness of interventions may be greater if longer timeframes are used. In particular, it has been argued that for population strategies, including youth-focused strategies that aim to influence long-term patterns of sexual behaviour, longer time horizons for evaluation are needed (Changalucha *et al.* 2003; Ross *et al.* 2003).

The context-specific nature of cost-effectiveness analysis

The limited body of evidence on the cost-effectiveness of different interventions implemented in different settings also makes it difficult to assess the generalizability of findings between settings. In particular, cost-effectiveness results are likely to be highly context specific. Intervention costs for similar interventions implemented in different settings will be influenced by many factors, including the degree of instrastructure, salary and transport cost variation between settings. An intervention's impact on HIV transmission will be influenced by many factors, including the coverage achieved by an intervention in a particular setting, the degree to which behaviour change can be achieved and sustained, and the extent to which the intervention's activities are complemented by other forms of prevention activity.

A key contextual factor influencing the impact and cost-effectiveness of an intervention is the underlying prevalence of HIV infection among the groups targeted by an intervention and their sexual partners.

To illustrate the degree to which HIV prevalence affects cost-effectiveness, Fig. 4.2 shows modelled projections of how the cost-effectiveness of

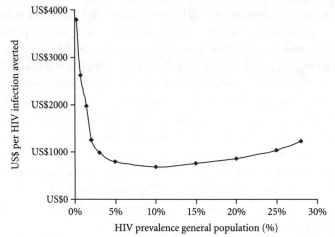

Fig. 4.2 Variation in estimates of cost-effectiveness of STI treatment by HIV prevalence in Hillbrow, Johannesburg.

Source: Terris-Prestholt *et al.* (2003). 'Are targeted HIV prevention activities cost-effective in high prevalence settings?' Results from Johannesburg, South Africa.

implementing brothel-based syndromic STI treatment for sex workers in Johannesburg varies by the prevalence of HIV infection in the general population (Terris-Prestholt *et al.* 2003). The curve is U-shaped, with cost-effectiveness being best at prevalence rates of between 5 and 15% (with the corresponding sex worker prevalence rates of between 27 and 60%). This is because at very low and very high HIV prevalences, the number of infections averted by the targeted STI intervention becomes smaller. This illustrates how targeted STI interventions are most cost-effective when the there is a large prevalence difference between the high-risk group and the general population. At higher general population prevalences, the main transmission is no longer between high-risk groups and the general population, and the cost-effectiveness is reduced. In this situation, non-targeted interventions may be equally cost-effective. At low general population prevalences, fewer HIV infections are averted because the dynamics of HIV infection are much slower at this stage of the epidemic. However, if the intervention failed to prevent the epidemic from progressing, then the cost-effectiveness would improve as the project was viewed over a longer timeframe.

This example illustrates how the cost-effectiveness of different interventions within a particular setting will change as the epidemic evolves in a particular setting. Consequently, the mix of interventions will need to change over the course of the epidemic, with priorities for intervention shifting between population subgroups, and from more targeted to broader population-focused interventions as the patterns of HIV incidence change over time (Kumaranayake and Watts 2000; Pisani *et al.* 2003).

This example illustrates one critical debate in priority settings for HIV prevention, which has centred around the degree to which interventions are targeted to groups most vulnerable to HIV infection, including commercial sex workers and their clients, and IDUs, or whether interventions aimed more broadly at the wider population should be prioritized (Ainsworth and Teokul 2000; Grosskurth *et al.* 2000; Jha *et al.* 2000). At the early stages of an epidemic, it is widely acknowledged that the greatest gains can be achieved by focusing resources on those most vulnerable to infection and/or those who have the greatest potential to contribute to the more widespread transmission of HIV infection. However, in settings where the HIV epidemic is more generalized, there is debate about the extent to which prevention resources should be used for targeted interventions, rather than invested in more population focused interventions.

Conclusions

One of the main challenges related to priority setting and resource allocation for HIV prevention efforts is the limited evidence base on the cost-effectiveness of different forms of intervention implemented in different settings, and at different stages of the HIV epidemic. The current evidence base on HIV prevention cost-effectiveness is limited, and there is need for further economic analysis of different forms of intervention. The analysis in this chapter also highlights that the available evidence is likely to be very context specific, with the generalizability of findings potentially being relatively limited. Since much of the analysis has used different approaches and timeframes, the comparability of findings between settings may also be different. Our analysis related to the matching of costs and effects suggests that the existing evidence base has been short term in nature, and used a variety of approaches to estimate intervention impact. A clearer specification of the context and the stages of the HIV epidemic in which each intervention is being implemented and the time horizons over which costs and effects are measured can be used to understand better the existing base and the potential biases in the findings, and to draw conclusions for policy. This longer timeframe may differentially impact and improve the cost-effectiveness of broader population-based interventions or may also improve targeted interventions. As the HIV epidemic evolves in different settings, future challenges for CEA include assessments of how most efficiently to share resources between targeted and more widespread infections; how to balance short- and long-term benefits of different forms of intervention; and how to capture and reflect the potential complementarities and synergies between different aspects of HIV prevention.

References

Ainsworth, M. and Teokul, W. (2000) Breaking the silence: setting realistic priorities for AIDS control in less developed countries. *Lancet* **356**, 35–40.

Aisu, T., Raviglione, M.C., van Praag E. *et al.* (1995). Preventive chemotherapy for HIV-associated tuberculosis in Uganda: an operational assessment at a voluntary counselling and testing centre. *AIDS* **9**, 267–273.

Changalucha, J., Ross, D., Everett, D. *et al.* (2003) *A randomised controlled trial of an adolescent sexual and reproductive health intervention programme in rural Mwanza, Tanzania: 3. Results: Biomedical outcomes (Abstract 699).* Presented at the 2003 ISSTDR (International Society for Sexually Transmitted Diseases Research) Congress, Ottawa.

Creese, A., Floyd, K., Alban, A. and Guinness, L. (2002) Cost-effectiveness of HIV/AIDS interventions in Africa: a systematic review of the evidence. *Lancet* **359**, 1635–1642.

Drummond, M.F., O'Brien, B., Stoddart, G.L. and Torrance, G.W. (1997) *Methods for the Economic Evaluation of Health Care Programmes.* Oxford Medical Publications, Oxford.

Foster, S. and Buve, A. (1995) Benefits of HIV screening of blood transfusions in Zambia. *Lancet* **346**, 225–227.

Garnett G. and Anderson R. (1995) Strategies for limiting the spread of HIV in developing countries: conclusions based on studies of the transmission dynamics of the virus. *Journal of Acquired Immune Deficiency Syndrome* **9**, 500–513.

Gibson, D.R., Flynn, N. and Perales, D. (2001) Effectiveness of syringe exchange programs in reducing HIV risk behavior and HIV seroconversion among injecting drug users. *AIDS* **15**, 1329–1341.

Gilson, L., Mkanje, R., Grosskurth, H. *et al.* (1997) Cost-effectiveness of improved treatment services for sexually transmitted diseases in preventing HIV-1 infection in Mwanza Region, Tanzania. *Lancet* **350**, 1805–1809.

Grosskurth, H., Mosha, F., Todd, J. *et al.* (1995) Impact of improved treatment of sexually transmitted diseases on HIV infection in rural Tanzania: randomised controlled trial. *Lancet* **346**, 530–536.

Grosskurth, H., Gray, R., Hayes, R., Mabey, D. and Wawer, M. (2000) Control of sexually transmitted diseases for HIV-1 prevention: understanding the implciations of the Mwanza and Rakai trials. *Lancet* **355**, WA8–WA14.

Henry, C. and Farmer, P. (1999) Risk analysis: infections and inequalities in a globalising era. *Development* **42**, 31–34.

Homan, R.K., Visness, C., Welsh, M. and Schwing, P. (1999) Estimated HIV prevention and costs for female condom introduction program in alternative target audiences. Powerpoint presentation.

Jacobs, B. and Mercer, A. (1999) Feasibility of hospital-based blood banking: a Tanzanian case study. *Health Policy and Planning* **14**, 354–362.

Jacobs, P., Calder, P., Taylor, M., Houston, S., Saunders, L.D. and Albert, T. (1999) Cost effectiveness of Streetworks' needle exchange program of Edmonton. *Canadian Journal of Public Health* **90**, 168–71.

Jamison, D.T., Mosley, H., Measham, A.R. and Bobadilla, J.L. (eds) (1993) *Disease Control Priorities in Developing Countries.* Oxford Medical Publications, Oxford.

Jha, P., Nagelkerke, J.D., Ngugi, E.N., Prasada Rao, J.V., Willbond, B., Moses, S. and Plummer, F.A. (2001) Public health. Reducing HIV transmission in developing countries. *Science* **292**, 224–225.

Korenromp, E.L., van Vliet, C. *et al.* (2000) Model-based evaluation of single-round mass treatment of sexually transmitted diseases for HIV control in a rural African population. *AIDS* **14**, 573–593.

Kumaranayake, L. and Walker, D. (2002) Cost-effectiveness analysis and priority setting: global approach without local meaning? In: Lee, K., Buse, K. and Fustkian, S. (eds), *Crossing Boundaries: Health Policy in a Globalising World.* Cambridge University Press, Cambridge, pp. 140–156.

Kumaranayake, L. and Watts, C. (2000) Economic costs of HIV/AIDS prevention activities in sub-Saharan Africa. *AIDS* **14** (Supplement 3), S239–S252.

Kumaranayake L. and Watts, C. (2001) Resource allocation and priority-setting of HIV/AIDS interventions: addressing the generalised epidemic in Sub-Saharan Africa. *Journal of International Development* **13**, 451–466.

Kumaranayake, L., Mangtani, P., Boupda-Kuate, A. *et al.* (1998) Cost effectiveness of a HIV/AIDS peer education programme among commercial sex workers (CSW): results from Cameroon. 1998. Poster number 33592, Geneva World AIDS Conference 1998.

Kumaranayake, L., Pepperall, J., Goodman, H., Mills, A. and Walker, D. (2000) *Costing Guidelines for HIV/AIDS Prevention Strategies.* UNAIDS Best Practice Collection-Key Materials.

Kumaranayake, L., Vickerman, P., Watts, C.H., Guinness, L., Yaremenko, A., Balakireva, O. and Artyukh, O. (2002) Cost-effectiveness analysis: aiding decision-making in HIV prevention in the Ukraine [http://www.britishcouncil.org.ua/english/governance/Finalre1.pdf]. The British Council.

Kumaranayake, L., Watts, C., Vickerman, P., Walker, D., Zviagin, V., Samoshkin, S. and Romantosov (2004) The cost-effectiveness of HIV preventive measures among injecting drug users in Svetlogorsk. *Addiction* **99**, 1565–1576.

Laufer, F.N. (2001) Cost-effectiveness of syringe exchange as an HIV prevention strategy. *Journal of Acquired Immune Deficiency Syndrome* **28**, 273–278.

MacDonald, M., Law, M.G., Kaldor, J.M., Hales, J. and Dore, G.J. (2003) Effectiveness of needle and syringe programmes for preventing HIV transmission. *International Journal of Drug Policy* **14**, 353–357.

Marseille, E., Kahn, J.G., Mmiro, F. *et al.* (1999) Cost effectiveness of single dose nevirapine regimen for mothers and babies to decrease vertical transmission in Sub Saharan Africa. *Lancet* **354**, 803–809.

McFarland, W., Kahn, J.G., Katzenstein, D.A., Mvere, D. and Shamu, R. (1995) Deferral of blood donors with risk factors for HIV infection saves lives and money in Zimbabwe. *Journal of Acquired Immune Deficiency Syndromes and Human Retrovirology* **9**, 183–192.

McLean, A.R. and Blower, S.M. (1993) Imperfect vaccines and herd immunity to HIV. *Proceedings of the Royal Society of London, Series B* **253**, 9–11.

Moatti, J.P., N'Doye, I., Hammer, S.M., Hale, P. and Kazatchkine, M. (2003) Antiretroviral treatment for HIV infection in developing countries: an attainable new paradigm. *Nature Medicine* **9**, 1449–1452.

Moses, S., Plummer, F.A., Ngugi, E.N. *et al.* (1991) Controlling HIV in Africa: effectiveness and cost of an intervention in a high-frequency STD transmitter core group. *AIDS* **5**, 407–411.

Murray, C. and Acharya, A. (1997) Understanding DALYs. *Journal of Health Economics* **16**, 703–730.

Murray, C., Evans, D., Acharya, A. and Baltussen, R. (2000) Development of WHO guidelines on generalised cost-effectiveness analysis. *Health Economics* **9**, 235–251.

Perucci, C.A., Arca, M. *et al.* (1992) A mathematical model to evaluate the impact of a multiple-strategy preventive programme on HIV infection. In: Paccaud, F., Vader, J.P. and Gutzwiller, F (eds), *Assessing AIDS Prevention*. Selected papers presented at the international conference held in Montreux, Switzerland, October 29–November 1, 1990. Birkhauser, Basel, pp. 57–68.

Pisani, E., Garnett, G.P., Brown, T., Stover, J., Grassly, N.C., Hankins, C.A., Walker, N. and Ghys, P.D. (2003) Back to basics in HIV prevention: focus on exposure. *British Medical Journal* **326**, 1384–1387.

Rhodes, T., Stimson, G.V., Crofts, N., Ball, A., Dehne, K. and Khodakevich, L. (1999) Drug injecting, rapid HIV spread, and the 'risk environment': implications for assessment and response. *AIDS* **13** (Supplement A), S259–S269.

Robinson, N.J., Mulder, D.W., Auvert, B. and Hayes, R. (1997) Proportion of HIV infections attributable to other sexually transmitted diseases in a rural Ugandan population: simulation model estimates. *International Journal of Epidemiology* 180–189.

Ross, D., Todd, J., Changalucha, J. *et al.* (2003) *A randomised controlled trial of an adolescent sexual and reproductive health intervention programme in rural Mwanza, Tanzania: 3. Results: Knowledge, attitudes and behaviour (Abstract 698)*. Presented at the 2003 ISSTDR (International Society for Sexually Transmitted Diseases Research) Congress. Ottawa.

Schwartlander, B., Stover, J., Walker, N., Bollinger, L., Gutierrez, J.P., McGreevey, W., Opuni, M., Forsythe, S., Kumaranayake, L., Watts, C. and Bertozzi, S. (2001) Resource needs for HIV/AIDS. *Science* **292**, 2434–2436.

Soderlund, N., Zwi, A., Kinghorn, A. and Gray, G. (1999) Prevention of vertical transmission of HIV: analysis of cost effectiveness of options available in South Africa. *British Medical Journal* **318**, 1650–1656.

Stringer, J.S.A., Rouse, D., Vermund, S.H., Goldenberg, R.L., Sinkala, S. and Stinnett, A. (2000) Cost-effective use of nevirapine to prevent vertical HIV transmission in sub-Saharan Africa. *Journal of Acquired Immune Deficiency Syndrome* **24**, 369–377.

Stringer, E.M., Sinkala, M., Stringer, J.S.A., Mzyece, E., Makuka, I., Goldenberg, R.L., Kwape, P., Chilufya, M. and Vermund, S.H. (2003) Prevention of mother to child transmission of HIV in Africa. *AIDS* **17**, 1377–1382.

Sweat, M., Gregorich, S., Sangiwa, G., Furlonge, C., Balmer, D., Kamenga, C. *et al.* (2000) Cost-effectiveness of voluntary HIV-1 counselling and testing in reducing sexual transmission of HIV-1 in Kenya and Tanzania. *Lancet* **356**, 113–121.

Terris-Prestholt, F., Delaney, S., Vickerman, P., Kumaranayake, L., Rees, H. and Watts, C. (2003) *Are targeted HIV prevention activities cost-effective in high prevalence settings? Results from Johannesburg, South Africa.* Presented at the 4th World Congress of the International Health Economics Association. San Francisco, USA, 2003.

UNAIDS (2004) *AIDS Epidemic Update.* December 2004. UNAIDS/WHO, Geneva.

Van Vliet, C., Holmes, K. *et al.* (1998) The effectiveness of HIV prevention strategies under alternative scenarios: evaluation with the STDSIM model. In: Ainsworth, Fransen and Over (eds), *Confronting AIDS: Evidence from the Developing World. Selected Background Papers for the World Bank Policy Research Report.* The European Commission.

Vickerman, P. and Watts, C. (2002) The impact of an HIV prevention intervention for injecting drug users in Svetlogorsk, Belarus: model predictions. *International Journal of Drug Policy* **13**, 149–164.

Voluntary HIV-1 Counselling and Testing Efficacy Study Group (2000) Efficacy of voluntary HIV-1 counselling and testing in individuals and couples in Kenya, Tanzania, and Trinidad: a randomised trial. *Lancet* **356**, 103–112.

Walker, D. (2003) Cost and cost-effectiveness of HIV/AIDS prevention strategies in developing countries: is there an evidence base? *Health Policy and Planning* **18**, 4–17.

Watts, C., Goodman, H. and Kumaranayake, L. (2000a) *Improving the Efficiency and Impact of Blood Transfusion Services in the Context of Increasing HIV Prevalence.* Health Policy Unit, London School of Hygiene and Tropical Medicine, London.

Watts, C., Vickerman, P., Kumaranayake, L., Cheta, C., Nama, M.N., Kwenthieu, G. and Del Amo, J. (2000b) *Impact and cost-effectiveness modeling of in-school youth programmes in sub-Saharan Africa.* Presented at the XIII International AIDS Conference in Durban, South Africa. Abstract [ThPeC5407].

Wawer, M.J., Gray, R.H., Sewankambo, N.K. *et al.* (1998) A randomized, community trial of intensive sexually transmitted disease control for AIDS prevention, Rakai, Uganda. *AIDS* **12**, 1211–1225.

Wawer, M.J., Sewankambo, N.K., Serwadda, D. *et al.* (1999) Control of sexually transmitted diseases for AIDS prevention in Uganda: a randomised community trial. Rakai Project Study Group. *Lancet* **353**, 525–535.

World Bank (1993) *World Development Report 1993.* Oxford University Press, Washington, DC.

Chapter 5

Modelling the cost-effectiveness of new interventions: how can technological change be incorporated?

Richard Grieve

Introduction

To allocate health care resources in an efficient way, policy makers require information on the costs and outcomes of competing health care interventions (Maynard and Kavanos 2000). However, published information on the cost-effectiveness of new interventions is often not available (Davies *et al.* 1994). To address this problem, an increasing number of economic evaluations are being commissioned and published (Elixhauser *et al.* 1998; Pritchard 1998). Many economic evaluations now use models as trials are of insufficient duration to estimate cost-effectiveness over the required time horizon (Buxton *et al.* 1997).

Although the rationale for models in this area is well established, serious concerns have been voiced about the assumptions which models make, and the uncertainty which surrounds their estimates (Sheldon 1996; Briggs 2000). The particular concern to be addressed in this chapter is that models usually assume that the way in which the disease is managed does not change over the model's projection period. If this assumption is incorrect, it may render the model's predictions inaccurate. This issue will be considered here with recourse to appropriate economic theory. Insights from theory will then be applied to a case study of an economic model for hepatitis C.

The chapter is divided into four sections: the first section describes the use of cost-effectiveness models, the second considers production function theory, the third examines the impact of technological change more empirically using the hepatitis C case study, and the last section discusses the findings and offers some conclusions.

Cost-effectiveness models

There is a general consensus amongst health economists that models are often required to provide information on the costs and outcomes of new interventions over a sufficiently long time horizon. Economic models have been used in the infectious disease literature for evaluating new treatments and prevention strategies. For example, in the human immunodeficiency virus (HIV) field, trials may measure the effect of new antiviral therapies on intermediate clinical outcome measures such as CD4 counts (Simpson *et al.* 2001; see also Kumaranayake *et al.* Chapter 4). Economic models may then use these trial data, together with epidemiological data on disease progression, to estimate costs and outcomes over the lifetime of patients.

Critics of economic models have suggested that they may not be appropriate for clinical decision making because of the uncertainties inherent in this form of analysis (Sheldon 1996). Briggs (2000) explained how different forms of uncertainty such as methodological and parameter uncertainty may arise when modelling cost-effectiveness. Methodological uncertainty arises when there is a disagreement over the appropriate technique to use for measuring key parameters. For example, health economists disagree as to which is the most appropriate method to use for valuing outcomes in economic evaluation (Mehrez and Gafni 1982; Torrance 1986; Donaldson 1990). Guidelines have suggested that methodological uncertainty can be highlighted by taking a particular methodological standpoint in the base case analysis and then adopting different methodological positions in the subsequent sensitivity analysis (Gold *et al.* 1996).

Parameter uncertainty refers to the sampling variability that surrounds the variables introduced into the model (Briggs 2000). For instance, while a model requiring a particular cost input may use one estimate of the mean cost for the population concerned, the model should recognize the sampling variability that surrounds this estimate. Probabalistic sensitivity analysis can incorporate this parameter uncertainty by using Monte Carlo simulation to sample from the probability distributions that surround the model estimates (Doubilet *et al.* 1985). The resulting uncertainty is then captured in the model's estimate of the relative cost-effectiveness of different health care programmes (Briggs 2000). Recent methodological guidelines for cost-effectiveness analyses now explicitly require analysts to consider this parameter uncertainty by using probabilistic sensitivity analysis (National Institute of Clinical Excellence 2004a).

Cost-effectiveness guidelines have given less consideration to uncertainty arising from changes in the way the disease is managed over time. In fact, most models assume that the physical inputs used in treating a particular condition remain fixed over the model's projection period. However, empirical evidence has shown that technological advances occur over time, which may be associated with increasing or decreasing health care costs (Scitovsky 1985; Johnson *et al.* 1998). For example, Johnson *et al.* (1998) showed that the expenditure on drug therapy for acute myocardial infarction increased in the UK during the 1980s. By contrast, the mean length of hospitalization in OECD countries has been falling over the last two decades, leading to potential reductions in hospitalization costs (Organization for Economic Co-operation and Development 2000). Such changes in health care costs according to technological change may have an important impact on cost-effectiveness analyses for chronic diseases. Here, if the disease is slowly progressive, as is the case with many infectious diseases, then important technological changes may occur over the model's projection period. Ignoring such developments could reduce the accuracy, credibility and usefulness of these cost-effectiveness models. The issues posed by potential technological progress for these models is now considered using production function theory.

What is a production function?

The production function specifies the technical relationship between inputs and outputs under the assumption of cost minimization (Heathfield and Wibe 1981). In this section, I consider insights that basic production function theory offers when designing and analysing cost-effectiveness models.

The production function provides a way of defining alternatives and specifying the range of technical possibilities that are open to producers. Considering the alternative methods of production may be especially important in industries such as health care where providers may often subscribe to what Victor Fuchs has termed the monotechnic view and believe that there is only one way of providing a service (Folland *et al.* 1987). In spite of this belief, research has shown there is great variability in the way in which particular health services are provided (Jensen and Morrisey 1986; Folland and Stano 1990; Phelps and Mooney 1993).

The combination of inputs used to produce output will be 'technically efficient' if the minimum level of factor inputs (e.g. doctors' time, nurses' time) are used to produce a particular level of output. Differences observed in the use of inputs across health care providers may therefore reflect differences in technical efficiency. The inputs required will change as output increases. The mix of inputs chosen for any given output will be economically efficient if the ratio of the marginal productivity of the inputs equals the ratio of their factor prices.

The expansionist path of production can then be derived for each level of output for each set of prices. The efficient combination of inputs will change if either the marginal productivity of the factor inputs or their relative prices change. This static representation does not consider the shifts that may occur if the technical properties of the production process change over time. There may be technological progress, for example from the development of a new drug or procedure. This may lead to completely different levels of factor inputs and outputs being chosen to maximize economic efficiency. If a long-term perspective is taken, technological change may occur—this may be defined as either substitution in the factor inputs used to produce particular levels of output, or shifts in the technology whereby completely different levels of input and output are chosen.

Unlike other forms of economic evaluation that may only take a short-term perspective (e.g. trial-based evaluations), economic models usually aim to take a long-term perspective and estimate costs and outcomes well into the future. In the long term, firms may substitute factor inputs or adopt new technology. Therefore, theory would suggest that the design of cost-effectiveness models should consider either of these different forms of technical change which may arise over the model's projection period. The issues posed by factor substitution and shifts in technology are now considered using a case study of an economic model developed for assessing new interventions in hepatitis C.

Case study: hepatitis C

Hepatitis C is an appropriate disease for assessing whether incorporating technological change is likely to be important for the results of cost-effectiveness analyses. Chronic hepatitis C is slowly progressive, and it is estimated that it can take over 30 years for patients infected with the disease to reach disease states, such as cirrhosis and liver cancer, which have a large impact on health care costs and quality of life (Poynard *et al.* 1997). The latent nature of the disease means that prospective studies cannot provide timely information on the cost-effectiveness of new interventions. Instead, economic evaluations in this area have often used Markov models to assess the relative costs and effects of new interventions over a time period not covered by randomised controlled trials (RCTs) (Dusheiko and Roberts 1995; Bennett *et al.* 1997; Kim *et al.* 1997; Shepherd *et al.* 2000, 2004; Shiell *et al.* 2002; Stein *et al.* 2002).

A Markov model divides the natural history of the disease into a series of health states. Information on the probability of progressing between the states and the costs and health-related quality of life (HRQoL) associated with each state is required to populate the model. Studies of the cost-effectiveness of antiviral therapies for hepatitis C have used Markov models and concluded that antiviral therapies (e.g. α-interferon and ribavirin) bring about sufficient gain in quality-adjusted life years (QALYs) to justify their costs (Dusheiko and Roberts 1995; Bennett *et al.* 1997; Kim *et al.* 1997; Shepherd *et al.* 2000, 2004; Shiell *et al.* 2002; Stein *et al.* 2002). Based on these models' results, decision-making agencies such as the National Institute of Clinical Excellence (NICE) have recommended that antiviral therapy should be made available for patients with moderate hepatitis C or cirrhosis (National Institute of Clinical Excellence 2000, 2004b). Although recent economic evaluations in this area have reported measures of uncertainty surrounding their results, they have usually just measured parameter uncertainty (Wright *et al.* 2006). In common with decision-analytical models in general, little attention has been given to technological change. The questions to be addressed therefore are: how can changes in technology be incorporated into the modelling process, and how might consideration of these issues alter the results and policy recommendations?

Model for mild hepatitis C

A Markov model was developed as part of a study assessing the cost-effectiveness of α-interferon and ribavirin for patients with mild chronic hepatitis C (Grieve and Roberts 2002). The model divided the natural history of the disease into a series of pre-defined health states (Fig. 5.1). The proportion of patients who responded to treatment was taken from previously

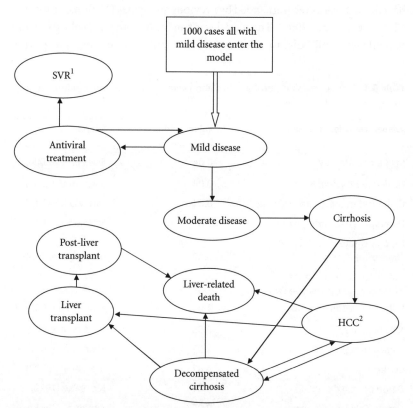

Fig. 5.1 Structure of cost-effectiveness model for treatment of mild chronic hepatitis C.

[1] SVR: Sustained Virological Response. [2] HCC: Hepatatic Cellular Carcinoma

published RCTs comparing combination therapy with placebo for patients with chronic hepatitis C. The evidence available from multinational trials suggested that following the intervention, 43% of patients have a sustained virological response (SVR) defined as a negative polymerase chain reaction (PCR) at least 6 months post-treatment (Poynard *et al.* 1998). There was also trial evidence to show that there was no further histological progression in those patients who had an SVR following antiviral therapy (Poynard *et al.* 1998). The model assumed that patients in the control group or patients who were treated but did not have an SVR faced the same annual probabilities of progressing through the disease (Table 5.1). As the patients move along the clinical path of the disease, they experience correspondingly worse HRQoL (Table 5.1). The values used for the probability of disease progression and the HRQoL associated with particular disease states were taken from the literature (Table 5.1).

The analysis period for the model was flexible, but in this case study results are presented over the patients' lifetime. All costs were discounted at 6% and benefits at 1.5% as recommended by previous guidelines (National Institute of Clinical Excellence 2002). The model was run for hypothetical cohorts of 1000 patients with mild disease with and without antiviral therapy. The outputs

Table 5.1 Annual transition probabilities and estimates of health-related quality of life (HRQoL) used in the model

Annual transition probability	Value used in base case	Source
Mild-moderate HCV	0.04	Shiell *et al.* (2000)
Moderate HCV-cirrhosis	0.04	Shiell *et al.* (2000)
Cirrhosis-decompensated cirrhosis	0.04	Fattovich *et al.* (1997)
Decompensated cirrhosis-HCC	0.01	Fattovich *et al.* (1997)
Decompensated cirrhosis-liver transplant	0.03	Bennett *et al.* (1997)
HRQoL for each health state (0 = dead, 1 = perfect health)		
Following SVR to antiviral therapy	1.00	Stein *et al.* (2002)
Mild hepatitis C	0.98	Stein *et al.* (2002)
Moderate hepatitis C	0.92	Stein *et al.* (2002)
Cirrhosis	0.82	Stein *et al.* (2002)
Decompensated cirrhosis	0.50	Kim *et al.* (1998)
Hepato Cellular Carcinoma	0.25	Kim *et al.* (1998)

from the model were QALYs and total health service costs for the treatment compared with the no treatment cohort. This enabled the model to estimate the incremental cost-effectiveness ratio (ICER) of using antiviral treatment compared with no treatment.

Cost estimates used in the model

To estimate the relative cost-effectiveness for new interventions, the model required information on the average cost of each disease stage. For some disease stages, such as liver transplantation, costs were available from the literature (Longworth *et al.* 2001). For mild and moderate disease, cirrhosis and decompensated cirrhosis, accurate costs were not readily available and so an empirical study was conducted to measure the costs. A sample of patients in each disease stage who had attended one of three large hepatology centres in London, Southampton and Newcastle were included in the study. Resource inputs for each case were measured retrospectively over the period 1993–2002, by extracting data from medical records. These data were combined with local unit cost data to give mean annual costs for each disease stage. The principal aim of this costing exercise was to provide cost data for use in the model. However, as part of the analysis, insights were gained into the extent to which technology change occurred in the study centres. So although full longitudinal analysis of the cost data was not possible, certain trends in the way care was produced were identified. These can be defined according to substitutions in factor inputs and shifts in technology.

Substitutions in factor inputs

The empirical data illustrated that potentially important substitutions were made in the inputs used to produce care. In particular, at the start of the observation period, antiviral therapy was monitored in out-patient clinics where patients were seen by a consultant or senior registrar. Each of these visits cost £65. When the unit cost data were combined with information collected on the frequency of visits and the other costs associated with monitoring, the overall cost of monitoring treatment was £1010. However, the data suggested that towards the end of the observation period, rather than attending an out-patient clinic for treatment monitoring, patients were more likely to visit the nurse. The unit cost of a nurse visit was £10, and the annual costs of monitoring with this form of care fell to £374. It was assumed that output was unaffected by the substitution of nurses for doctors and that this switch led to an improvement in economic efficiency.

The second example of an input substitution over the observation period came from the move to perform certain procedures on a day case rather than an in-patient basis. In the early period of analysis, liver biopsies and diagnostic endoscopies were done on an in-patient basis and cost on average £381 and £319, respectively. However, towards the end of the observation period it became more common for the procedures to be performed as day cases. The costs of these procedures were considerably lower; the unit cost of a liver biopsy fell to £265 and for a diagnostic endoscopy to £97. Assuming that output levels were unaffected, then the switch to day case procedures would again be regarded as a move towards economic efficiency.

Shifts in technology

The previous scenarios have all emphasized a change in input combinations within the same technological process. However, the empirical data suggested there was some evidence of a complete shift in certain technologies. For example, the treatment of hepatocellular carcinoma (HCC) over the early part of the observation period was by chemoembolization. However, new techniques are now available for treating this condition, for example laser ablation of the liver. The move to treating HCC by laser ablation rather than chemoembolism represents a complete shift in the technology rather than a mere substitution of one factor input for another. Laser ablation requires a particular type of magnetic resonance imaging (MRI) scanner, highly trained radiologists and nurses, and particular consumables and drugs. Such technological change is only feasible in the long term. The unit costs of the procedure are much higher for laser ablation at over £4000 per procedure compared with £373 for chemoembolization. However, although the procedure costs are higher, the procedure may lead to better quality care which could mean that fewer recurrent procedures are required and the patients' survival improves.

The development of more effective new antiviral therapies is also an example of a technological development. These more effective therapies have a higher unit cost, for example a 48 week course of α-interferon and ribavirin costs £8849 whereas a corresponding course of pegylated interferon and ribavirin costs £15 648 (British Medical Association and the Royal Pharmaceutical Society of Great Britain 2001). The question for the model to address is whether adopting this higher cost but more effective intervention is a cost-effective way of treating patients with mild disease?

Assessing the impact of these changes in technology on the cost-effectiveness of treating mild hepatitis C

In the base case scenario, the standard assumption that there were no changes in technology over the model's projection period was made. The ICER of

Table 5.2 Unit costs used in each scenario to illustrate technological changes

Input	Base case scenario	Substitution scenario		Shift in technology scenario	
		Day case for in-patient	Doctor–nurse substitution	New HCC procedure	Move to pegylated interferon[1]
Preparation for treatment	£676	**£560**	£676	£676	£676
48 weeks antiviral therapy	£8849[2]	£8849	£8849	£8849	**£15 648**
Treatment monitoring	£1010	£1010	**£374**	£1010	£1010
Liver biopsy	£381	**£265**	£381	£381	£381
Diagnostic endoscopy	£319	**£97**	£319	£319	£319
Therapeutic endoscopy	£432	**£210**	**£432**	£432	£432
Intervention for tumour	£373	£373	£373	**£4437**	£373

Parameters which change for a particular scenario compared with the base case scenario are shown in bold.

[1] In this scenario, it is assumed that the only the cost of the intervention change, in practice, pegylated interferon may be associated with lower monitoring costs, but currently few data are available to support this.

[2] α-Interferon and ribavirin are the intervention in the base case scenario.

antiviral treatment for patients with mild hepatitis C was then calculated. The mild hepatitis C model was designed with sufficient flexibility to assess the effect of changes in the production process. The impact of making different assumptions about these technical changes was assessed using sensitivity analysis based on different scenarios. For each scenario, the assumptions used about the state of the technology and the accompanying unit costs are listed in Table 5.2. For example, in the base case scenario, it was assumed that the patients in the treatment cohort received α-interferon and ribavirin, which was monitored by doctors at out-patient clinics, all procedures were done on an in-patient basis and HCC was treated by chemoembolization. Each of these assumptions was varied in the subsequent scenarios and the impact on the key model outputs was estimated.

Results

The results are presented as an average for the hypothetical cohort of 1000 cases in the treatment and control groups. In the base case scenario, the mean lifetime cost for the cases in the control group was £14 620 compared with £18 679 in the treatment group, so the incremental costs of treatment were £4060 (Table 5.3). There was an average gain of 1.13 QALYs for the treatment cohort, and the ICER was £3594 per QALY. This ratio is below the threshold beneath which new interventions are usually regarded as relatively cost-effective (National Institute of Clinical Excellence 2004a), so an analysis based on the assumptions used in this scenario could conclude that combination therapy was, on average, cost-effective for patients with mild hepatitis C.

Table 5.3 Average annual costs of different disease stages and model output for each scenario

	Base case scenario	Substitution scenario		Shift in technology scenario	
		Day case for in-patient	Doctor–nurse substitution	New HCC procedure	Move to pegylated interferon[1]
Disease stage					
Treatment and monitoring	£8986	**£8870**	**£8531**	£8986	**£15 918**
Costs of chronic disease	£809	**£711**	£809	£809	£809
Costs of cirrhosis	£1630	**£1518**	**£1630**	£1630	£1630
Costs of decomp disease	£7844	**£7759**	**£7844**	£7844	£7844
Costs of HCC	£9519	**£9402**	£9519	**£9123**	£9519
Model output					
Lifetime costs of illness (no treatment)	£14 620	**£13 191**	£14 620	**£14 611**	£14 620
Lifetime costs of illness (with treatment)	£18 679	**£18 289**	**£18 225**	£18 677	**£24 260**
Incremental costs of treatment	£4060	**£5098**	**£3605**	**£4066**	**£9640**
QALYs gained from treatment	1.13	1.13	1.13	1.13	1.52
Incremental Costs per QALY	£3594	**£4512**	**£3191**	**£3599**	**£6358**

Parameters which change for a particular scenario compared with the base case scenario are shown in bold.

[1] In this scenario, it is assumed that the only the cost of the intervention change, in practice, pegylated interferon may be associated with lower monitoring costs, but currently there is little evidence available to support this.

Substitutions of factor inputs

If nurses rather than doctors are assumed to monitor treatment, then the average monitoring costs fall from £8986 to £8870 (Table 5.3). The lifetime costs for the treated cohort therefore fall slightly to £18 289. Under this scenario, all other costs are unchanged so the lifetime costs of illness for the no treatment cohort remain on average £14 620. The incremental costs of the treatment therefore fall to £3605, and the ICER to £3191 per QALY. So if nurses substitute for doctors, the intervention becomes slightly more cost-effective.

If the common procedures for hepatitis C are performed on a day case rather than an in-patient basis, then lifetime costs fall slightly for the treatment cohort. However, the greatest reduction in costs is for the no treatment cohort as more patients in this group progress to disease stages where procedures are needed. This means that, compared with the base case scenario, the incremental costs of treatment and the ICER both increase.

Technological change

Moving to laser ablation rather than chemoembolization for treating HCC increases the costs of managing this aspect of liver disease. However, the impact on lifetime costs for patients with hepatitis C is small. Hepatitis C is a slowly progressive disease and the majority of patients never have HCC, and if they do it is well into the future. In our model, future costs are subject to a discount rate of 6% so the net present value of these costs is low compared with more immediate costs such as the management of mild disease. The data collected suggested that laser ablation of the liver may improve the quality of care and mean that patients require fewer recurrent procedures for HCC, which offsets some of the additional costs. However, in this scenario, it is assumed that there is no corresponding gain in survival. However, there was no evidence available in the literature on survival following laser ablation of the liver compared with chemoembolization for treating HCC. The estimates therefore provide a conservative estimate of the impact of adopting this technology.

Another technological change considered was the development of new antiviral therapies for treating mild disease. In the base case scenario, patients were treated with standard α-interferon and ribavirin, then in this scenario pegylated interferon is used in combination with ribavirin. Although the intervention costs are higher (Table 5.2), a higher proportion of patients have an SVR following treatment with pegylated interferon and ribavirin rather than standard interferon and ribavirin (56% compared with 43%) (Fried *et al.* 2001; Manns *et al.* 2001). The higher SVR means that fewer patients progress to the severe disease states and the QALYs gained from the intervention rise from 1.13 in the base case scenario to 1.52 in the pegylated interferon scenario. However, there is a corresponding increase in the incremental costs of treatment from £4066 to £9640, and the cost-effectiveness ratio rises from £3594 to £6358. So although this technical change, unlike the others considered, does have a substantive impact on the ICER, the estimated cost-effectiveness ratio is still well below the decision makers cut off point for treatment.

The analysis has so far considered the impact of each technological change in turn using one-way sensitivity analysis. However, policy makers might also be interested in simultaneously considering the impact of all the changes. This can be evaluated using multiway sensitivity analysis. If it is assumed that nurses instead of doctors monitor treatment, procedures are done on a day case rather than an in-patient basis, laser ablation is used for HCC and pegylated interferon is used for treating mild disease, then the overall effect is to increase the ICER from £3594 to £8705.

Discussion

This study examined the impact of changes to the production process on the results of cost-effectiveness models. The brief review of production function theory suggested that two forms of technological change needed considering: the impact of substituting factor inputs and the effect of shifts in the technology available to providers. Economic theory indicated that if economic models take a long-term perspective, then technological changes are likely to occur over the model's projection period, and should be considered.

These theoretical insights were applied to a hepatitis C model which, because of the slowly progressive nature of the disease, required a long time horizon. The results showed that none of the changes in the technological process altered the conclusion that antiviral therapy for patients with mild hepatitis C was, on average, relatively cost-effective. This suggests that the results from cost-effectiveness analyses may be reasonably robust to changes in technology. However, further studies are needed to test this before general conclusions can be drawn. Certain issues, which arose from the empirical work presented here, could inform the design of these studies.

The model presented was designed to incorporate different assumptions about the degree of technical change. Some scenarios, for example incorporating the use of day case rather than in-patient procedures, simply required the cost inputs used in the model to be changed. However, for other technical changes such as the move to a new procedure for treating liver cancer, more fundamental changes to the model structure were needed. The challenge facing the analyst is to design the model with the flexibility needed to be able to incorporate a series of changes in the production process. The model could then be revisited as changes in technology emerge which affect its inputs and estimates. Commentators have argued that health technology assessment is not a one-off process, rather the process needs to be iterative with estimates continually revised as new information emerges (Sculpher *et al.* 1997) A cost-effectiveness model designed with flexibility and foresight would therefore seem to be an appropriate mechanism for assessing cost-effectiveness in an iterative way.

Cost-effectiveness models could make more use of existing information on the potential changes to the production process. In this study, longitudinal data were collected on the resources used in managing hepatitis C for a cohort of patients attending three UK teaching hospitals. Formal longitudinal analyses of the resource inputs were not possible due to the constrained time-frame of the study. However, preliminary analysis showed that there were certain trends in the use of inputs over time for the teaching hospitals surveyed. The trends observed covered both substitutions (doctors for nurses, day case for in-patient care) and shifts in technology (laser treatment for chemoembolization, pegylated interferon as antiviral treatment). The assumption used in the sensitivity analysis was that these recent trends in production processes in teaching hospitals provided a reasonable basis for predicting the future change in the production of hepatology services more generally. This relies on the widely held premise that technological innovations at teaching hospitals, after some time delay, may be implemented more generally (Drummond *et al.* 1994).

In the scenario analysis, it was assumed that each technical change was adopted completely over the whole timeframe of the model. So, for example, for the move from day case to in-patient care, it was assumed that in the day case scenario, certain procedures were all done on a day case basis for years 1–50. This may well overestimate the likely uptake (and hence the effect) of techno-logical change as there will always be hospitals that do not adopt the change in technology or adopt the changes later, and individual patients for whom the change is not appropriate or efficient.

In many studies, even basic longitudinal data on the use of technologies are not available to the modeller looking to incorporate technological change. However, this does not mean that the potential for change should be ignored. One alternative way of examining technological change would be to ask experts to estimate the likely change in the use of technologies over time. The views of key decision makers could be used in the same way that they have been for other inputs into cost-effectiveness models. Although the use of expert opinion has been criticized for limiting the validity of models (Mandelblatt *et al.* 1996), it could still be useful for assessing the value of collecting more information on technological advances. If expert opinion is the only way in which data on new technologies can be incorporated into the analysis, then at least this should be done as rigorously as possible. For instance, a range of experts with different disciplinary perspectives, from various parts of the health care system concerned, should be sampled (Mandelblatt *et al.* 1996). This is necessary to ensure that a range of values can be stipulated for the rate of technological dissemination.

In the general health economics literature, several studies have estimated the rate of change of various technologies and the level of substitution between certain inputs (see, for example, Jensen and Morrisey 1986). Using these insights from the literature offers another potential way of proxying future changes in technology. However, for our case study, there were certain difficulties surrounding the use of the published literature for this purpose. First, many of the studies looking at substitutions, for example between nurses and doctors, are several years old, and may be difficult to use for predicting future changes. Secondly, information may not be available from the literature on the particular production processes used in the model. For example, the general literature on the relative use of day case and in-patient procedures may not apply to the relative use of these different modes of delivering procedures for patients with hepatitis C.

One problem with estimating the impact of technological change is that the rate at which the new technologies are adopted is uncertain. The diffusion of new technology is likely to vary across health care providers partly because of uncertainty regarding the cost-effectiveness of the new technology (Folland and Stano 1990). National agencies have been set up to regulate the rate of technological change. Models therefore need to try to incorporate recommendations from these agencies in the modelling process. The hepatitis C model now needs to be updated in light of the changing recommendations on the use of antiviral therapy for patients with more severe disease. During the early stages of model development, there was little evidence to suggest that antiviral therapy was cost-effective for patients with moderate hepatitis C or cirrhosis and so the model compared antiviral treatment with a 'do nothing' alternative. However, during the course of model development, the NICE decided that, based on recently published studies, antiviral treatment was cost-effective and should be available for patients with moderate hepatitis C and cirrhosis (National Institute of Clinical Excellence 2002, 2004b). This change in policy has to be recognized by subsequent models assessing the cost-effectiveness of antiviral treatment at a mild disease stage. The appropriate comparator, certainly in England and Wales, is no longer 'no treatment' but 'antiviral treatment for those who reach moderate disease'. If the model was adapted to incorporate this change in recommendations, the ICER for treating patients with mild disease under the base case assumptions rises to £7257. Once again, the cost-effectiveness model needs to be flexible to allow changes, in this case from policy makers' recognition of a technical advance, to be incorporated into the analysis.

An additional form of uncertainty that may surround estimates of the cost-effectiveness of interventions for preventing infectious disease concerns the indirect effect of the intervention on the rate of infection amongst the general population. This form of uncertainty is not considered here, but is the subject of the chapter in this book by Edmunds. The focus in this chapter has been on the implications of technological change for the likely cost-effectiveness of the new interventions. This form of uncertainty should be considered alongside more recognized sources of variation in cost-effectiveness such as parameter uncertainty and methodological uncertainty.

This case study was presented for the 'average' patient with mild hepatitis C. This group was characterized as being aged 40 at diagnosis, 50% of whom were genotype 1. Varying these patient characteristics is likely to change either the probability of responding to treatment or the rate of progression to advanced stages of the disease (Poynard *et al.* 1997, 1998). So, for example, if the model is run for the patients who are genotype non–1, the SVR following α-interferon and ribavirin treatment rises to 67% and the ICER falls to £1203, whereas for patients who are genotype 1 the SVR was only 28% and the corresponding cost-effectiveness ratio is £7622. This illustrates the importance of presenting the uncertainty surrounding other inputs to the production function, such as patient characteristics, rather than focusing solely on those relating to the providers' inputs to the production process.

To conclude, the use of cost-effectiveness models is becoming an established analytical method especially for evaluating treatment and prevention strategies for infectious diseases. The main advantage of using decision-analytical models in this context is that they are able to project costs and outcomes over a sufficient timeframe. Production function theory suggests that if a long-term perspective is adopted, then a range of changes to the production process may occur. Although, for the example presented, the empirical impact of incorporating such changes was small, it may still be useful to consider technological change when modelling cost-effectiveness. By showing they can take account of technological progress, cost-effectiveness models can demonstrate a broader understanding of the uncertainty that surrounds their results. This could help make such models more credible and useful for health care decision making, both in infectious diseases and more generally.

References

Bennett, W.G., Beck, R., Inoue, Y. *et al.* (1997) Estimates of the cost-effectiveness of a single course of interferon 2b in patients with histologically mild chronic HCV. *Annals of Internal Medicine* **127**, 855–865.

Briggs, A.H. (2000) Handling uncertainty in cost-effectiveness models. *Pharmacoeconomics* **17**, 479–500.

British Medical Association and the Royal Pharmaceutical Society of Great Britain (2001) *British National Formulary*. BMJ Books, London.

Buxton, M.J., Drummond, M.F., Van Hout, B.A. *et al.* (1997) Modelling in economic evaluation: an unavoidable fact of life. *Health Economy* **6**, 217–227.

Davies, L., Coyle, D., Drummond, M. and the EC Network on the Methodology of Economic Appraisal of Health Technology (1994) *Social Science and Medicine* **38**, 1601–1607.

Donaldson, C. (1990) Willingness to pay for publicly provided goods: a possible measure of benefit. *Journal of Health Economy* **9**, 103–118.

Doubilet, P., Begg, C.B., Weinstein, M.C. *et al.* (1985) Probabilistic sensitivity analysis using Monte Carlo simulation: a practical approach. *Medical Decision Making* **5**, 157–177.

Drummond, M. (1994) Evaluation of health technology: economic issues for health policy and policy issues for economic appraisal. *Social Science and Medicine* **38**, 1593–1600.

Dusheiko, M. and Roberts, J.A. (1995) Treatment of chronic type B and C hepatitis with interferon alfa: an economic appraisal (special article). *Hepatology* **22**, 1863–1872.

Elixhauser, A., Halpern, M., Shimier, J. *et al.* (1998) Health care CBD and CEA from 1991 to 1996: an updated bibliography. *Medical Care* **36**, MS1–MS9.

Fattovich, G., Giustina, G., Gegos, F. *et al.* (1997) Morbidity and mortality in compensated cirrhosis type C: a retrospective follow-up study of 384 patients. *Gastroenterology* **112**, 463–472.

Folland, S. and Stano, M. (1990) Small area variations: a critical review of propositions, methods and evidence. *Medical Care Review* **47**, 419–465.

Folland, S., Goodman A. *et al.* (1987) *The Economics of Health and Health Care*. Prentice Hall, New Jersey.

Fried, M.W., Shiffman, M.L., Reddy, R.K. *et al.* (2001) Pegylated (40 kDa) interferon alfa-2a in combination with ribavirin: efficacy and safety results from a phase III, randomized, actively-controlled multicenter study [abstract]. *Gastroenterology* **120**, A55.

Gold, M.R., Siegel, J.E. *et al.* (1996) *Cost-effectiveness in Health and Medicine*. Oxford University Press, New York.

Grieve, R. and Roberts, J. (2002) Economic evaluation for hepatitis C. *Acta Gastro-enterologica Belgica* **65**, 104–109.

Heathfield, D.F. and Wibe, S. (1981) *An Introduction to Cost and Production Functions*. MacMillan Education, London.

Jensen, G.A. and Morrisey, M.A. (1986) The role of physicians in hospital production. *Review of Economics and Statistics* **68**, 432–442.

Johnson, S., Whynes, D., Brown, N. *et al.* The cost-effectiveness of advances in technology in the treatment of acute myocardial infarction between 1982 and 1992. Paper presented to the Health Economics Study Group Meeting, Galway, Ireland, July 1998.

Kim, R.W., Poterucha, J.J., Hermans, J.E. *et al.* (1997) Cost-effectiveness of 6 and 12 months of interferon-α therapy for chronic hepatitis C. *Annals of Internal Medicine* **127**, 866–874.

Longworth, L., Young, T., Ratcliffe, J. *et al.* (2001) *An Assessment of the Cost-effectiveness of Liver Transplantation for Three Disease Groups. Preliminary Report to the Department of Health*. Department of Health, London.

Mandleblatt, J.S., Fryback, D.G., Weinstein, M.C. *et al.* (1996) Assessing the effectiveness of health interventions. In: **Gold M.R., Siegel J.E.** *et al.* (eds), *Cost-effectiveness in Health and Medicine*. Oxford University Press, New York, pp. 150–152.

Manns, M.P., McHutchinson, J.G., Gordon, S.C. *et al.* (2001) Peginterferon alfa-2b plus ribavirin for initial treatment of chronic hepatitis C: a randomised trial. *Lancet* **358**, 958–965.

Maynard, A. and Kanavos, P. (2000) Health economics: an evolving paradigm. *Health Economy* **9**, 183–190.

Mehrez, A. and Gafni, A. (1982) Quality-adjusted life years, utility theory, and healthy-years equivalents. *Medical Decision Making* **2**, 449–462.

National Institute of Clinical Excellence (2000) *Guidance on the Use of Ribavirin and Interferon Alpha for Hepatitis* C. NICE, London.

National Institute of Clinical Excellence (2002) *Guidance for Manufacturers and Sponsors. Technology Appraisal Process Series No 5*. NICE, London.

National Institute of Clinical Excellence (2004a) Guidance for manufacturers and sponsors. www.nice.org.uk/pdf/technicalguidanceformanufacturersandsponsors.pdf (accessed June 2004).

National Institute of Clinical Excellence (2004b) *Guidance on the Use of Interferon Alpha (Pegylated and Non Pegylated) and Ribavirin for the Treatment of Chronic Hepatitis C*. NICE, London.

Organization for Economic Co-operation and Development (2000) *OECD Health Data 2000*. OECD, Paris.

Phelps, C.E. and Mooney, C. (1993) Variations in medical practice use, causes and consequences. In: **Arnoud, R.J., Rich, R.F.** and **White, W.D.** (eds), *Competitive Approaches to Health Care Reform*. The Urban Institute Press, Washington, DC.

Poynard, T., Bedosa, P. and Opolon, P. (1997) Natural history of liver fibrosis progression in patients with chronic hepatitis C. *Lancet* **349**, 825–832.

Poynard, T., Marcellin, P. and Lee, S.S. *et al.* (1998) Randomised trial of interferon alpha2b plus ribavarin for 48 weeks or for 24 weeks versus interferon alpha2b plus placebo for 48 weeks for treatment of chronic infection with hepatitis C virus. International Hepatitis Interventional Therapy Group (IHIT). *Lancet* **532**, 1426–1432.

Pritchard, C. (1998) *Trends in Economic Evaluation*. OHE Briefing No. 36. Office of Health Economics, London.

Scitovsky, A. (1985) Changes in the costs of treatment of selected illnesses, 1971 to 1981. *Medical Care* **23**, 1345–1207.

Sculpher, M., Drummond, M.F. and Buxton, M.J. (1997) The iterative use of economic evaluation as part of the process of health technology assessment. *Journal of Health Services Research and Policy* **2**, 26–30.

Sheldon, T. (1996) Problems of using modelling in the economic evaluation of health care. *Health Economics* **5**, 1–11.

Shepherd, J., Waugh, N. and Hewitson, P. (2000) Combination therapy (interferon alfa and ribavirin) in the treatment of chronic hepatitis C: a rapid and systematic review. *Health Technology Assessment* **4**, No. 33.

Shepherd, J., Brodin, H., Cave, C., Waugh, N., Price, A. and Gabbay, J. (2004) Pegylated interferon α-2a and -2b in combination with ribavirin in the treatment of chronic hepatitis C: a systematic review and economic evaluation. *Health Technology Assessment* **8**, No. 39.

Shiell, A., Brown, S. and Farrel, G.C. (1999) Hepatitis C: an economic evaluation of extended treatment with interferon. *Medical Journal of Australia* **171**, 189–193.

Simpson, K.N., Voit, E., Goodman, R. *et al.* (2001) Estimating the social and economic benefits of pharmaceutical innovation: modeling clinical trial results in HIV-disease. *Investing in Health: The Social and Economic Benefits of Health Care Innovation* **14**, 175–196.

Stein, K., Rosenberg, W. and Wong, J. (2002) Cost-effectiveness of combination therapy for hepatitis C: a decision analytic model. *Gut* **50**, 253–258.

Torrance, G.W. (1986) Measurement of health state utilities for economic appraisal: a review. *Journal of Health Economics* **5**, 1–30.

Wright, M., Grieve, R., Roberts, J., Main, J. and Thomas, H. (2006) Health benefits of anti-viral therapy for mild chronic hepatitis c: randomised control trial and economic evaluation. *Health Technology Assessment* (in press).

Chapter 6

Complexity and the attribution of cost to hospital-acquired infection

Nicholas Graves and Diana Weinhold

Introduction

Estimates of the cost of hospital-acquired infection (HAI) have been used for two purposes. Haley (1998) argues they are required to create 'political urgency' and raise the profile of the various infections patients may acquire during their hospital stay. Also, champions for infection control activities use the estimates to argue that incremental investment in effective prevention programmes, which incur their own cost, are justified and might well lead to net benefits for the health care system (see Sperry and Craddock 1968; Sencer and Axnick 1975; Haley 1978; Lambert and Fabry 1985; Haley 1986; Lambert 1987; Currie and Maynard 1989; Miller *et al.* 1989; Olsen 1990; Plowman *et al.* 1997, 2001).

The challenge is to isolate, precisely, the increase in length of stay and the marginal resources used because of hospital infection. Many methods have been proposed, and these are reviewed in the second part of this chapter. The methods have evolved since Clarke's (1957) investigation of the bed wastage due to *Staphylococcus aureus* in patients' wounds. However, Clarke did highlight an issue that plagues the most sophisticated attempts to tease out the cost of hospital infection. She argues.... 'The average length of stay in hospital of patients whose wounds were infected with *Staph. aureus* was found to be 5 days longer than the average length of stay of patients whose wounds were not so infected. However, many patients stayed in hospital for more than the usual length of time for reasons not connected with staphylococcal infection. These patients then, owing to their long stay in hospital, acquired *Staph. aureus* in their wounds'.

It seems that while hospital infection prolongs length of stay, a longer length of stay increases the risk of infection. This two-way relationship causes a serious bias in statistical regression models where cost or length of stay is the outcome and the incidence of hospital infection is an explanatory term. A feature of regression modelling is that the explanatory variables are causally related to the outcome of interest. They should explain or predict the outcome, rather than the converse. It is the endogenous nature of length of stay and HAI that gives rise to the bias. A novel procedure for correcting for these endogenous variables is discussed in the third part of this chapter. In the final part, we summarize the complexity in the relationship between hospital infection and length of stay.

Existing methods for the attribution of cost to HAI

(Note, all costs are reported in US$ dollar 2002 prices.)

Haley (1998) reviewed the different methods used for attributing extra days and costs to hospital infection. We follow his schema with one exception, we replace 'Stratification with indirect standardization' with 'Regression analysis on cohort data' (see Box. 6.1).

The crude weighting method relies on a constant factor to predict excess length of stay due to hospital infection. If mean length of stay was 10 days for uninfected patients and this is multiplied by a constant of 1.5, we conclude

---

Box 6.1 Classification of methods used to estimate the number of days and costs that are attribute to nosocomial infections

I. Crude weighting

II. Direct attribution
    A. Clinician's subjective judgement
    B. Variation from a predicted value
    C. Standardized case review protocol

III. Comparative attribution
    A. Unmatched group comparison
    B. Matching of multiple characteristics
    C. Matching on summary measures of confounding

IV. Regression analysis on cohort data

V. Randomized trial

Source: Adapted from Haley (1998, p. 253).

From Haley, R.W. (1998). Cost-Benefit Analysis of Infection Control Activities. In *Hospital Infections* by P. Brachman and J. Bennett. Reproduced with kind permission by Lippincott, Williams & Wilkins.

that infected patients stay for 15 days, with the extra 5 days being the cost of the infection. Dixon (1978) used this method, estimating the combined cost of community and HAI, in the USA, to be US$11 billion and responsible for engendering 10% of all hospital bed days. Using this method, Haley (1978) estimated the cost of HAI to be US$2.33 billion. The precision of this method depends on the constant factor.

Direct attribution requires some assessment of each infected patient to identify by how much infection prolonged the stay, and the extra resources used as a consequence of the infection. These judgements were made by a physician in studies conducted by Scheckler (1978), who estimated the cost of a case of surgical wound infection to be US$3899, and Haley et al. (1981), who estimated the cost of a lower respiratory tract infection (LRTI) in three sepa-rate hospitals to be US$2571–US$2868, of a surgical wound infection to be US$$989–US$1829, a urinary tract infection to be US$$296–US$395 and a of a bloodstream infection to be US$98–US$5430. Critics of this method argue the decision is subjective and the results are unlikely to be reproducible from observer to observer or across different time periods (McGowan, 1982). Freeman and McGowan (1984) and Haley et al. (1980) conclude that this method is likely to underestimate, as they believed physician surveyors judged extra cost conservatively.

The variation from a predicted value method requires the expected length of stay, assuming the patient would not acquire an infection, to be deducted from the actual length of stay, if they did. Clarke (1957) used this method and found that patients with infections in their surgical wounds remained in hospital for an extra 5 days, and Goetz et al. (1988) found that patients with surgical wound infections remained in hospital an extra 5–48 days. This method relies on the estimates of the expected cost or length of stay.

The standardized case review protocol was developed by Wakefield et al. (1987) in response to criticisms of the direct attribution methods discussed. Trained staff worked to carefully prepared protocols, they assess each day of the patient's hospital stay according to whether it was: attributable to the reason for admission; jointly attributable to the reason for admission and the HAI; or attributable to the HAI alone. The method has been tested by Gertman and Restuccia (1981) and Rishpon et al. (1986) and found to produce high levels of interviewer agreement, but the estimates depend on the quality of the data included in the patient's records.

The first of the comparative approaches, unmatched group comparison, is the least sophisticated. The length of stay, or hospital cost, of those with and without infection are compared and the gross difference attributed to infec-tion. This unmatched group comparison is likely to suffer from what Haley (1998) describes as severity (of illness) bias. The source of this bias is true confounding, which occurs when a variable is associated with the outcome, length of stay or cost, and the incidence of HAI. This problem arises because patients who go on to acquire a hospital infection are likely to stay longer and so incur greater cost than those who do not, regardless of their infection risks. They might be older, sicker, be admitted to different specialties or have different co-morbidities. For the rest of the chapter, the terms 'severity bias' and 'confounding' are used interchangeably.

In an attempt to control for severity of illness bias, researchers conducted cohort studies in which patients with HAI were matched with uninfected patients on key factors thought likely to explain the differences in cost or length of stay. Davies and Cottingham (1979) estimated cost at US$3951 for a surgical site infection; Rubinstein *et al.* (1982) estimated the cost of a surgical wound infection at US$2403 and a case of a patient with multiple sites of infection at US$3353. Coello *et al.* (1993) and Green and Wenzel (1977) both studied surgical patients and found the cost of wound infection to be US$2382 and US$2044, respectively.

The number of matching variables used in these studies varied from one to eight and included age, sex, admitting speciality, primary surgical procedure, social class, year of discharge, indices of obesity and smoking status. Although a popular approach, researchers matching on multiple characteristics face a trade-off. The more variables used for matching, the more accurate is the cost estimate; however, finding uninfected controls for all infected patients becomes more difficult. As the number of matching variables increases, some patients, for whom no match can be found, are excluded. It appears that reducing severity bias may introduce a selection bias due to the exclusion of otherwise eligible patients for whom no match can be found. If common factors determine participation in the research and the likelihood of acquiring the disease or outcome then selection bias may arise (Rothman and Greenland 1998). Both severity and selection bias will make regular appearances in the rest of the chapter.

Haley (1998) suggests that even when patients are matched perfectly on multiple factors, the severity of illness, infection risk and expected length of stay may still vary between those with and without infection. He calls for summary measures over and above the usual matching factors that capture these differences between patients. He paid special attention to DRGs, as a mechanism for achieving this, but we argue that some relatively simple measures of the severity of chronic illness, obtained on admission before the infection is acquired, may be a useful control. For example, Elixhauser *et al.* (1998) attempted to segregate certain co-morbidities from other aspects of the patient's condition that predicted length of stay, costs and mortality. Although the number of co-morbidities has been used as a control variable by Plowman *et al.* (2001), it was not important in their model. It might be that the type of co-morbidity, or combination, rather than the number of co-morbidities plays a more important role in explaining variation in cost outcomes. Williams (1992) suggests low serum albumin as a crude but reliable indicator of general health status, although care should be taken as the level can fluctuate over the period of the in-patient stay. Another useful indicator of chronic disease severity may lie in the pharmaceutical profile of the patient. Von Korff *et al.* (1992) used data on the pharmacy products consumed by patients to identify a chronic disease score. It was found to be stable over time, correlated with other health status measures and physicians' assessment, and also predicted length of stay and mortality after controlling for age, gender and health care visits. Currently, nothing is known of whether these measures will be appropriate to control for severity bias, and their inclusion will increase the chance of selection bias if used in cohort studies with matching.

An alternative method for exploring the relationship between cost and HAI is the use of regression analysis. This statistical procedure can be used to quantify the relationship between the outcome of 'cost' or 'length of stay' and a single explanatory variable, hospital infection. A more relevant approach is the inclusion of multiple explanatory variables thus simultaneously controlling for multiple confounders [see Katz (2003) for a good introduction]. Selection bias is avoided as no patients are excluded, and severity bias can be minimized by the inclusion of as many explanatory variables and confounders as are appropriate. This method provides a measure of effect, or association, between the outcome and one or more of the explanatory variables. Confidence intervals provide a measure of the precision of this estimate.

Using this approach, Dominguez *et al.* (2001) found that the cost of infection in a paediatric intensive care **unit was US$50 361 per case, Hyryla and Sintonen (1994) found a 4-fold increase in the length of stay of patients with infections in their surgical wounds, and Plowman *et al.* (2001) found that patients with hospital infection had their stay prolonged by 2.8 times at a cost of US$4170. To control for severity bias, these researchers included values for the following explanatory variables in their models: age, risk of mortality, mortality, number and type of co-morbidities, diagnosis, length of pre-operative stay, sex, admission type and speciality.

Hollenbeak *et al.* (2002) compared four methods for analysing the results of a study into the cost of infections in surgical wounds following coronary artery bypass surgery. The methods used were: unmatched comparison; matching on multiple factors; linear regression; and a procedure they describe as Heckman's two-stage model. The attributable cost was very similar for three of the four methods used, between US$19 579 and US$20 103, but the two-stage model provided a much lower estimate of the attributable cost, US$14 211. In particular, the researchers additionally controlled for a risk index derived from the following risk factors for infection: diabetes; obesity; steroid therapy; prolonged mechanical ventilation; and extended pre-operative stay. They argued that these factors would also independently increase cost and so act as a true confounder. Presumably, the purpose of including this risk index on the right hand side of the regression model was to minimize the normally unobserved severity bias.

The final method for attributing cost to hospital infection, reviewed by Haley (1998), is by randomized controlled trial (RCT). Patients are randomized into two groups, with one receiving an intervention to reduce the risk of infection, and the other receiving a placebo. The purpose is to identify significant differences in the outcome of interest, hospital infection. Because the patients are randomly assigned, the confounders are also randomly assigned; the only difference in cost should be those that result from differences due to the rates of infection (McGowan 1982; Altman and Dore 1990). Mugford *et al.* (1989) conducted a meta-analysis of RCTs of antibiotic prophylaxis administered to patients undergoing caesarean section. With the routine use of antibiotics, the odds of wound infection were reduced by between 50 and 70%. The additional average cost of wound infection was estimated to be US$1735 and the introduction of routine antibiotic prophylaxis was found to reduce the average costs of postnatal care by between US$3152 and US$9455 per 100 caesarean sections. Stone *et al.* (1979) randomized 463 patients undergoing elective surgery to receive cefazoline prophylaxis or placebo. Patients in the placebo group had 25 more hospital infections and spent 428 more post-operative days in hospital, an average of 17.1 extra days per infection. In theory, this method should prevent confounding (severity bias) and, as long as drop-outs and non-compliers are randomly assigned between the arms, selection bias.

Despite this, the face validity of the results reported by Stone *et al.* (1979) was questioned by Haley (1998) who argued the attributable costs were the highest reported in the literature. There are other problems with this method. Because a relatively small number of patients acquire an infection, large numbers of patients have to be recruited, making RCTs expensive. In addition, Black (1996) argues that because many effective interventions are already common practice, it might be unethical to substitute a placebo for an intervention that produces benefits.

This concludes our review of the existing methods that attribute cost to infection. In particular, we have discussed severity and selection bias. In the next section, we discuss some preliminary work that builds on the regression analysis method, but additionally tackles another source of complexity in the relationship between hospital infection and cost, namely the two-way relationship between incidence of infection and length of stay discussed in the introduction.

Addressing the problem of endogenous variables in models of infection and cost

Regression analysis avoids selection bias while allowing the inclusion of unlimited variables to control for severity bias. However, regression models are likely to suffer from the additional bias arising from endogenous variables. In particular, if the incidence of hospital infection causes increased length of stay and length of stay is a risk factor for infection, these two variables are endogenous, i.e. values for both variables are determined within the model, and are likely to bias the estimate of the cost of hospital infection.

Graves *et al.* (2005) addressed this question and proposed a solution. They modelled the cost of infection using a subset of the data collected by Plowman *et al.* (2001). All patients over 65 years, admitted to the 'general medicine' and 'care of the elderly' services, with or without a hospital-acquired LRTI were selected. They found LRTI was a significant and important predictor of hospital cost, and showed the primary channel was via the effect on length of stay. In light of overwhelming clinical evidence that length of stay is an important risk factor for HAI (see, for example, Garibaldi *et al.* 1981; Haley *et al.* 1981; Hooton *et al.* 1981; Axelrod and Talbot 1989; Arbo *et al.* 1993; Glynn *et al.* 1997; de Boer *et al.* 1999), their conclusion was that LRTI and length of stay were determined endogenously. In the context of regression analysis, endogeneity of any of the regressors introduces serious bias. The authors adopted an instrumental variables estimation strategy to control the endogenous variables. This required the identification of variables correlated with the incidence of LRTI, but unrelated to length of stay except through their relationship with LRTI. They chose whether or not a patient had a nasogastric tube inserted and whether or not the patient required oxygen therapy. Both of these were risk factors for LRTI but not independently associated with length of stay, and thus they were valid instruments. The authors then modelled the incidence of LRTI as a function of the instrumental variables as well as an additional set of control variables. As the predicted LRTI from this regression is entirely a function of variables that are not determined by length of stay, this instrumented measure of LRTI, which we can call $LRTI_{IV}$, is not endogenously determined. While the incidence of $LRTI_{IV}$ may cause an increase in the length of stay, variation in $LRTI_{IV}$ cannot, by construction, be caused itself by variation in length of stay. By using $LRTI_{IV}$ instead of the uninstrumented LRTI in a regression, they effectively eliminate endogeneity bias from the regression analysis.

In practice, the incidence of LRTI is a categorical variable that takes the value 1 if an infection is observed, and 0 otherwise. Accordingly, the predicted value of LRTI as a function of exogenous and instrumental variables, $LRTI_{IV}$, is estimated using a probit model and constitutes, in effect, an estimated probability of infection. The values for $LRTI_{IV}$ indicated that 93.4% of patients had a risk of less than 10% and the remaining patients had a risk greater than or equal to 10% but less than 40%. The final model of total cost regressed on controls and $LRTI_{IV}$ provided an estimate of the expected increase in total hospital costs from an (exogenous) increase in the probability of getting an infection.

They found that for every 10% decrease in the ex ante probability of acquiring an $LRTI_{IV}$, expected costs fell by £693 (about US$985) per patient. Dealing with estimated risk in this fashion can be confusing, so it is important to keep in mind that a risk reduction of 10% in a patient whose ex ante risk is estimated to be 10% constitutes something approaching a 100% reduction of risk for that particular patient! Since this is virtually impossible, with costs probably increasing exponentially as risk is marginally reduced, the costs of achieving such a reduction are likely to be much higher than one might think at first glance. Among the few higher risk patients, if the risk of LRTI were reduced from 40 to 20% (i.e. a 50% reduction in risk for those patients), the expected total savings in hospital costs would be £1386 (US$1970) per patient. We can see from this exercise that there is no single estimate of cost savings for a given reduction in the risk of infection; the savings will vary from patient to patient depending on their initial risk level. This is intuitive; the expected cost savings of cutting the risk in half for a high-risk patient will be much greater than the cost savings of cutting the risk in half for a low-risk patient. Similarly, the expected savings from avoiding infection in high-risk patients will be much higher than a similar outcome in low-risk patients.

Plowman et al. (2001) used the same data (but OLS rather than IV regression analyses) and estimated the cost of an LRTI to be £3050 (about US$4500) for admissions to general medicine services and £1765 (about US$2650) for admissions to care of the elderly services. Comparison with the result of Graves et al. (2005) is difficult as the Plowman estimates considered the coefficient estimate on the 'yes or no' infection outcome and interpreted it as the additional cost of an infection. Graves et al. (2005) derived a bias-free continuous variable, yet no patient had a 100% ex ante risk of infection. It may be considered an artificial exercise to consider the cost savings from avoiding an infection that you 'know' would have occurred. However, if you performed that exercise and calculated the savings by avoiding an infection in someone with an ex ante probability of 100%, you find that in the study of Graves *et al.* (2005), the savings were substantially larger, at £6930 (about US$9850), than has been previously estimated in the literature.

The conventional wisdom has been that the endogeneity between length of stay and LRTI should bias the traditional estimates upwards, not downwards, so this result seems puzzling. However, it is important to recognize that endogeneity bias can be quite complex, and predicting in advance the direction of the bias is not as straightforward as it seems. In general, without completely understanding the processes driving the data, it is not possible to predict the direction of the bias. Perhaps in this case the endogeneity bias is actually decreasing the conventional estimates.

To illustrate this point, we generate a simple data set that shares some of the key properties of the actual data set. It was derived from the assumptions that the likelihood of getting an LRTI increased with length of stay and the length of stay increased whenever a patient acquired an infection. A naïve regression with endogeneity bias and then the instrumental variable (IV) model were applied to the simulated data and the actual data.

For the simulated data, we found exactly the results that conventional wisdom would have suggested. Estimates from the IV model were lower than those from the naïve, biased model. When the assumptions about the underlying data-generating process are correct, the IV estimation works as expected. However, we found a different pattern when they used the actual data for the 'naïve' and 'IV' specifications. As can be seen from Table 6.1, the IV model estimate is quite a bit larger than the naïve OLS estimator for the actual data. Maybe it was the properties in the underlying data that were driving the results rather than the estimation strategy.

The primary conclusion is that the relationship between length of stay and risk of infection could be much more complex than the simple feedback mechanism conventional wisdom may have assumed. Furthermore, given the underlying complexity of the endogeneity, it is impossible to guess in advance whether simple OLS estimates will produce estimates biased upwards or downwards.

Table 6.1 Comparison of estimates from simulated and real data

Stay	Naïve	IV model
Simulated data	18.30 (15.24)	15.69 (2.07)
Actual data	26.30 (17.42)	44.08 (5.35)

t-statistics are given in parentheses.

Conclusions

Within the environment of increasing demand for health care and increasing expenditures, efficiency in resource allocation is paramount. It is important to identify and measure sources of excess cost within the hospital environment so that cost saving measures can be implemented where appropriate. The minimization of the costs of hospital infection and control programmes contributes to efficiency.

In order to identify the cost-effectiveness of different approaches to infection control, an accurate estimate of the true cost of HAIs is required, and consequently a good deal of academic research has been devoted to these ends. This chapter has reviewed the different methods that have been used. We conclude that a promising method is the IV regression approach that controls for the most commonly identified sources of bias: selection bias, severity bias and endogeneity bias.

A regression analysis can avoid the selection bias of more traditional matching studies by including all patients in the study. Alternatively, if some patients are missing from the analysis but are known to exist, there are well known statistical methods, such as a Heckman selection bias correction procedure, that may be effective for eliminating the resulting biases.

In addition, regression analysis is ideally suited to the task of correcting for severity bias. If a researcher can measure the degree of severity, or can find variables that are correlated with severity, then these measures can be included as control variables.

If suitable instrumental variables can be identified, then the two-stage instrumental variables procedure described in this chapter can be used to correct for endogenous variables. This approach appears to be the only method reported in the literature that makes headway in terms of correcting endogenous variables. To date only one study of HAIs (Graves *et al.* 2005) has been conducted that uses this approach, and more work needs to be done in refining our understanding of how to interpret the estimates. Furthermore, more effort needs to be put into the identification of additional suitable instruments so that the first-pass study of Graves *et al.* (2005) can be expanded, duplicated and verified.

References

Altman, D.G. and Dore, C.J. (1990) Randomisation and baseline comparisons in clinical trials. *Lancet* **335**, 149–153.

Arbo, M.J., Fine, M.J. *et al.* (1993) Fever of nosocomial origin: etiology, risk factors, and outcomes. *American Journal of Medicine* **95**, 505–512.

Axelrod, P. and Talbot, G.H. (1989) Risk factors for acquisition of gentamicin-resistant enterococci. A multivariate analysis. *Archives of Internal Medicine* **149**, 1397–1401.

Black, N. (1996) Why we need observational studies to evaluate the effectiveness of health care. *British Medical Journal* **312**, 1215–1218.

Clarke, S.K.R. (1957) Sepsis in surgical wounds, with particular reference to *Staphlyococcus aureus*. *British Journal of Surgery* **44**, 592–596.

Coello, R., Glenister, H. *et al.* (1993) The cost of infection in surgical patients: a case control study. *Journal of Hospital Infections* **25**, 239–250.

Currie, E. and Maynard, A. (1989) *The Economics of Hospital Acquired Infection, Discussion Paper 56.* Centre for Health Economics, University of York.

Davies, T. and Cottingham, J. (1979) The cost of hospital infection in orthopaedic patients. *Journal of Infection* **1**, 330–338.

de Boer, A.S., Mintjes de Groot, A.J. *et al.* (1999) Risk assessment for surgical-site infections in orthopedic patients. *Infection Control and Hospital Epidemiology* **20**, 402–407.

Dixon, R. (1978) Effect of infections on hospital care. *Annals of Internal Medicine* **89**, 749–753.

Dominguez, T.E., Chalom, R. *et al.* (2001) The impact of adverse patient occurrences on hospital costs in the pediatric intensive care unit. *Critical Care Medicine* **29**, 169–174.

Elixhauser, A., Steiner, C. *et al.* (1998) Comorbidity measures for use with administrative data. *Medical Care* **36**, 8–27.

Freeman, J. and McGowan, J.E. (1984) Methodologic issues in hospital epidemiology: III. Investigating the modifying effects of time and severity of underlying illness on estimates of cost of nosocomial infection. *Review of Infectious Diseases* **10**, 1118–1141.

Garibaldi, R.A., Britt, M.R. *et al.* (1981) Risk factors for post-operative pneumonia. *American Journal of Medicine* **70**, 677–680.

Gertman, P.M. and Restuccia, J.D. (1981) The appropriateness evaluation protocol: a technique for assessing unnecessary days of hospital care. *Medical Care* **19**, 855.

Glynn, A., Ward, V. *et al.* (1997) *Hospital Acquired Infection: Surveillance Policies and Practice.* Public Health Laboratory Service, London.

Goetz, A., Yu, V.L. *et al.* (1988) Surgical complications related to insertion of penile protheses with emphasis on infection and cost. *Infection Control and Hospital Epidemiology* **9**, 250.

Graves, N., Weinhold, D. and Roberts, J.A. (2005) Correcting for bias when estimating the cost of hospital acquired infection: an analysis of lower respiratory tract infections in non-surgical patients. *Health Economics* **14**, 756–761.

Green, J. and Wenzel, R.P. (1977) Postoperative wound infection: a controlled study of the increased duration of hospital stay and direct costs of hospitalization. *Annals of Surgery* **185**, 264–268.

Haley, R.W. (1978) Preliminary cost-benefit analysis of hospital infection control programs (The SENIC Project). In: Daschner, F. (ed.), *Proven and Unproven Methods in Hospital Infection Control.* Gustav, Fisher and Verlag, Stuttgart, pp. 93–96.

Haley, R.W. (1986) *Managing Hospital Infection Control for Cost-effectiveness: A Strategy for Reducing Infectious Complications.* AHA, USA.

Haley, R.W. (1998) Cost-benefit analysis of infection control activities. In: Brachman, P. and Bennett, J. (eds), *Hospital Infections.* Pippincott-Raven, Philadelphia, pp. 249–267.

Haley, R.W., Schaberg D. *et al.* (1980) Estimating the extra charges and prolongation of hospitalization due to nosocomial infections: a comparison of methods. *Journal of Infectious Diseases* **141**, 248–257.

Haley, R.W., Hooton, T.M. *et al.* (1981a) Nosocomial infections in US hospitals 1975–76. Estimated frequency by selected characteristics of patients. *American Journal of Medicine* **70**, 947–959.

Haley, R.W., Schaberg, D. *et al.* (1981b) Extra charges and prolongation of stay attributable to nosocomial infections: a prospective inter-hospital comparison. *American Journal of Medicine* **70**, 51–58.

Hollenbeak, C.S., Murphy, D. *et al.* (2002) Nonrandom selection and the attributable cost of surgical-site infections. *Infection Control and Hospital Epidemiology* **23**, 177–182.

Hooton, T.M., Haley, R.W. *et al.* (1981) The joint associations of multiple risk factors with the occurrence of nosocomial infection. *American Journal of Medicine* **70**, 960–970.

Hyryla, M.L.J. and Sintonen, H. (1994) The use of health services in the management of wound infection. *Journal of Hospital Infections* **26**, 1–14.

Katz, M.H. (2003) Multivariable analysis: a primer for readers of medical research. *Annals of Internal Medicine* **138**, 644–650.

Lambert, D.C. (1987) The cost of nosocomial infection and it's prevention. Projection and limitations of an economic analysis. *Aggressologie* **28**, 1123.

Lambert, D.C. and Fabry, J. (1985) Cost-benefit and cost-effectiveness methods and evaluation of additional costs due to a hospital infection. 26(173).

McGowan, J.E. (1982) Cost and benefit – a critical issue for hospital infection control. *American Journal of Infection Control* **10**, 100–108.

Miller, P.J., Farr, B.M. *et al.* (1989) Economic benefits of an infection control program: case study and proposal. *Reviews of Infectious Diseases* **11**, 284–288.

Mugford, M., Kingston J. *et al.* (1989) Reducing the incidence of infection after caesarean section: implications of prophylaxis with antibiotics for hospital resources. *British Medical Journal* **299**, 1003–1006.

Olsen, M.M. (1990) Continuous, 10 year wound surveillance: results, advantages, and unanswered questions. *Archives of Surgery* **125**, 794.

Plowman, R.P., Graves, N. *et al.* (1997) Hospital Acquired Infection. Office of Health Economics, London.

Plowman, R.P., Graves, N. *et al.* (2001) The rate and cost of hospital-acquired infections occurring in patients admitted to selected specialties of a district general hospital in England and the national burden imposed. *Journal of Hospital Infections* **47**, 198–209.

Rishpon, S., Lubasch, S. *et al.* (1986) Reliability of a method of determining the necessity of hospitalization days in Israel. *Medical Care* **24**, 279.

Rothman, K.J. and Greenland, S. (1998) Precision and validity in epidemiologic studies. In: Rothman, K.J. and Greenland, S. (eds), *Modern Epidemiology*. Lippincott-Raven, Philadelphia.

Rubinstein, E., Green, M. *et al.* (1982) The effect of nosocomial infections on the length and costs of hospital stay. *Journal of Antimicrobial Chemotherapy* **9** (Supplement A), 93–100.

Scheckler, W.E. (1978) Septicaemia and nosocomial infections in a community hospital. *Annals of Internal Medicine* **89**, 754–756.

Sencer, D.J. and Axnick, N.W. (1975) Utilization of cost/benefit analysis in planning prevention programs. *Acta Medica Scandinavica, Supplement* **576**, 123.

Sperry, H.E. and Craddock, J. (1968) It pays to spend money for infection control. *Modern Hospital* **111**, 124–128.

Stone, H.H., Haney, B.B. *et al.* (1979) Prophylactic and preventive antibiotic therapy: timing, duration and economics. *Annals of Surgery* **189**, 691–699.

Von Korff, M., Wagner, E.H. *et al.* (1992) A chronic disease score from automated pharmacy data. *Journal of Clinical Epidemiology* **45**, 197–203.

Wakefield, D.S., Pfaller, M.A. *et al.* (1987) Use of the appropriateness evaluation protocol for estimating the incremental costs associated with nosocomial infections. *Medical Care* **25**, 481–488.

Williams, T.F. (1992) Serum albumin, aging and disease. *Journal of Clinical Epidemiology* **45**, 205–206.

Chapter 7

Decision analysis of strategies to deal with non-compliance with TB treatment

João G Q Costa, Laura C Rodrigues, Andreia C Santos and Maurício L Barreto

Introduction

Non-compliance in tuberculosis (TB) treatment is a major cause of concern because it increases the chance of drug resistance and of spreading the disease to others. Non-compliance requires resources that would not be used if the patient had followed the treatment. A patient who abandons the treatment and eventually comes back to start a new treatment has to be enrolled in a longer and more expensive drug scheme. In this way, the resources consumed in the first treatment are wasted and new resources have to be spent on the same patient. One of the reasons why the World Health Organization (WHO) supports DOT (directly observed treatment) is the increase in compliance achieved by this strategy, but DOT has been questioned as not feasible in many contexts.

This work presents a simulated comparison between strategies of dealing with interruption of TB treatment. The simulation takes place in two steps. First, the strategies of tracing a proportion of the patients that do not come to the health centres on the day of their appointments (defaulters) are compared with a strategy which aims at tracing 100% of defaulters. Some strategies approximate to the status quo in Salvador (Brazil), where the TB control programme tries to trace only a small proportion of defaulters. The second step compares the alternative of enrolling all the defaulters in a DOT scheme with another alternative of enrolling in DOT only those who do not return to treatment after being traced by the most cost-effective tracing strategies among the four tested in the first part. The comparisons are performed using decision analysis tools. Based on cost of treatment, cost of tracing activities and presumed success of tracing activities (described by the number of avoided defaulters among those that interrupt treatment), it is clear that the best strategy is to try to trace all defaulters. Considering estimations of cost of treating a patient in the DOT scheme, the strategy which covers with DOT only the defaulters that do not return after being traced is the most cost-effective.

Anecdotal reports say that in some urban settings in Brazil where there is only one health centre to cover a large population with high TB incidence rates, it is impossible for health workers to visit the households and supervise all patients being treated. Apart from that, there is a high demand for health workers in several programmes and activities being carried out in health centres. On the other hand, if patients are required to come to the health centre to receive the drugs on a daily basis, they are likely to default given the distance and travel costs and the time they could spend in income generation activities. The current level of defaulters in Brazil, around 11.7% (SINAN/MS, 2001), is attributed to patients' lack of the resources needed to come to the health centre just once a month to collect their monthly pack of drugs. It has been reported that some centres established a routine of covering travel expenses and supplying food in order to enhance patients' attendance and compliance.

Although largely recommended for presenting lower rates of defaulting, high rates of success (Chaulk 1998) and lower hospitalization (Weis 1999) and less acquired multidrug resistance (Burman 1997; Yew 1999) when compared with self-administered therapy, there are still uncertainties regarding the cost-effectiveness of the universal implementation of DOT (Moore 1996; Chaulk 1998) and the questionable results of its 'authoritarian' surveillance procedure (Zwarenstein 1998), and further evaluation is required (Migliori et al. 1999).

Snyder and Chin (1999) observed that the cost-effectiveness of DOT was sensitive to the rate of default and relapse. DOT would generate cost savings only when the default and relapse rates were more than 32.2 and 9.2%, respectively. These authors conclude that for default rates lower than the referred one, DOT implementation should be decided considering availability of resources and competing programme priorities.

Therefore, targeting specific high-risk defaulters can be a more cost-effective strategy than a universal implementation of DOT. In the Brazilian context, the extension of DOT to the successfully treated patients under the self-administered regime would represent an important waste of scarce resources. There is nevertheless the need to find ways to target the still high number of defaulters and ensure their adherence to the treatment.

New initiatives to identify other less expensive schemes (for patients and health services) that could achieve high rates of compliance are therefore needed. An alternative way of dealing with non-compliance would require means and actions to make sure that each patient is traced and receives the attention necessary, and be brought back to treatment and stay until the end.

The strategies with the lowest cost-effectiveness ratio could then be justified and implemented in a comprehensive way.

According to Brazilian official publications (SINAN/MS, 2001) 11.7% of the patients interrupt their treatment before it is completed. A number of these patients may come back if traced, but normally tracing activities are not extensive and there is no effort to trace a large proportion of those patients. The patients that do not show up on the day of their monthly appointment are likely to be classified as defaulters and have their files closed. Where the tracing work should start, in most cases it actually ends.

What happens to these defaulters? It is expected that 25% of defaulters are cured without treatment (World Health Organization 2004a). It is also expected (according to local studies) that 18% of the defaulters return to treatment voluntarily in the same year they defaulted (Costa *et al.* 2000). Given these proportions, and considering that some patients will die, it is estimated that around 50% of defaulters remain ill and contagious. This scenario calls for an urgent evaluation of cost and effectiveness of tracing strategies.

According to anecdotes collected among staff involved with tracing activities in health centres, once traced, found and properly instructed, defaulters tend to come back and adhere to the treatment up to its completion. It is expected that around 80% of the visited defaulters return to the treatment. If a large proportion of defaulters could be brought back to treatment with a single visit, DOT would be only recommended for those with a high risk of remaining non-compliant after being visited. This work therefore simulates and compares the cost-effectiveness of tracing strategies and the cost-effectiveness of strategies of implementing DOT in connection with the results of the tracing initiatives.

Objectives

The objectives of this study were to compare the expected costs and expected effectiveness of strategies of tracing TB patients that do not comply with the prescribed treatment and to compare two strategies of assigning them to DOT schemes.

Methods, approaches and measures

The study is organized in two steps. First, the cost-effectiveness of defaulter tracing strategies which target 20, 30, 50 and 100% of the defaulters is tested. The second part compares the alternative of enrolling all the defaulters in a DOT scheme with the alternative of enrolling in DOT only those who do not return to treatment after being traced by the most cost-effective tracing strategies among the four tested in the first part.

The strategies in both parts are modelled using decision analysis tools. Two decision trees have been designed. In the first tree (Fig. 7.1), each of the four branches represents a tracing strategy which aims at 20, 30, 50 and 100% of the defaulters, respectively. The second tree (Fig. 7.2) represents the two DOT strategies.

A number of assumptions are adopted in order to make the simulation feasible.

1. Five per cent of the defaulters are not found in spite of the effort dedicated to tracing them. This estimate was obtained in fieldwork carried out for this study. A systematic attempt to trace defaulters found 95% and considered 5% lost to follow-up despite repeated attempts to find them.

2. Once the patient is found, according to the reported experience of staff members involved with the activity, the chances of getting them back to treatment are high. In this work, it was assumed that 80% of the traced patients come back to treatment. Nevertheless, for the second tree, a sensitivity analysis is carried out testing this assumption. In the sensitivity analysis, this percentage is tested in the range of 10–80%.

3. Once found and brought back to the treatment, the patients get back to the point of the interruption and adhere to the treatment up to completion (no further interruption is introduced in the model).

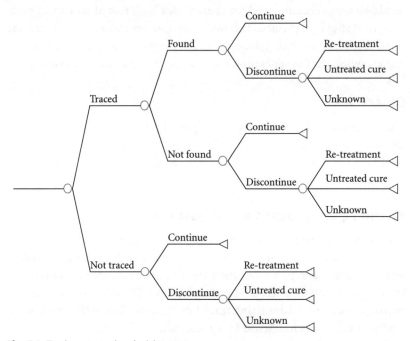

Fig. 7.1 Tracing strategies decision tree.

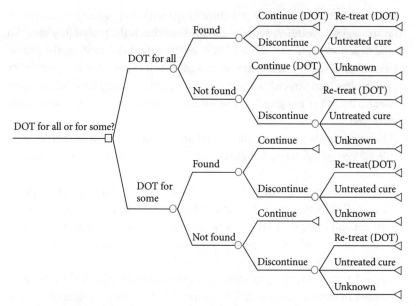

Fig. 7.2 Decision tree: DOT for all or some defaulters.

4. It is also assumed that 25% of untreated patients achieve a cure, based on the literature.

For the patients traced and brought back to treatment, this work considers that the treatment costs are the same as for a patient who does not interrupt it. For patients that do not return, the costs of an abandoned treatment is a weighted mean estimated considering the proportion of abandonment per month of occurrence. For patients that do not come back when traced but return later and start another treatment, the costs include the costs of the abandoned treatment plus the costs of the new treatment. As 12% of the reported cases initiate their treatment with a hospital admission, 12% of an admission cost is added to the estimated costs. Regarding the tracing costs, no economy of scale was considered; therefore, it is assumed that the cost of tracing a defaulter is the same for all strategies.

A sensitivity analysis is carried for some of the adopted assumptions.

Results

Table 7.1 presents the unit costs employed in the simulations. The costs are based on public sector wages, public sector evaluation of value of facilities, and market prices of materials and services in Salvador/Brazil in 1999. The costing methodology and techniques are described in details in Costa *et al.* (2005).

Figure 7.1 depicts the basic structure of the defaulter-tracing model for all four strategies. The difference between the branches is the probability assigned to the first nodule. In the 'tracing 100% of the defaulters' strategy, the probability assigned to the nodule named 'traced' is 1; it means that the probability of a defaulter being traced is 1. For the 'tracing 30%' strategy, for instance, the probability 0.3 is assigned to the nodule 'traced' and 0.7 to the nodule 'not traced'.

The other probabilities in the model are the same for all four strategies. Table 7.2 presents these probabilities and the range used for sensitivity analysis purpose.

The cost assigned to each end node is the sum of the respective appropriate unit cost. For instance, for a patient who was traced, did not continue the treatment and came back later to start a re-treatment, the respective total cost would be the sum of the tracing cost plus the cost of the abandoned treatment plus the cost of the re-treatment.

Regarding the measure of effectiveness, except for the end nodes with unknown outcomes (for which it is assumed that the patient remains ill), it is

Table 7.1 TB control programme activities and unit cost

Activity/treatment	Unit cost
Standard treatment	171.00
Interrupted treatment	74.00
Re-treatment	180.00
Defaulter tracing	7.18
DOT (home visitors and transport)	54.00

Table 7.2 Probabilities and sensitivity analysis ranges

Events	Probability	Sensitivity analysis
Being traced	$0.2 \geq P \leq 1$	$0.2 \geq P \leq 1$
Being found	0.95	–
Continuing treatment if found	0.8	$0.1 \geq P \leq 0.8$
Continuing treatment if not found	0.05	–
Continuing treatment if not traced	0.05	–
Re-treatment after discontinuing	0.18	–
Untreated cure	0.3	–
Finishing DOT treatment	0.9	–

assigned an effectiveness equal to 1 for all end nodes, which means that the patients are presumed cured. An effectiveness of 0 is assigned to end nodes with unknown outcomes.

Table 7.3 presents the results of the cost-effectiveness analysis. Strategy 100% presents the highest cost (£162.8), the highest effectiveness (0.876) and the lowest cost-effectiveness ratio (£185.78). None of the strategies strictly dominates any of the others. The incremental cost-effectiveness, £143.61 per additional defaulter cured, is the same for all strategies (which indicates a linear relationship across strategies). As the incremental cost-effectiveness is lower than the cost-effectiveness ratio of all strategies, this gives support to the implementation of the 100% strategy. The 100% strategy presents the highest effectiveness, and thus the lowest number of unknown outcomes or patients who remain ill and will presumably come back in the future to start a new treatment. If the costs of future treatment (and the costs of treating the secondary cases infected by them) are incorporated in the model, this will make the 100% strategy even more cost-effective and recommendable. Considering the future cost equal to the cost of a re-treatment and introducing it into the model, it makes the 100% strategy strictly dominate all the others, which gives a clear indication for its recommendation.

The second tree depicted in Fig. 7.2 presents two alternative approaches to provide DOT to all traced and found defaulters, or to provide DOT only to those who are traced and found but do not return to treatment after they are contacted.

The cost of DOT (Table 7.1) includes only the salary of the community agent (which is derived by taking into account the number of other activities the agent undertakes in the communities) and the cost of transport (the agent uses public transport). The cost of treatment remains the same (including drugs, consultation, examinations, etc.) for a patient enrolled or not in a DOT scheme. It is assumed that 90% of the patients in the DOT scheme adhere to the treatment and achieve a cure. All those who start a DOT re-treatment are assumed to finish the treatment and achieve a cure.

Table 7.3 Cost-effectiveness analysis (Fig. 7.1)

Strategy	Cost	Marginal cost	Effectiveness	Marginal effectiveness	C/E
20%	£120.3		0.580		£207.33
30%	£125.6	£5.3	0.617	0.037	£203.50
50%	£136.2	£10.6	0.691	0.074	£197.08
100%	£162.8	£26.6	0.876	0.185	£185.78

Table 7.4 Cost-effectiveness analysis (Fig. 7.2)

Strategy	Cost	Marginal cost	Effectiveness	Marginal effectiveness	C/E
DOT for some	£165.1	0.8765	£188		
DOT for all	£216.7	£51.5	0.9259	0.0494	£234

The results of the cost-effectiveness analysis are presented in Table 7.4. As shown in the table, the strategy DOT for all is more effective but is also costlier and presents a higher cost-effectiveness ratio. The incremental cost-effectiveness is £1043, which suggests that given the high cost per additional unit of effect (defaulter cured), the implementation of such a strategy depends on availability of resources.

Discussion

The global targets for TB control consist of detecting 70% of the cases and curing 85% of these by 2005. In its effort to achieve such targets, the WHO has launched DOT as a model for worldwide TB control. According to the WHO Report 2004 (World Health Organization, 2004b), up to 2002 DOT was introduced in 180 out of 210 countries. Nevertheless, the coverage achieved by country varies from 10 to 90% of the population. From the 4.08 million cases reported in 2005, 26% (1.04 million) were notified by non-DOT control programmes. A few high-burden countries (India, China, the Russian Federation, Brazil and Bangladesh) are responsible for 75% of the cases identified by non-DOT programmes. In India, half of the cases were identified and treated in non-DOT programmes, and in Brazil and the Russian Federation, around 88% of the cases were not treated under the DOT strategy.

There is always tension between recommending a global strategy and adjusting it to local context. A strategy which is tailored for each context might lose identity, credibility and implementation momentum. On the other hand, a strategy that is globally defined regardless of local needs or experiences is likely to be criticized for its 'one-size-fits-all' approach, therefore losing momentum and credibility too. Solving this dilemma is a complex task planners of global strategies have to face.

Lienhardt and Ogden (2004) have discussed evidence from several sources that social context factors have profound influence on the ability of control programmes to implement DOT policy effectively. Thus these authors question the appropriateness of applying a universal paradigm for global TB control. In support of such criticism, some trials have identified that in fact there is no evidence that DOT is more cost-effective than a non-DOT programme. Khan *et al.* (2002) have found that a non-DOT programme was more cost-effective (although not statistically significant) in Pakistan, a country where 90% of the cases are treated under DOT. If a non-DOT programme achieves comparatively the same results as DOT, the country would save many resources by adopting a non-DOT strategy. On the other hand, Vassall *et al.* (2002) found that once integrated in the primary health care system in Egypt and Syria, DOT was more cost-effective.

Brazil has a vast health system which provides universal and free health care for its citizens. TB drugs are delivered free of charge for all patients, and private pharmacies are forbidden to sell TB drugs. Patients can only receive their treatment in the public system. According to the WHO Report 2004 (World Health Organization 2004b), only 11% of the TB cases were treated under DOT in Brazil. Nevertheless, the country has shown a very low level of interruption of treatment, which seems to explain the little effort spent on introducing DOT throughout the country. Even without widespread DOT, Brazil is close to the 2005 target of curing 85% of identified cases. According to the SINAN/MS (2001), 72.2% of the identified patients have been cured. In this sense, with additional effort in implementing the combination of default tracing and DOT for some, as suggested in the simulation reported in this chapter, Brazil could be very close to the WHO target.

An implication of the simulation carried out in this chapter is that attention should be paid to the contextual factors; in particular, the specificities of the country health system should be considered in adjusting DOT to the local characteristics. In the simulation model, considering the future cost of patients who discontinued treatment after being traced, and assuming in the end that all patients are treated and cured, the results of the sensitivity analysis indicate that the probability of continuing the treatment (DOT for some scheme) after being contacted is the crucial variable. If 20% or fewer defaulters return to the treatment (non-DOT) after being contacted, the strategy of DOT for all dominates and should be recommended. If 40% or more defaulters are brought back to the treatment (non-DOT) after being traced and contacted, the non-DOT strategy dominates. (Threshold analysis indicates 0.44 as the probability above which DOT for all changes from dominant to dominated by DOT for some strategy.) This discussion suggests that more research is needed into how to make effective adjustments of the DOT strategy suitable to the local needs and characteristics.

Conclusion

It is more cost-effective to trace 100% of defaulters rather than to trace just a fraction (20, 30 or 50%) of the defaulters. These results seem to be consistent and are fairly acceptable as it is clear that the costs of tracing are very small compared with the costs of the abandoned treatment plus re-treatment.

Considering the high expected level of adherence to the treatment by traced defaulters (80%), giving DOT to some patients is more cost-effective than giving it to all. The defaulters who do not come back to the treatment after being contacted are the ones who should be targeted and enrolled in a DOT scheme.

The conclusion of this work suggests that health managers can improve TB control programme performance by adopting cost-effective strategies such as systematic default tracing and a selective DOT scheme.

References

Burman, W., Dalton, C.B., Cohn, D.L., Butler, J.R. and Reves, R.R. (1997) A cost-effectiveness analysis of directly observed therapy vs self-administered therapy for treatment of tuberculosis. *Chest* 112, 63–70.

Chaulk, C.P. and Kazandjian, V.A. (1998) Directly observed therapy for treatment completion of pulmonary tuberculosis: Consensus Statement of the Public Health Tuberculosis Guidelines Panel. *Journal of the American Medical Association* 279, 943–948.

Costa, J.G.Q., Santos, A.C. and Barreto, M.L. (2000) Pacientes com mais de uma notifição de tuberculose: implicações para o controle. *Boletim de Pneumologia Sanitária* 8, 41–45.

Costa, J.G., Santos, A.C., Rodrigues, L.C., Barreto, M.L and Roberts, J.A. (2005) Tuberculosis in Salvador, Brazil: costs to health system and families. *Revista de Saude Publica* 39, 1–6.

Khan, M.A. *et al.* (2002) Costs and cost-effectiviness of different DOT strategies for the treatment of tuberculosis in Pakistan. *Health Policy and Planning* 17, 178–186.

Lienhardt, C. and Ogden, J.A. (2004) Tuberculosis control in resource-poor countries: have we reached the limits of the universal paradigm? *Tropical Medicine and International Health* 9, 833–841.

Migliori, G.B., Ambrosetti, M., Besozzi, G., Farris, B., Nutini, S., Saini, L., Casali, L., Nardini, S., Bugiani, M., Neri, M. and Raviglione, M.C. (1999) Cost-comparison of different management policies for tuberculosis patients in Italy. AIPO TB Study Group. *Bulletin of the World Health Organization* 77, 467–476.

Moore, R.D., Chaulk, C.P., Griffiths, R., Cavalcante, S. and Chaisson, R.E. (1996) Cost-effectiveness of directly observed versus self-administered therapy for tuberculosis. *American Journal of Respiratory and Critical Care Medicine* 154, 1013–1019.

SINAN (Sistema de Informação de Agravos de Notificação-Ministerio da Saude-Brazil) (2001) (http://dtr2001.saude.gov.br/svs/epi/Tuberculose/tuberculose_00.htm

Snyder, D.C. and Chin, D.P. (1999) Cost-effectiveness analysis of directly observed therapy for patients with tuberculosis at low risk for treatment default. *American Journal of Respiratory and Critical Care Medicine* 160, 582–586.

Vassall, A. *et al.* (2002) Cost-effectiviness of different treatment strategies fro tuberculosis in Egypt and Syria, *International Journal of Tuberculosis and Lung Diseases* **6**, 1083–1090.

Weis, S.E., Foresman, B., Matty, K.J., Brown, A., Blais, F.X., Burgess, G., King, B., Cook, P.E. and Slocum, P.C. (1999) Treatment costs of directly observed therapy and traditional therapy for *Mycobacterium tuberculosis*: a comparative analysis. *Internaional Journal of Tuberculosis and Lung Disease* **3**, 976–984.

World Health Organization (2004a) *TB/HIV, a Clinical Manual*, 2nd edon. WHO, Geneva.

World Health Organization (2004b) *WHO Report 2004—Global Tuberculosis Control*. WHO, Geneva.

Yew, W.W. (1999) Directly observed therapy, short-course: the best way to prevent multidrug-resistant tuberculosis. *Chemotherapy* 45 Supplement **2**, 26–33.

Zwarenstein, M., Schoeman, J.H., Vundule, C., Lombard, C.J. and Tatley, M. (1998) Randomised controlled trial of self-supervised and directly observed treatment of tuberculosis. *Lancet* **352**, 1340–1343.

Chapter 8

The economic evaluation of HAI

Rosalind Plowman

Introduction

Economic evaluation is concerned with the assessment of the costs and consequences of alternative practices, thus enabling the comparison of alternative interventions in order to obtain the maximum health gain for a given expenditure, or the lowest expenditure for a given health gain (Drummond *et al.* 1987).

In the context of hospital-acquired infection (HAI), it is clear from the literature that HAIs affect a substantial number of patients every year (Emmerson *et al.* 1996; Plowman *et al.* 2001b). Whilst it is unlikely that all infections can be prevented (Ayliffe 1986), a proportion could be prevented through improvements in infection control practice (Haley *et al.* 1985). Evidence from the study of the efficacy of nosocomial infection control (SENIC) conducted in the USA indicated that hospitals with an organized hospital-wide infection control programme which included intensive surveillance, the feedback of results to those who need to know, one infection control nurse per 250 beds and the involvement of an infection control physician or microbiologist on average achieved a 32% reduction in infection rates over time (Haley 1986). This evidence informed guidance issued by the Department of Health in 1995, which stated that about 30% of HAIs could be prevented through improvements in infection control (Department of Health and Public Health Laboratory Service 1995).

More recently, the National Audit Office (NAO) in England conducted a survey of National Health Service (NHS) hospitals in which they asked infection control teams (ICTs) whether they believed a 30% reduction in rates could be achieved in their NHS Trust; 39% thought this could be achieved, 49% thought the estimate was too high, and the remaining 12% either did not know or did not answer the question. The NAO survey also asked ICTs to estimate what proportion of infections they considered to be preventable in their Trust. The responses varied from less than 5% to over 35%. The average percentage reduction across all NHS Trusts, adjusted for the number of beds in the hospitals that responded, was 15% (Report by the Comptroller and Auditor General 2000). Whilst this is a subjective assessment of the proportion of HAIs that are preventable, it does demonstrate that there is a strong belief that a proportion of infections can be prevented. Evidence from studies which have assessed the incidence of HAI over time in response to various interventions provides harder evidence that a proportion can be prevented

The prevention of HAIs is not, however, cost free. Economic evaluation is thus concerned with estimating the costs associated with these infections, and the cost of activities that aim to prevent infection and their economic consequences, thus providing valuable data that can contribute to decisions about the allocation of resources to infection control.

The literature relating to the economic evaluation of HAIs has been reviewed. The literature was identified through a series of consecutive searches, carried out during the period 1993–March 2003, using the computerized bibliographic databases Medline and PubMed, supplemented by reference follow-up, hand searching of selected journals and consultation with experts in the field. The search was limited to papers published in English during the period 1975–March 2003, and further limited to studies conducted in the developed countries of Europe, Canada, Australia and the USA.

The chapter begins with an overview of the processes and techniques of economic evaluation and discusses these in the context of HAI. Studies that have assessed the economic burden of HAI and the benefits of investment in prevention activities will then be reviewed and a framework for assessing the costs and benefits of preventive activities presented.

Economic evaluation

Economic evaluations take a number of different forms including the following approaches: cost of illness (COI), cost-effectiveness, cost utility and cost-benefit analysis. Drummond (1987), when describing the various techniques available, classifies them into two distinct groups based on whether they enable a partial or full economic evaluation.

Economic evaluations which do not include a comparator and fail to include both costs and consequences may be considered partial evaluations. They may be limited to a description of the outcome, or the costs, or include both costs and outcomes but no comparator.

COI or burden of illness studies are examples of partial economic evaluations. These studies are limited to an assessment of the costs associated with a particular illness. They aim to identify, measure and value the direct, indirect and intangible costs of a particular illness. The approach represents one of earliest forms of economic evaluation (Fein 1971).

COI studies became increasingly popular in the 1950s and 1960s (Fein 1971), then their popularity declined, with many questioning their value. In the past, COI studies have been conducted to demonstrate the economic burden of a disease and thus facilitate comparison of the burden of different diseases and assist in decision making regarding prioritizing health care and the subsequent allocation of resources. However, it has been argued that data limited to the burden of disease have little value and may be misleading. By definition, these studies are limited to the cost of the disease and do not attempt to look at the potential effectiveness or cost of interventions to prevent or treat the illness, and the benefits that might result. As such, COI studies do not provide direct guidance on the allocation of resources (Drummond 1992).

Byford *et al.* (2000) argue that without data on both the cost and the effectiveness of prevention activities, informed decisions about the allocation of resources cannot be taken. The situation might arise when a decision is taken to allocate more resources to the treatment or prevention of a particular disease simply because it is more expensive than the others that are being considered. However, without knowledge of the cost of the activities being considered and their effectiveness, the decision might result in additional resources being used for little health gain. (Byford *et al.* 2000)

Similarly, illnesses that impose a relatively small burden, but are easily preventable, may be overlooked. Byford *et al.* (2000) cite the example of phenylketonuria, a disease which has a relatively low incidence and imposes a relatively small burden on society, but which is easily preventable at low cost, resulting in substantial health gains for the individuals concerned. Byford *et al.* (2000) thus argue that the results of some COI studies may divert the attention of policy decisions makers away from areas where improvements and health gains can be made at low cost.

Despite these limitations, COI studies do provide valuable data. Whilst the results do not represent the net benefits of investment, they do represent the resources that might become available if the disease did not exist. The results represent the potential benefits that might arise in terms of costs avoided and can be used to evaluate intervention strategies. The results of COI studies can highlight the magnitude of a problem and identify items that are most costly, thus facilitating managers' attempts to improve efficiency. They may also be influential in setting the agenda for policy initiatives and for initiating further evaluative studies (Rice 1995). In the context of HAI, a review of the literature indicates that a number of COI studies have been conducted.

Drummond *et al.* (1987) term economic evaluations that assess both the costs and consequences of two or more alternatives as full economic evaluations. Using this definition, cost-effectiveness analysis, cost utility analysis and cost-benefit analysis are all techniques that might be used in a full economic evaluation (see also Chapters 1 and 2).

The economic evaluation of HAI

Studies that have considered the economics of HAI vary in scope. Many are partial evaluations adopting a COI approach, whereas others have used techniques such as cost-effectiveness and cost-benefit analysis. Economic modelling, utilizing data from a variety of data sources, has also been conducted.

Estimates of the economic burden of HAI

A number of studies have assessed the economic burden of HAI. Tables 8.1–8.6 provide an overview of studies conducted between 1975 and 2002, that have assessed the burden of HAI to the hospital sector and the estimates derived. Table 8.1 presents estimates of the economic impact of all types of HAI and Tables 8.2–8.6 present estimates of the economic impact of specific types of infection.

The estimates presented demonstrate that the estimated impact of HAI varies considerably not only with site of infection, but also with study. The observed variations can be attributed in part to methodological and case mix differences.

Methodological differences include variation in the range of costs included, the methods used to attribute resources to HAI and the methods used to value resources. Other methodological differences relate to the definitions of HAI used, and the methods used to identify HAIs.

Variations in the case mix studied include important differences in the types of patients studied and the treatment regimes received. For example, some studies include a broad case mix of patients whereas others focus on a particular patient group defined by operative procedure or specialty (see Grieve and Weinhold Chapter 5). Treatment patterns also vary with hospital and over time. For example, patients are discharged home at an earlier point in their recovery today than a few years ago. This changing treatment pattern affects the cost estimates and prohibits valid direct comparisons between the results of studies conducted at different times.

Despite these differences, some common themes emerge from the literature. Before considering these, some of the key methodological differences and issues that emerge from the literature will be discussed.

The range of costs resulting from HAI

The acquisition of an infection in hospital may affect costs to the health care sector, community care services, affected patients, those who care for them, the economy and the environment. For example, HAIs may result in additional costs to the hospital sector, general practitioners, district nursing services, community midwifery services and a range of other health and community care services. Patients' health status may be reduced and they may incur personal expenditure on items such as drugs and dressings and suffer financial losses from a reduction in earning capacity in either the short or long term. Informal carers may also lose work or leisure time. Production losses may result from delayed or non-return to work and environmental costs may ensue, e.g. the treatment of HAIs may result in an increase in the use of dressings, which have to be destroyed (Daschner 1989).

The range of costs to be included in an evaluation of the burden of HAI will depend on the viewpoint to be taken. If a societal viewpoint is adopted, then all costs should be included, whereas if the viewpoint of the health service is adopted, then the range of costs may be limited to those that impact on the health service. Studies that have estimated the economic burden of HAI tend to limit the range of costs included to those that fall on the hospital sector. There are, however, a few exceptions, for example, Elliston *et al.* (1994), in a small study involving 71 patients who had a surgical wound, examined the incidence of surgical wound infections (SWIs) presenting after discharge and their impact on community health care services; Kirkland *et al* (1999) in their study of SWIs in surgical patients admitted to a hospital in the USA extended their cost analysis to include the costs associated with re-admission to hospital within 30 days of discharge; and Hyryla *et al.* (1994) considered the implications of HAI for the Finnish social security system.

Attributing resources to HAI

Studies have generally used one of three key methods to attribute costs to the presence of infection: the concurrent method, comparative method and comparative method with matching (see Haley *et al.* 1980; McGowan 1981, 1982; Haley 1992 for a detailed discussion of these methods).

With the concurrent method, a suitably qualified individual reviews patient records and identifies which resources were used as a result of an infection. Given the subjective nature of assessment of resources attributed to infection, the validity and reliability of the approach have been questioned (McGowan 1982). It has also been suggested that physician reviewers may be reticent about attributing the use of resources to HAI, and so costs were likely to be underestimated (Haley 1980). Some of these difficulties were overcome in a study by Wakefield *et al.* (1987). Trained personnel reviewed medical records, using a carefully prepared protocol—'the appropriateness evaluation protocol'—to assess whether each in-patient day was (i) attributable to the reason

Table 8.1 An overview of studies that have assessed the impact of HAIs (all sites) on hospital length of stay and costs (1975–2002)

First author and date of publication	Year of study	Country	Types of patients studied	Type of hospital	No. of hospitals	No. of HAIs included in analysis	Additional days in hospital	Additional hospital costs
Haley (1980)	1975	USA	All admissions	Not stated	1	120	13.4	US$1018
Haley (1980)	1975	USA	All admissions	Not stated	1	58	16.1	US$1224
Haley (1980)	1975	USA	All admissions	Not stated	1	183	17.0	US$1292
Haley (1980)	1975	USA	All admissions	Not stated	1	183	4.8	US$576
Scheckler (1978)	1978	USA	All admissions	Community teaching hospital	1	123	3.0	US$636
Haley (1981)[1]	1975–6	USA	All admissions	Mixed	3	256	4.5	US$590
Davies (1979)	1978	UK	Orthopaedic	District general hospital	1	29	17.0	£775
Rubenstein (1982)	1979	Israel	General surgical and orthopaedic	University affiliated	1	90	7.9	US$787

Coello (1993)	1988	UK	General surgical, orthopaedic and gynaecology patients who had a surgical procedure	District general hospital	1	67	8.2	£1041
Vegas (1993)	1990	Spain	General and digestive surgical patients	Not stated	1	52	11.4	US$4449
Erbaydar (1995)	1992–94	Turkey	General surgical	University tertiary hospital	1	223	17.0	–
Erbaydar (1995)	1992–94	Turkey	General surgical	University tertiary hospital	1	151	10.6	–
Plowman (1999)	1993–94	England	General surgical, general medicine, orthopaedics, urology, gynaecology, care of the elderly, ENT, obstetrics (caesarean sections only)	District general hospital	1	309	11	£2917

Table 8.2 An overview of studies that have assessed the impact of hospital acquired UTIs on hospital length of stay and costs (1975–2002)

First author and date of publication	Year of study	Country	Types of patients studied	Type of hospital	No. of hospitals	No. of HAIs included in analysis	Additional days in hospital	Additional hospital costs
Haley (1986)	1975–6	USA	All admissions	Mixed	3	177[1]	1.0	US$593[2]
Scheckler (1978)	1978	USA	All admissions	Community hospital	1	35	0.6	US$146
Davies (1979)	1978	UK	Orthopaedic	District general hospital	1	9	13.0	£617
Rubenstein (1982)	1979	Israel	General surgical and orthopaedics	University affiliated	1	90	5.1	US$510
Coello (1993)	1988	UK	General surgical, orthopaedic and gynaecology patients who had a surgical procedure	District general hospital	1	36	3.6	£467

Hillan (1995)	Not stated	UK	Patients who had a caesarean section	University teaching hospital	1	65	0.8	–
Plowman (1999)	1993–94	England	General surgical, general medicine, orthopaedics, urology, gynaecology, care of the elderly, ENT, obstetrics (caesarean sections only)	District general hospital	1	107	5	£1122
Tambyah (2002)	1997–98	USA	Adult patients scheduled to be catheterized for >24 h taking part in a trial of different types of catheter	University teaching hospital	1	235	*	US$589

* Only one patient was considered to have an extended LOS attributable to a hospital-acquired catheter associated UTI. The patient had a BSI Secondary to the CAUTI.

Table 8.3 An overview of studies that have assessed the impact of hospital-acquired SWIs on hospital length of stay and costs (1975–2002)

First author and date of publication	Year of study	Country	Types of patients studied	Type of hospital	No. of hospitals	No. of HAIs included in analysis	Additional days in hospital	Additional hospital costs
Haley (1986)	1975–6	USA	All admissions	Mixed	3	110*	7.0	US$2734
Scheckler (1978)		USA	All admissions	Community teaching hospital	1	26	6.5	US$1329
Rubenstein (1982)	1979	Israel	General surgical and orthopaedic	Not stated	1	19	12.9	US$1290
Mugford (1989)	1987	UK	Patients who had a caesarean Section	University teaching hospital	1	41	1.3	£716
Coello (1993)	1988	UK	General surgical, orthopaedic and gynaecology patients who had a surgical procedure	District general hospital	1	12	10.2	£1456
Poulsen (1994)	1985–8	Denmark	Surgical	University teaching hospital	1	291	5.7	–
Hyryla (1994)	1988–90	Finland	Surgical patients whose infection warranted compensation	All types	All	1100	33.2	–
O'Donoghue (1992)	1990	UK	Orthopaedic patients	District general hospital	1		17.0	£2220

Vegas (1993)	1990	Spain	General and digestive surgical patients	–	1	30	14.3	US$5617
Hillan (1995)	not stated	UK	Patients who had a caesarean section	University teaching hospital	1	42	3.6	–
Taylor (1995)	1992	Canada	Surgical patiens admitted to selected specialties who underwent clean or clean-contaminated surgery*	University hospital	1	68	19.5	–
Kirkland (1999)	1991–95	USA	Surgical	Community hospital	1	255	6.5	US$3089
Plowman (1999)	1993–94	England	General surgical, general medicine, orthopaedics, urology, gynaecology, care of the elderly, ENT, obstetrics (caesarean sections only)	District general hospital	1	38	7	£1594
Whitehouse (2002)	2000	USA	Orthopaedic	University teaching hospital and a community hospital	2	59	1.0	–

* General surgery, orthopaedic surgery, thoracic surgery, neurosurgery, Department of Obstetrics and Gynaecology patients

Table 8.4 An overview of studies that have assessed the impact of hospital acquired LRTIs on hospital length of stay and costs (1975–2002)

First author and date of publication	Year of study	Country	Types of patients studied	Type of hospital	No. of hospitals	No. of HAIs included in analysis	Additional days in hospital	Additional hospital costs
Scheckler (1978)	1978	USA	All admissions	Community hospital	1	17	3.8	US$878
Dixon (1978)	Not stated	USA	All admissions	Mixed	Not stated	Not stated	4.0	US$832
Haley (1986)	1975–76	USA	All admissions	Mixed	3	64	6	US$4947
Kappstein (1992)	1988–89	Germany	Ventilated patients–ICU	University hospital	1	34	10.13 ICU days	US$8800
Hillan (1995)	Not stated	UK	Patients who had a caesarean section	University teaching hospital	1	23	2.5	–
Plowman (1999)	1993–94	England	General surgical, general medicine, orthopaedics, urology, gynaecology, care of the elderly, ENT, obstetrics (caesarean sections only)	District general hospital	1	48	8	£2080

Table 8.5 An overview of studies that have assessed the impact of hospital-acquired blood stream infections on hospital length of stay and costs (1975–2002)

First author and date of publication	Year of study	Country	Types of patients studied	Type of hospital	No. of hospitals	No. of HAIs included in analysis	Additional days in hospital	Additional hospital costs
Wey (1988)	1983–86	USA	All admissions	University teaching hospital	1	34	30.0	–
Pittet (1994)	1998–90	USA	Surgical intensive care	University teaching hospital	1	81	14.0	£33 268
Pittet (1994)	1998–90	USA	Surgical intensive care	University teaching hospital	1	41 (survivors)	24.0 (per survivor)	£40 890
Plowman (1999)	1993–94	England	General surgical, general medicine, orthopaedics, urology, gynaecology, care of the elderly, ENT, obstetrics (caesarean sections only)	District general hospital	1	4	4	£6209
Orsi (2002)	1994–95	Italy	Surgical	University teaching hospital	1	105	19.1	16 356 Euro
Orsi (2002)	1994–95	Italy	Surgical	University teaching hospital	1	105	19.9	–

Table 8.6 An overview of studies that have assessed the impact of multiple HAIs on hospital length of stay and costs (1975–2002)

First author and date of publication	Year of study	Country	Types of patients studied	Type of hospital	No. of hospitals	No. of HAIs included in analysis	Additional days in hospital	Additional hospital costs
Rubenstein (1982)	1979	Israel	General surgery and orthopaedics	Not stated	1	8	18	US$1800
Coello (1993)	1988	UK	General surgery, orthopaedic and gynaecology who had	District general hospital	1	9	26	£3362
Plowman (1999)	1993–94	England	General surgical, general undergone a surgical procedure medicine, orthopaedics, urology, gynaecology, care of the elderly, ENT, obstetrics (caesarean sections only)	District general hospital	1	57	29	£8631

for admission; (ii) jointly attributable to the reason for admission and the HAI; or (iii) attributable to the HAI alone. This approach has been found to be both repeatable and valid (Rishpon *et al.* 1986; Gertman and Restuccia 1991; Wakefield *et al.* 1992). However, the approach requires detailed and accurate hospital records.

The comparative method involves assessing the cost of resources used by infected and uninfected patients, and then attributing the differences between the costs observed to the presence of an infection. This method therefore assumes that the two groups (infected and uninfected patients) are the same in all respects except for the presence or absence of an HAI. This is clearly not the case. There may be many factors, other than HAI, which differ between these two groups.

The comparative method with matching attempts to control for factors other than HAI that might differ between the two patient groups. Infected patients are matched with one or more uninfected patients on the basis of factors thought to have an impact on resource use. Studies have generally matched patients using a range of factors including: age, sex, diagnosis, number of co-morbidities and type of operation. The resources used by patients and controls are then compared, and the differences in costs attributed to the HAI. Haley (1991) notes that it is important that the differences between the cost incurred by infected and uninfected patients are first determined for individual patients, and then summed (or averaged) to determine the total (or average) costs attributable to infection. Haley (1991) notes that a common mistake in studies of this type is to break the matching, and simply compare the total costs incurred by infected patients with the costs incurred by uninfected patients. This approach is invalid and may lead to biased estimates of the costs attributable to HAI.

This comparative method with matching approach is hampered by practical difficulties associated with finding suitable control patients. Many studies have been unable to match all infected patients with uninfected controls. Haley *et al.* (1980), in a review of matched studies conducted between 1953 and 1975, found considerable variation in the percentage of infected patients successfully matched with uninfected patients. Successful matching of infected patients with uninfected patients ranged from a low of 32% up to 100%.

Freeman *et al.* (1979) notes that the ability to find matched uninfected patients depends on the size of the pool of uninfected patients and the number of matching characteristics. The absence of a suitable pool of uninfected patients may necessitate a reduction in the number of matching parameters, thus reducing the comparability of the infected and uninfected groups, and/or the exclusion of unmatched infected patients from the analysis, which, in some cases, may limit the analysis to an unrepresentative subset of infected patients. Both responses may have an impact on the accuracy of the estimates of the costs attributable to HAI (Haley 1991).

In 1980, Haley *et al.* (1980) compared the concurrent and comparative method by using both to study the same population. Haley found that the closer the matching, the lower the estimate of the number of additional days attributable to infection. However, regardless of the level of matching, the comparative method appeared to overestimate the number of days attributable to HAI compared with the results derived using the concurrent method. At the same time, it was acknowledged that the concurrent method may underestimate the cost of HAI. The physician-epidemiologist tended to attribute extra days to HAI only if they were clearly the consequences of an HAI.

Haley (1991) suggests that one of the problems with studies utilizing the comparative approach is that matching parameters such as age, sex, service, first diagnosis and first operation do not adequately control for differences between infected and uninfected patients, which may have an impact on resource use. Matching should ensure that prior to the acquisition of an infection, infected and uninfected patients have the same predicted length of stay and level of resource use. Haley argues that diagnostic related groups are the best predictor of length of stay, and that this should be included in such studies, together with the number of discharge diagnoses. This latter measure increased the predictive power of the diagnostic group on length of stay and level of resources used. Together, these factors explain 34% of the variance in length of stay (Haley, 1991).

Estimating the cost of resources attributable to HAI

Economists measure costs as the benefit forgone by using resources in one way rather than in another; more precisely, the next best alternative use. In the context of HAI, it is probable that resources used to care for patients with an HAI would, in the absence of the infection, have had alternative uses. The benefits forgone represent the opportunity costs of HAI.

Deriving estimates of the opportunity costs of HAI presents difficulties. The most common method used to estimate the value of resources used in one way, as opposed to another, is by applying monetary prices. However, prices will only approximate the opportunity costs if markets are 'perfect'. For a number of reasons, markets are not 'perfect'. There are problems associated with uncertainty, imperfect information, externalities and the number of firms given the size of the market (Dawson 1994). Furthermore, few health care systems generate prices and, when they do, for example charges in the US health system, they may not reflect the cost of resources. For example, cost shifting may be present as a result of hospitals shifting their charges for under-reimbursed costs to those payers for whom they can recover more than their costs (Finkler 1982; Haley 1992) To overcome these difficulties, some studies, particularly those conducted in the USA, have applied a cost-to-charge ratio in an endeavour to convert charges to costs. This measure is generally the ratio of the sum of the total hospital expenditure per annum to the sum of patient charges per annum. The cost-to-charge ratio typically lies between 0.6 and 0.8 (Haley 1991). This approach overcomes some of the bias associated with applying charges; however, the estimate derived is a somewhat crude estimate of total costs attributable to HAI and, as a result of cost shifting, may not be accurate for individual patients and departments (Haley 1991). This latter criticism can be overcome to a degree by stratifying the resources and associated charges attributable to HAI by individual departments, and applying a department-based cost-to-charge ratio to these charges.

Dawson (1994) argues that the costs derived from the UK health sector are usually the result of mechanistic accounting conventions designed to recover expenditure rather than reflect resource use. For example, the allocation of overheads and capital charges is made by convention. These costs are a significant proportion of total costs (Magee and Osmolski 1978).

In many studies, average unit costs are applied. For example, the number of additional days a patient with an HAI remains in hospital is determined and an average cost per bed day applied. This approach may also introduce bias. Average costs depend upon the function of the total quantity produced. The average cost per bed day is a function of the total number of bed days produced and the aggregate costs, so average cost estimates derived from hospitals operating at different levels of capacity will differ. Furthermore, daily costs will differ over the period of hospitalization. For example, Hollingsworth *et al.* (1993) found that patients admitted to hospital with a fractured neck of femur incurred relatively high daily costs during the first few days in hospital, after which they decreased. This pattern of daily costs is likely to vary by type of patient, specialty and presence of an infection acquired in hospital.

An alternative approach to those identified above is the cost accounting approach, or what Haley (1991) has described as 'micro costing. This involves determining the actual cost of delivering the identified services. It provides more accurate and valid estimates of the costs attributable to HAI but is time consuming, costly and difficult to conduct.

An alternative measure is the number of additional days patients remain in hospital as a result of HAI. Haley argues that this is a harder measure of the cost of HAI as it is subject to less variation from year to year than charges which are subject to inflationary pressures. Studies generally provide estimates of both the number of additional days in hospital and the costs incurred. A few studies have also presented data on the number of antibiotic days and the number of investigations (e.g. Coello *et al.* 1993).

Estimates of the economic burden of HAI to the hospital sector

The economic burden of HAI presented in Tables 8.1–8.6 varies considerably with the site of infection and also within any specialty. Whilst in part this can be attributed to methodological and case mix differences as indicated above, some common themes emerge from the literature and are discussed below.

Infections of the urinary tract are generally the least expensive, while infections of the bloodstream and chest, and infections at multiple sites are the most expensive.

The results presented in Tables 8.1–8.6 indicate marked variations in the estimates of the impact of different types of infections. Estimates of the number of days that may be attributable to a urinary tract infection (UTI) vary from 1 to 13 days. In contrast, estimates of the impact of SWIs range from a low estimate of 1.3 additional days in a study limited to women who had a caesarean section (Mugford *et al.* 1989) to 33.2 additional days in a study which involved patients whose infection warranted compensation from the Finnish Social Security system (Hyryla and Sintonen 1994). Estimates of the impact of bloodstream infections on hospital length of stay range from 4 to 14 extra days, and estimates of the impact of chest infections vary from 2.5 to 10.3 additional days. Finally, estimates of the impact of HAIs at more than one site vary from 18 to 29 additional days.

Costs have also been found to vary considerably by patient group. This may reflect differences in the type of infection occurring in the selected patient group which have different resource implications in different patient groups. Infections in intensive care patients are particularly resource intensive. For example, Pittet *et al.* (1994) estimated that bloodstream infections occurring in intensive care unit patients cost US$40 000 per survivor.

Some studies have disaggregated the cost estimates and have examined the distribution of the in-patient costs. For example, Coello *et al.* (1993) estimated the costs associated with an extended length of hospital stay, antibiotics, microbiology tests and radiological investigations: 93% of the total additional cost incurred by surgical patients with an HAI could be attributed to an extended length of stay (Coello *et al.* 1993). Plowman *et al.* (1999) included a very detailed assessment of costs and found that hospital overheads, capital charges and cost of management time accounted for 33% of the additional costs incurred, nursing care accounted for 42%, medical care 6%, operations and consumables 6%, paramedicas and speciaist nurses 4%, antimicrobials 2%, other drugs 3%, microbiology tests 1%, and other tests and investigations 3%.

The national burden of HAIs

National estimates of the burden of HAI are also presented in the literature. Based on estimates derived from a single district general hospital in England, Plowman *et al.* (1999) estimated that HAIs cost the hospital sector in England at least £931 million per annum. UTIs, which were estimated to have a relatively low cost per case, were, as a result of their relatively high incidence, found on aggregate to be the most costly single site infection (£124.million). Estimates for a number of other countries are also presented in the literature (Losos *et al.* 1984; Haley 1985; Department of Health and Public Health Laboratory Service 1988; Coello *et al.* 1993). All point to the substantial burden HAIs place on the health sector.

Assessment of benefits of prevention

Studies that have assessed the benefits of prevention vary in scope and study design. They can be broadly categorised into those that have assessed the gross benefits of prevention, that is they have not taken into account the costs of achieving reduction in rates; those that have taken into account the costs of prevention and assessed the net benefits of prevention; and those that have looked at the cost of carrying out selected ineffective 'prevention' activities.

Estimates of the gross benefits of prevention

The results of the recent NAO survey of ICTs at acute NHS Trusts in England indicated that on average ICTs considered that an estimated 15% of HAIs could be prevented. Applying this figure to the most recent estimate of the national burden these infections place on the health sector in England, the NAO estimated that a 15% reduction in infection rates would result in the release of resources valued at £150 million (Report by the Comptroller and Auditor General 2000). This estimate represents the gross benefits of prevention. The net benefits of prevention would be dependent on the costs of achieving a 15% reduction in rates.

Estimates of the net benefits of prevention

Studies that have estimated the net benefits of prevention can be broadly categorized into those that have assessed the benefits of an effective infection control programme, those that have focused on the costs and benefits of prophylactic antibiotics and those that have assessed the costs and benefits of selected infection control practices.

Studies assessing benefits of an effective infection control programme

A number of US estimates of the potential benefits of investing in an ICT and infection control programme are found in the literature. In 1975, the US Centre for Disease Control estimated the cost and benefits of an infection control programme implemented in a 250 bed hospital. These estimates were subsequently revised in 1979, and further adjusted to 1985 prices in 1986 (Haley 1986). The cost of establishing and maintaining an infection control programme in 1985 prices was estimated to be US$60 000. This estimate includes the cost of employing an infection control nurse, a part time physician consultant and part-time clerical support, and the cost of consumables and overheads. Earlier work indicated that HAIs cost the average 250 bed hospital in the US $1 million per year. Consequently, a 6% reduction in the costs associated with infection would pay for the cost of the infection control programme and any further reductions would result in greater returns for the investment. A number of other similar models have also been presented in the literature (Dixon 1987; Currie and Maynard 1989; Miller *et al.* 1989; Wenzel 1995).

Studies assessing costs and benefits of antimicrobial prophylaxis

A number of studies have assessed the costs and benefits of antimicrobial prophylaxis (Hojer 1978; Kaiser *et al.* 1983; Shapiro *et al.* 1983; Jones and Chawala 1984; Persson *et al.* 1988; Mugford *et al.* 1989; Davey *et al.* 1995) and a review article by McGowan (1991) discusses issues relating to the assessment of the costs and benefits of this form of prevention. Many of these studies have found that the benefits, measured in terms of a reduction in the incidence of HAI and the associated costs, outweigh the costs of the intervention, although the level of benefits differs with alternative regimens (Persson *et al.* 1988; McGowan 1991; Davey *et al.* 1995)

Studies assessing the costs and benefits of specific prevention activities

In addition to the above, some studies have assessed the costs and benefits of specific infection control practices. For example, Slater *et al.* (2001) estimated the potential savings of employing a vascular catheter-care specialist nurse for the surgical intensive care unit within a US hospital, as a means of tackling the problem of catheter-associated bloodstream infections. The costs of employing the nurse were compared with the potential savings that might accrue if one infection per month was prevented. The potential benefits in terms of the estimated value of resources released if one infection per month was prevented were found to be greater than the costs of employing the nurse. A specialist nurse was subsequently employed. Within 9 months of employment, 18 fewer blood steam infections than the previous year had been identified. Assuming that on average each bloodstream infection utilizes hospital resources valued at US$6000 per infection, this represented gross savings estimated at US$108 000 and estimated net savings of at least US$58000.

Plowman *et al.* (2001a) developed a model for estimating the costs and benefits associated with the routine use of silver alloy-coated urinary catheters as a means of preventing hospital-acquired catheter-related UTIs. The results of their model indicated that in England, a 14.6% reduction in UTIs in catheterized medical patients and an 11.4% reduction in surgical patients would cover the cost of this intervention, and any further reductions would result in net benefits.

Estimates of cost savings resulting from not carrying out 'prevention' activities which have little or no positive effect

A number of studies have looked at the appropriateness of allocation of resources to infection control practices considered to have little or no positive preventative effect. For example, Lawrence *et al.* (1989) assessed the costs of routine pre-operative urine testing and subsequent treatment of asymptomatic bacteriuria in patients admitted for elective non-prosthetic knee surgery. The results indicated that routine screening and treatment cost US$1.5 million per SWI prevented.

Daschner (1984) provides a summary account of a number of changes that were made to infection control policy and practice in a hospital in Germany and the estimated cost savings. The aim was to move to more cost-effective practice and away from infection control 'rituals' with little or no proven efficacy. For example, in the absence of an epidemic, routine environmental culturing and screening of staff for staphylococci was discontinued as was twice daily meatal care with PVP-iodine, changing of intravenous infusion sets every 24 hours and the use of in-line filters as a means of reducing urinary tract and bloodstream infections. These other changes were made in response to research findings. The estimated cost savings to the hospital sector as a result of these and other changes in practice over a 6 year period between 1977 and 1982 was 5 522 471 DM.

A framework for assessing the net benefits of investment in infection control

In the absence of studies that have assessed the costs and benefits of investment in specific infection control studies, simple economic models to demonstrate the net benefits of investment in infection control practices can be developed.

Models of the net benefits of investment in prevention activities have been derived from information on infection rates; the cost of the infection control practice to be evaluated and its efficacy (assuming 100% compliance); the cost of alternative strategies which would need to be introduced to maximize compliance and the level of compliance they are expected to achieve; and the magnitude, type and distribution of economic burdens that may have resulted had the HAIs not been prevented.

Data on infection rates can be difficult to obtain and have been gleaned from a variety of sources including hospital records, the literature and national surveillance schemes. Data on the cost of selected infection control practices and the cost of strategies to enhance compliance with a given practice can generally be relatively easily estimated, and data on the cost of the burden that may have resulted had the HAIs not been prevented can be obtained from published studies. However, data on the efficacy of interventions and strategies that aim to enhance compliance and hence effectiveness are a little more difficult to obtain. Whilst a number of studies have demonstrated the effectiveness of surveillance and feedback of results to the appropriate personnel (Haley *et al.* 1985; Merle *et al.* 2002), with the exception of studies that have assessed the efficacy of specific antibiotics, there is a marked lack of information on the efficacy of specific infection control activities. Lack of information on the effectiveness of infection control practices was highlighted by Thames Valley University, when drafting infection control guidelines for the prevention of HAIs (EPIC 2000). When drafting these guidelines, prevention activities were categorized according to the quality of the supporting evidence.

- ◆ Category 1 included activities where there were generally consistent findings from a range of evidence derived from well designed experimental studies.

- ◆ Category 2 included activities for which evidence of effectiveness was based on a single acceptable study, or a weak or inconsistent finding in multiple acceptable studies.

- ◆ Category 3 included those activities for which there was limited scientific evidence that did not meet all the criteria of 'acceptable studies', or an absence of directly applicable studies of good quality. This included published or unpublished expert opinion. The majority of the activities fell within category 3 (Pratt *et al*, 2001).

In the absence of rigorous data on the efficacy of a particular intervention, models can be developed which assess the potential benefits of prevention assuming different levels of effectiveness. Information on the break-even point given different levels of effectiveness can subsequently be derived from these models. That is the point at which the potential benefits cover the cost of the intervention, and any further reduction in rates results in net benefits. This information can subsequently be used to inform decision making regarding investment in the activity assessed.

Figure 8.1 provides a framework for assessing the costs and benefits of an intervention to reduce HAI.

The starting point is the number of admissions to the specialties of interest (cell 1). These patients are then subdivided into the specialty groups of interest (cells 2–3 in Fig. 8.1). The estimated number of HAIs that might occur in these patients are then determined based on the specialty-specific incidence rates (cells 4–7). Estimates of the economic impact these infections place on the hospital sector are then derived by multiplying the number of HAIs by an appropriate estimate of the additional cost of these infections (cells 8–9) and the number of extra days patients remain in hospital (cells 10–11).

The potential gross benefits (value of resources and the number of days released for alternative use) are then derived for varying levels of effectiveness (0–100%), and the net benefits derived by subtracting the cost of the intervention from the estimated gross benefits. Finally, the costs of the intervention can be plotted against the benefits that might accrue assuming different levels of effectiveness and the cut-off point where potential benefits are equal to the costs of the intervention identified. Any further reduction in rates would result in net benefits (Fig. 8.2).

Sensitivity analysis can subsequently be conducted to assess the impact that varying the incidence of HAIs and the cost per case has on the results obtained.

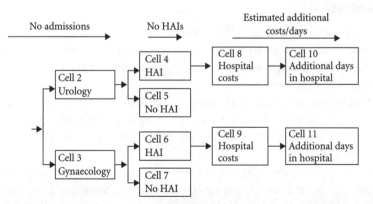

Fig. 8.1 The structure of an economic model to assess the costs and benefits of an intervention to prevent HAIs.

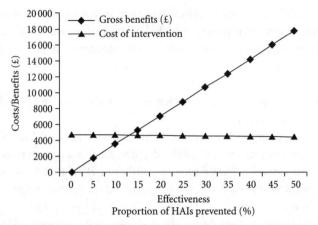

Fig. 8.2 Estimated costs and benefits of an intervention to prevent HAIs.

Models developed in this way represent a flexible tool which can readily be adapted to the specific needs of the user. Using this approach, the costs and benefits of a range of interventions can be estimated and the results used to inform decision making, in relation to infection control policy and practice. The results may be of particular interest to infection control nurses and doctors who wish to demonstrate the burden of HAIs and the benefits associated with investing in specific infection control practices. However, it should be noted that the validity of the model developed will be dependent on how realistic the structure of the model is and how accurately the estimates of the parameters used reflect what is happening in the patient group of interest. (See also Grieve Chapter 5 for a discussion of the need to accommodate changes in techniques and processes.)

Conclusion

The economic evaluation of HAI presents a number of methodological difficulties. To date, studies have tended to focus on the assessment of the burden of HAI and relatively few have assessed the costs and benefits of investment in infection control activities.

Studies that have assessed the economic burden of HAIs vary in scope and in terms of the methods used. However, despite these differences, it is evident that the burden imposed is substantial, and that the economic impact varies with type of infection and admission specialty.

Some of these infections can be prevented. Studies that have assessed the benefits of prevention activity again vary in scope. Some are limited to the assessment of the gross benefits of prevention, whereas others take into account the costs of achieving a reduction in infection rates, and assess the net benefits.

Studies that have assessed the gross benefits of infection control activities point to the substantial benefits that may result, in terms of both the magnitude of the resources released for alternative use and improved patient outcomes.

Studies that have taken into account the costs of achieving a reduction have similarly demonstrated that in many cases the benefits exceed the cost of achieving a reduction in infection rates. The results of studies that have assessed the costs and benefits of investment in infection control activities can be used to inform infection control activities and the level of resources invested in infection control.

References

Ayliffe, G.A.J. (1986) Nosocomial infection—the irreducible minimum. *Infection Control* 7 (Supplement 2), 92–95.

Byford, S., Torhgerson, D. and Raftery, J. (2000) Cost of illness studies. *British Medical Journal* **320**, 1335.

Coello, R., Glenister, H., Fereres, J., Bartlett, C., Leigh. D., Sedgwick, J. *et al.* (1993) The cost of infection in surgical patients: a case control study. *Journal of Hospital Infection* **25**, 239–250.

Currie, E. and Maynard, A. (1989) *Economics of Hospital Acquired Infection*. Discussion Paper 56. Centre for Health Economics, University of York.

Daschner, F.D. (1984) The costs of hospital acquired infection. *Journal of Hospital Infection* **5** (Supplement A), 27–33.

Daschner, F. (1989) Cost-effectiveness in hospital infection control—lessons for the 1990s. *Journal of Hospital Infection* **13**, 325–336.

Davey, P., Lynch, B., Malek, M., Byrne, D. and Thomas, P. (1992) Cost-effectiveness of single dose cefotaxime plus metronidazole compared with three doses each of cefuroxime plus metronidazole for the prevention of wound infections after colorectal surgery. *Journal of Antimicrobial Chemotherapy* **30**, 855–864.

Davey, P.G., Parker, S.E., Crombie, I.K. and Jaderberg, M. (1995) The cost-effectiveness of amoxicillin/clavulanic acid as antibacterial prophylaxis in abdominal and gynaecological surgery. *PharmacoEconomics* **7**, 347–356.

Dawson, D. (1994) *Costs and Prices in the Internal Market*. University of York, York.

Department of Health and Public Health Laboratory Service (1988) *Hospital Infection Control: Guidance on the Control of Infections in Hospitals*. PHLS, London.

Department of Health and Public Health Laboratory Service (1995) *Hospital Infection Control: Guidance on the Control of Infections in Hospital*. Prepared by the Hospital Infection Working Group of the Department of Health and Public Health Laboratory Service. Department of Health, London.

Dixon, R. (1978) Effect of infections on hospital care. *Annals of Internal Medicine* **89**, 749–753.

Dixon, R. (1987) Costs of nosocomial infections and benefits of infection control programmes. In: Wenzel, R.P. (ed.), *Prevention and Control of Nosocomial Infections*. Williams and Wilkins, Baltimore, pp. 19–25.

Drummond, M. (1992) Cost-of-illness studies. A major headache? *PharmacoEconomics* **2**, 1–4.

Drummond, M. and Davies, L.F. (1991) Evaluation of the costs and benefits of reducing hospital infection. *Journal of Hospital Infection* 18 (Supplement 18), 85–93.

Drummond, M.F., Stoddart, G.L. and Torrance, G.W. (1987) *Methods for the Economic Evaluation of Health Care Programmes.* Oxford Medical Publications, Oxford.

Elliston, P.R.A., Slack, R.C.B., Humphreys, H. and Emmerson, A.M. (1994) The cost of postoperative wound infection. *Journal of Hospital Infection* **28**, 241–242.

Emmerson, A.M., Entstone, J., Griffin, M., Kelsey, M.C. and Smyth, E.T.M. (1996) The second national prevalence survey of infection in hospitals—overview of the results. *Journal of Hospital Infection* **32**, 175–190.

EPIC (2000) *National Evidence-based Guidelines for Preventing Hospital-acquired Infections: Standard Principles.* Thames Valley University.

Erbaydar, S., Akgun, A., Eksik, A., Erbaydar, T., Bilge, O. and Bulut, A. (1995) Estimation of increased hospital stay due to nosocomial infections in surgical patients: comparison of matched groups. *Journal of Hospital Infection* **30**, 149–154.

Fein, R. (1971) On measuring economic benefits of health programmes. In: *Medical History and Medical Care. A Symposium of Perspectives.* Nuffield Provincial Hospital Trust, London, pp. 183–219.

Finkler, S.A. (1982) The distinction between costs and charges. *Annals of Internal Medicine* **96**, 102–109.

Freeman, J., Rosner, B.A. and McGowan, J.E. (1979) Adverse effects of nosocomial infection. *Journal of Infectious Diseases* **140**, 732–740.

Gertman, P. and Restuccia, J. (1981) The appropriateness evaluation protocol: a technique for assessing unnecessary days of hospital care. *Medical Care* **19**, 855–871.

Haley, R. (1985) Incidence and nature of endemic and epidemic nosocomial infections. In: Bennett, J.V. and Brachman, P. (eds), *Hospital Infections.* Little, Brown & Co., Boston.

Haley, R.W. (1986) *Managing Hospital Infection Control for Cost-effectiveness: A Strategy for Reducing Infectious Complications.* American Hospital Publishing, Chicago.

Haley, R.W. (1991) Measuring the costs of nosocomial infections: methods for estimating economic burden on the hospital. *American Journal of Medicine* 91 (Supplement 3B), 32s–38s.

Haley, R.W. (1992) Cost benefit analysis of infection control activities. In: Brachman, P.S. and Bennett, J.V. (eds), *Hospital Infections*, 3rd edn. Little, Brown, Boston, pp. 507–532.

Haley, R.W., Schaberg, D., Von Allmen, S. and McGowan, J. (1980) Estimating the extra charges and prolongation of hospitalization due to nosocomial infections: a comparison of methods. *Journal of Infectious Diseases* **141**, 248–257.

Haley, R.W., Schaberg, D., Crossley, K., Von Allmen, S. and McGowan, J. (1981) Extra charges and prolongation of stay attributable to nosocomial infections: a prospective interhospital comparison. *American Journal of Medicine* **70**, 51–58.

Haley, R.W., White, J.W., Culver, D.H., Meade Morgan, W., Emori. T.G., Munn. V.P. *et al.* (1985) The efficacy of infection surveillance and control programmes in preventing nosocomial infections in US hospitals. *American Journal of Epidemiology* **121**, 182–205.

Hillan, E. (1995) Postoperative morbidity following caesarean delivery. *Journal of Advanced Nursing* **22**, 1035–1042.

Hojer, H. (1978) The effect on total anti-microbial consumption and hospitalization time after prophylactic treatment with doxycycline in colorectal surgery. *Acta Chirugica Scandinavica* **144**, 175–179.

Hollingsworth, W., Todd, C., Parker, M., Roberts, J.A. and Williams, R. (1993) Cost analysis of early discharge after hip fracture. *British Medical Journal* **307**, 903–906.

Hyryla, M.L.J. and Sintonen, H. (1994) The use of health services in the management of wound infection. *Journal of Hospital Infection* **26**, 1–14.

Jones, J.D. and Chawala, A. (1984) Patient costs in the prevention and treatment of post-caesarean infections. *American Journal of Obstetrics and Gynaecology* **149**, 363–366.

Kaiser, A.B., Roach, A.C., Mulherin, J.L.J. *et al.* (1983) The cost-effectiveness of anti-microbial prophylaxis in clean vascular surgery. *Journal of Infectious Diseases* **147**, 1103.

Kappstein, I., Schulgen, G., Beyer, U., Geiger. K., Schumacher, M. and Daschner, F.D. (1992) Prolongation of stay and extra cost due to ventilator-associated pneumonia in an intensive care unit. *European Journal of Clinical Microbiology and Infectious Disease* **11**, 504–508.

Kirkland, K., Briggs, J., Trivette, S., Wilkinson, W. and Sexton, D. (1999) The impact of surgical-site infections in the 1990s: attributable mortality, excess length of hospitalization, and extra costs. *Infection Control and Hospital Epidemiology* **20**, 725–730.

Lawrence, V., Gafni, A. and Gross, M. (1989) The unproven utility of the preoperative urinalysis: economic evaluation. *Journal of Clinical Epidemiology* **42**, 1185–1192.

Magee, C.C. and Osmolski, R.J. (1978) *A Comprehensive System of Management Information for Financial Planning, Decision Making and Control in the Hospital Service.* Royal Commission on the NHS, London.

McGowan, J.E. (1981) Cost and benefit in control of nosocomial infection: method for analysis. *Review of Infectious Diseases* **3**, 790–797.

McGowan, J.E. (1982) Cost and benefit—a critical issue for hospital infection control. *American Journal of Infection Control* 100–108.

McGowan, J.E. (1991) Cost and benefit of peri-operative antimicrobial prophylaxis Methods for economic analysis. *Review of Infectious Diseases* **13** (Supplement 10): S879–S889.

Merle, V., Germain, J., Bugel, H., Nouvellon, J., Czernichow, P. and Grise, P. (2002) Nosocomial urinary tract infections in urologic patients: assessment of a prospective surveillance program including 10,000 patients. *European Urology* **41**, 483–489.

Miller, P.J., Farr, B.M. and Gwaltney, J.M. (1989)Economic benefits of an infection control program: case study and proposal. *Reviews of Infectious Diseases* **11**, 284–288.

Mugford, M., Kingston, J. and Chalmer, I. (1989) Reducing the incidence of infection after caesarean section: implications of prophylaxis with antibiotics for hospital resources. *British Medical Journal* **299**, 1003–1006.

O'Donoghue, M. and Allen, K. (1992) Costs of an outbreak of wound infections in an orthopaedic ward. *Journal of Hospital Infection* **22**, 73–78.

Orsi, G., Di Stefano, L. and Noah, N. (2002) Hospital-acquired laboratory confirmed bloodstream infection: increased hospital stay and direct costs. *Infection Control and Hospital Epidemiology* **23**, 190–197.

Persson, U., Montgomery, F., Carlsson, A., Lindgren, B. and Ahnfelt, L. (1988) How far can prophylaxis against infection in total joint replacement offset its cost? *British Medical Journal* **296**, 99–102.

Pittet, D., Tarara, D. and Wenzel, R.P. (1994) Nosocomial bloodstream infection in critically ill patients. excess length of stay, extra costs and attributable mortality. *Journal of the American Medical Association* **271**, 1598–1601.

Plowman, R. M., Graves, N., Griffen, M., Roberts, J. A., Swan, A., Cookson, B., Taylor, L., (1999) The socio-economic burden of hospital acquired infection. PHLS London.

Plowman, R., Graves, N., Esquivel, J. and Roberts, J.A. (2001a) An economic model to assess the cost and benefits of an intervention to reduce the risk of catheter related nosocomial urinary tract infections. *Journal of Hospital Infection* **48**, 33–42.

Plowman, R., Graves, N., Griffin, M., Roberts, J.A., Swan, T., Cookson, B. and Taylor, L. (2001b) The rate and cost of hospital acquired infections occurring in patients admitted to selected specialties of a district general hospital in England and the national burden imposed. *Journal of Hospital Infection* **47**, 198–209.

Poulsen, K.B., Bremmelgaard, A., Sorensen, A.I., Raahave, D. and Petersen, J.V. (1994) Estimated costs of postoperative wound infections. *Epidemiology of Infection* **113**, 283–295.

Pratt, R., Pellowe, C., Loveday, H., Robinson, N. and Smith, G. (2001) Epic guideline development team. The Epic Project: developing national evidence-based guidelines for preventing healthcare associated infections. *Journal of Hospital Infection* **47** (Supplement), S3–S66.

Report of the Comptroller and Auditor General (2000) The *Management and Control of Hospital Acquired Infection in Acute NHS Trusts in England*. The Stationery Office, London.

Rice, D. (1995) Cost of illness studies, fact or fiction. *Lancet* **334**, 1519–1520.

Rishpon, S., Lubrash, S. and Epstein, L. (1986) Reliability of a method of determining the necessity of hospitalisation days in Israel. *Medical Care* **24**, 279.

Rubenstein, E., Green, M., Modan, M., Amit, P., Bernstein, L. and Rubenstein, A. (1982) The Effect of nosocomial infections on the length and costs of hospital stay. *Journal of Antimicrobial Chemotherapy* **9** (Supplement A), 93–100.

Scheckler, W.E. (1978) Hospital costs of nosocomial infections: a prospective three month study in a community hospital. *Infection Control* **1**, 150–152.

Shapiro, M., Schoenbaum, S.C., Tager, I.B., Munoz, A. and Polk, B.F. (1983) Benefit-cost analysis of antimicrobial prophylaxis in abdominal and vaginal hysterectomy. *Journal of the American Medical Association* **249**, 1290–1294.

Slater, F. (2001) Cost-effective infection control success story: a case presentation. *Emerging Infectious Diseases* **7**, 293–294.

Tambyah, P., Knasinski, V. and Maki, D. (2002) The direct costs of nosocomial catheter-associated urinary tract infection in the era of managed care. *Infection Control and Hospital Epidemiology* **23**, 27–31.

Taylor, G., Kirkland, T., McKenzie, M., Sutherland, B. and Wiens, R. (1995) The effect of surgical wound infection on post-operative stay. *Canadian Journal of Surgery* **38**, 149–153.

Vegas, A., Jodra, V. and Garcia, M. (1993) Nosocomial infection in surgery wards: a controlled study of increased duration of hospital stays and direct cost of hospitalization. *European Journal of Epidemiology* **9**, 504–510.

Wakefield, D.S., Pfaller, M.A., Hammons, G.T. and Massanari, R.M. (1987) Use of the appropriateness evaluation protocol for estimating the incremental costs associated with nosocomial infections. *Medical Care* **25**, 481–488.

Wakefield, D.S., Pfaller, M., Ludke, R.L. and Wenzel, R.P. (1992) Methods for estimating days of hospitalisation due to nosocomial infections. *Medical Care* **30**, 373–376.

Weinstein, M., Read, J., MacKay, D., Kresel, J., Ashley, H., Halvorsen, K. *et al.* (1986) Cost-effective choice of antimicrobial therapy for serious infections. *Journal of General Internal Medicine* **1**, 351–363.

Wenzel, R. (1995) The economics of nosocomial infections. *Journal of Hospital Infection* **31**, 79–87.

Wey, S., Mori, M., Pfaller, M., Woolson, R. and Wenzel, R. (1988) Hospital-acquired candidemia. The attributable mortality and excess length of stay. *Archives of Internal Medicine* **148**, 2642–2645

Whitehouse, J., Friedman, N., Kirkland, K., Richardson, W. and Sexton, D. (2002) The impact of surgical-site infections following orthopaedic surgery at a community hospital and a university hospital: adverse quality of life, excess length of stay, and extra costs. *Infection Control and Hospital Epidemiology* **23**, 183–189.

Chapter 9

The socio-economic burden of influenza: costs of illness and 'willingness to pay' in a publicly funded health care system

Punam Mangtani and Amishi Shah

Introduction

Epidemic or seasonal influenza poses a serious health risk to those persons who are elderly and frail. Effective vaccines exist which provide important reductions in morbidity (Govaert *et al.* 1994) as well as hospitalizations and mortality (Mangtani *et al.* 2004). In the UK, vaccination against influenza is recommended to all persons with certain underlying diseases, such as lung and heart disease. In 2000, the policy for influenza vaccination was changed to include all persons over the age of 65. A study to determine the socio-economic burden of influenza was carried out at that time. This was part of an economic and epidemiologic evaluation of influenza and pneumococcal vaccination in adults.

Cost of illness studies

Socio-economic burden of illness or cost of illness (COI) studies are often the first step in the economic evaluation of interventions to prevent or control illness. A COI study is a useful tool as it provides an account of how the costs of an illness are distributed not only amongst individuals but also within health services (Kuchler and Golan 1999). Decision makers tend to find COI studies useful for heightening awareness of the problem and the potential health and financial returns that might be recouped if the disease was prevented. Such evidence thus highlights the need for further information about managing the disease and for effective medicines and prevention strategies (Szucs 1999). For instance, estimations of the avoidable costs of epidemic influenza are useful because they can be used to justify allocation of resources to reduce illness by vaccination. There are costs to the health sector for care of the patient, general practitioner (GP) visits, hospital beds, use of laboratory facilities, and medicines. There are costs to society arising from the loss of productivity of those who are ill and those who need to take time off work or normal activities to care for them. Finally, there are costs to the individual incurred in accessing health care and out of pocket expenses that arise as a result of the illness and payments incurred to compensate for the individual's impaired ability to carry out normal daily functions.

The COI approach may, however, over- or underestimate the value placed on the intervention so it cannot be used to provide estimates of individual or social welfare (Mishan 1975). Far too many intangible and non-marketed goods contribute to well being to define welfare accurately in cost terms (Kuchler and Golan 1999). COI also presents a problem when used as a measure of disease severity since disease is often most severe in the poorest persons, whose resulting lost earnings would be less than those of rich persons. Thus, COI would suggest that a disease that strikes rich people was more important than a disease that predominantly affected the poor; as such it cannot be used to determine priorities.

Willingness to pay surveys

An alternative way of assessing the burden of illness is to carry out a willingness to pay (WTP) survey or contingent valuation study. As opposed to COI studies, which take a wealth-maximizing approach, WTP studies can put individuals' values on intangibles such as pain and suffering, i.e. take a social welfare-maximizing approach (Kuchler and Golan 1999). This method estimates the burden of disease by measuring what people are willing to pay to avoid it (Clifford et al. 1977). The approach involves questioning the individual about the maximum amount he or she would pay for an intervention, or the minimum they would be willing to accept in order to forgo the intervention (Arrow et al. 1993).

Especially in publicly funded health care systems, where the economic market cannot or does not function well, the WTP method is thought to be useful to elicit the value of certain health care programmes (Clifford et al. 1977). It is a relatively new technique in health economics, having been adapted from its more widespread use in transport and the environment. WTP is rooted in welfare economics where two value judgements are assumed: first that 'social welfare should comprise individuals' welfare and that individuals should be considered the best source of information on their own welfare' (Clifford et al. 1997); and, secondly, that it can give a direct monetary value of such intangible benefits as: satisfaction from the existence of a service even if it is never used (option value), e.g. the existence of an out of hours service or a reduction in risk that is experienced when others are vaccinated (Birch et al. 1999; Coast et al. Chapter 11).

Estimates of the social value of a loss of life are available from non-health care settings (Bateman *et al.* 2002). For instance, the Health and Safety Executive (HSE) conducted empirical valuations of injuries using surveys of WTP to avoid statistical harm. The value of a fatality was estimated to be £766 000 per life saved at 1995/96 prices and £821 656 at 1998/99 price levels. Though no risk aversion was noted, i.e. there appeared to be no extra premium for a loss of life where there was little control, e.g. a rail accident compared with driving a car, in a study by Jones-Lee (quoted in Railway Safety 2002). Based on an expert appraisal of the 'willingness to pay' literature, the US Food and Drugs Administration also used a value of £561 120 per life saved to assess the potential welfare benefits of public spending. This value came to £66 800 per year of life saved in 1999 prices, after discounting by 7%, based on the years of life gained for a middle-aged man estimated as living a further 8.4 years (US Food and Drug Administration 1999). The value of an extra year to older people may be even higher. Moore and Viscusi (1998) explored the issue of whether workers at different ages reveal different WTP for job risks using the more indirect revealed preference methods for valuing life. They found that for a worker expecting to live for 35 more years, a 1 year life extension was estimated as being only worth US$11 000 now. However, a 1 year life extension was worth US$400 000 for an older worker with a life expectancy of 5 years.

However, WTP values of actions to prevent morbidity are not so readily available. As with revealed preference studies, most refer only to the value of preventing conditions stemming from environmental, transport or occupational hazards (but see Bhatia and Fox-Rushby Chapter 10). The WTP approach would be particularly useful for evaluating the contribution influenza vaccine is considered to make to social welfare because it provides a means of understanding the value of the vaccine in a situation where both risk of the respiratory illness and the outcome of the illness are uncertain (Birch *et al.* 1999).

WTP allows the benefit of the programme to be expressed as a monetary value, making it easier to compare with the total costs of the programme, and so assess if the programme is worth the cost. The main controversy is, however, the ability to obtain valid results. It is an open research issue (Johannesson 1996). Like COI, the amount people are willing to pay is affected by what they can afford to pay. This, however, can be easily dealt with by analyses that adjust for such confounding. There are a number of other methodological difficulties in measuring WTP, for example within- and between-person differences in risk perception, and making sure the information is clear and believable especially in a publicly funded health care system. They are examined further here.

Methods used to assess the value of an influenza vaccination programme (WTP) and COI from influenza-like illness

The UK Medical Research Council General Practice Framework was used to identify 10 volunteer practices in England where cases and non-cases could be identified using computerized records (Mangtani *et al.* 2005). Only those practices that recorded full morbidity events were included. Cases of influenza-like illness and pneumonia were identified from computerized GP records which are known to be highly sensitive (Hassey *et al.* 2001). A clinical diagnosis rather than an organism-specific diagnosis was acceptable given the nature of the study. A random sample of non-cases from the same practices of similar ages with replacement was also obtained. The sample size was based on being able to detect a 2-fold difference in WTP, e.g. more than £5 in patients who had had an influenza-like illness compared with patients who did not with 80% power and 90% confidence.

Design of WTP instrument

People have different levels of information about illnesses and their implications. To avoid such information bias, we prepared brief descriptive accounts of the illness and its consequences and the effectiveness of the prevention methods (see Box 9.1).

The design was based on Centers for Disease Control's (CDC) information sheets to patients. It was pre-tested in face to face interviews and in postal format with five and 10 volunteers, respectively, and revised accordingly.

WTP was obtained from patients who replied that they would have the influenza vaccine after the brief description of the disease and the efficacy of

---

Box 9.1 Structure of the WTP instrument carefully formulated question with the following aspects included

Definition of the condition
The risk of getting it
Clinical picture
Natural history
What control measures are available
How effective are they
Any side effects

the vaccine. Participants were asked to answer hypothetically how much they would be willing to pay for the vaccine by ticking an amount on a categorical scale.

This 'payment card' method was used at the time that a comparison with the NOAA (National Oceanographic and Atmospheric Administration) recommended 'yes/no referendum' approach was being conducted. The starting point used was £5, which was roughly the price of prescriptions in the UK at the time. We could have made it more realistic by asking for a vote (as in environmental evaluations) that would mean extra taxes but this was considered less appropriate in this age range. In the introduction, we used the statements: 'No intention of asking you to pay', 'Remember that you are not going to be asked to pay'.

A separate willingness to accept question was also piloted using the following statement 'if there was not enough vaccine to go round so that you could not have the vaccine, how much "compensation" do you think would leave you as well off as if you had had the vaccine?'

Sources of COI data and cost vectors

All subjects were posted a questionnaire which asked about general health including health in the last 2 weeks, any underlying chronic illness, use of health and social services in the last 3 months, the value of vaccination to them using the WTP instrument, and, in the cases, the socio-economic burden to them and carers from an influenza-like illness.

All participants were asked to complete a short form 12 (SF-12) health survey questionnaire, which provides a physical and mental health summary score (Jenkinson *et al.* 1997). The questionnaire also included a Townsend's Disability Scale, which is an index frequently used in the UK in elderly populations (Bowling 1997). Socio-economic status indicators were also included using questions about accommodation, employment and income.

Townsend's Disability Scale is a measure of disability that asks about activities of daily living (Bowling 1997). It consisted of eight questions asking about difficulty with daily tasks such as cutting toenails, dressing, cooking, light housework, using stairs, washing, walking 50 yards and shopping. The difficulty with each activity was given equal weighting. 'No difficulty' is scored as 0, 'some difficulty' is scored as 1, and 'unable to do it' is scored as 2. The scores were then summed in Stata with the overall range being 0–16. Persons with a score of 0 were allocated as having no disability, 1–2 as slightly affected, 3–6 as some disability, 7–10 as appreciable disability, and 11–16 as severely disabled.

The SF-12 health survey is a shorter version of the well-known 36-item short-form (SF-36), which is a generic measure of subjective health status.

The SF-12 consists of 12 questions about general well being, and results in two summary scores, the Physical Component Summary Scale (PCS) score and the Mental Component Summary Scale (MCS) score (Jenkinson et al. 1997). The scores are generated so that the means of each will be 50 and the standard deviation 10. Broadly, a score between 40 and 50 indicates a mild disability, 30–40 moderate disability, and below 30 severe disability (Ware et al. 1994).

Cost of illness cared for by the GP in the community

To obtain costs of a patient with influenza cared for in the community by the GP, the following questions regarding their illness were asked of patients: symptoms and duration of symptoms, health services use during illness (e.g. visits to casualty or out-patient clinic), use of other services used regularly or during the illness (i.e. home carer, meals on wheels, etc.) and any assistance given by friends and relatives during the illness. Direct costs—out of pocket expences—such as over the counter drugs and tissues were not asked about since the level of detail required was not possible in a short postal survey.

Information was also abstracted from the GP notes by research nurses and used in preference to information provided by the patient regarding: presence of chronic medical condition, vaccination status, prescriptions, use of health services in the last 3 months and, for cases, details regarding their illness including GP contacts and results of any laboratory tests or X-rays.

The direct costs included were: number of visits to the GP in the surgery, visits with GP at home, telephone conversations with GP, visits to casualty, hospital out-patient clinic visits, laboratory tests, drugs prescribed and chest X-rays. Indirect costs were estimated using the number of days confined to bed, days at home unable to carry out regular activities, distance to GP surgery and hospital, and assistance from partners, friends or relatives. Health service unit costs were obtained from the Personal Social Services Research Unit (PSSRU) who publish unit costs of health and social care derived from programme cost returns to the Department of Health for 1998/99 (Netten et al. 2000).

Accompanied and unaccompanied transport costs were determined by subtracting the mean number of times when a friend or relative accompanied the patient from the mean of the total number of visits. Costs of accompanying the patient were determined from the Automobile Association's estimates of cost per mile for use of a private car. Unaccompanied transport costs to the GP were determined as the cheapest bus fare. Unaccompanied transport to casualty or to the hospital, which resulted in an admission, was considered as ambulance use.

Leisure and work time forgone by the patient when ill and any carer changing their routine to care for them have some costs but are more difficult to determine. If a carer had to take time off work or cancel arrangements to look after an ill patient at home, an opportunity cost at least at the level of household production/housework was assumed (Posnett and Jan 1996; Brouwer *et al.* 1999). Ill patients in hospital or at home not able to do normal activities were considered to have an opportunity cost to the patient at least as leisure time forgone. The same opportunity cost would also apply to any carer who changed their routine to help the patient during their illness but did not have to cancel planned arrangements or take time off of work. The costs are likely to be an underestimate as carers may not consider that they had to cancel planned arrangements if they were retired or already unemployed. If the patient was ill in bed at home, but there was no carer, it was assumed that any household production lost in that time would be made up later so that the opportunity cost to the patient would at least be that of leisure time lost. If the patient was not in bed but not able to do normal activities, this was also seen as leisure time lost. The average income of pensioners in 1998/9 was used as the value of the opportunity cost of leisure time forgone (Pensioners' Income Series 2001).

Cost of illness requiring hospital admission

To estimate direct costs of a hospital admission for influenza, unpublished routine data on the average number of bed days for an acute respiratory admission as the primary diagnosis in over 64 year olds were obtained from national Hospital Episode Statistics (HES) data for 1995–2000 inclusive. Unpublished tabulations aggregating the records of care under different consultants were used, i.e. separate finished consultant episodes were aggregated for the same admission. Most of these admissions occur in winter when pressure on bed days is most acute. The average cost of the hospital stay per day used could therefore be considered conservative. The cost of a day as a thoracic medicine patient was between that of a geriatric admission and an infectious disease admission.

The indirect costs of a hospitalized patient were based on the mean number of days informal carers looked after patients admitted to care of the elderly in a study of acute admissions to a district general hospital in 1994 (Plowman *et al.* 2001). Conservative assumptions were made that the carer did not need to cancel arrangements or take time off work so that the unit cost was the cost per day of leisure time lost. It was also assumed that if a carer was needed, the patient lost the same amount of leisure time and was costed as such.

Results

A total of 118 eligible patients in the influenza season of 1998/99 were ascertained out of a practice population of 18 877 not in nursing/rest homes. This gave an incidence of influenza-like illness of 6.25 per 1000 population aged

65–84 years old. Out of the 118 patients, 85 replied, giving a response rate of 72%. Finally, out of 184 non-cases who replied, 80% were the first eligible randomly selected from the practices' age-sex register.

Participant characteristics

The majority of patients who had had an influenza-like illness had an uncomplicated illness (71.8%). The most common complication was developing pneumonia, which occurred in 9.4% of the flu cases, followed by exacerbation of asthma (8.2%).

Underlying illness and yearly income appeared to be similar in the two groups. There was slightly more disability among the patients who had had influenza compared with non-cases according to the Townsend Disability Score and SF-12 MCS scores (Table 9.1).

Table 9.1 Characteristics of the sample

	Non-cases		Influenza cases		P-value
	n	%	n	%	
Sex					0.926
Male	90	48.9	40	47.1	
Female	94	51.1	45	52.9	
Age					0.716
65–69.9	60	32.6	32	37.6	
70–74.9	46	25	16	18.8	
75–79.9	51	27.7	24	28.2	
80–84.9	27	14.7	13	15.3	
Underlying illness					0.468
None	80	43.5	31	36.5	
One	84	45.6	38	44.7	
More than one	20	10.9	16	18.8	
Yearly income					0.792
£0–5199	26	16.9	9	12.7	
£5200–£10 399	75	48.7	36	50.7	
£10 400–£15 599	31	20.1	16	22.5	
£15 600–£20 799	10	6.5	5	7.0	
£28 000+	12	7.8	5	7.0	
Townsend Disability Score					
No disability	93	58.1	32	44.4	<0.001

Table 9.1 (continued)

	Non-cases		Influenza cases		P-value
	n	%	n	%	
Slightly affected	33	20.6	12	13.4	
Some disability	14	8.7	17	23.6	
Appreciable disability	15	9.4	8	11.1	
Severe disability	5	3.1	3	4.2	
SF-12					
MCS score					
Severe disability	3	2.0	4	7.3	<0.001
Moderate disability	13	8.8	15	27.3	
Mild disability	28	19.0	14	25.4	
No disability	103	70.1	22	40	
PCS score					
Severe disability	9	6.1	3	5.4	0.117
Moderate disability	35	23.8	15	27.3	
Mild disability	33	22.4	20	36.4	
No disability	70	47.6	17	30.9	
Accommodation					
Owned	147	80.3	68	80	0.021
Rented from local council	29	15.8	8	9.4	
Rented from housing association	3	1.6	5	5.9	
Rented privately	3	1.6	4	4.7	
Other	1	0.5	0	0	
Live alone	7	31.32	54	28.6	
Living circumstances					
Live with spouse/partner	11	62.09	56	66.7	0.800
Live with children	7	3.85	2	2.4	
Live with other relatives/friends	4	2.2	2	2.4	
Live alone	1	0.55	0	0	
Central heating					
Central heating in all rooms	152	83.52	73	86.9	0.965
Central heating in some rooms	19	10.44	8	9.5	
No central heating	11	6.04	3	3.6	

The proportion of cases in one or more high risk groups was slightly, but not statistically, significantly higher than in the sample of 184 age-, sex- and practice-matched non-cases (63.5% compared with 56%). The distribution of risk is consistent with the fact that people aged at least 65 years old at higher risk are more likely to attend with influenza-like illness (Govaert *et al.* 1994).

Costs of illness

Costs of illness in the community seen by a GP (not requiring hospital care)

Although patients were asked about formal care, only two out of the sample of 85 patients presenting to GPs with influenza-like illness reported using any formal carers, home helps, home nurses, etc. Formal care was also not used more during their illness. Three out of the 84 with complete cost data had been hospitalized. In order to reduce the skewness in cost due to these patients, they were excluded from the cost analyses.

The total indirect cost in our study of time ill in bed and not in bed but not able to do normal activities with carer time involved was £327. This represented 85% of the total costs of illness with an influenza-like illness coming to a GP in this age group see (Table 9.2).

Table 9.2 Summary of direct cost per medically attended patient in the community with influenza-like illness

Items	Unit cost in £ in 1998/99		All cases $n = 81$	
	Cost vectors	Arithmetic mean	Cost	%
Costs to GP or social services				
GP surgery visit	18.00	0.87	15.72	
GP home visit[1]	54.00	0.48	25.97	
Phone call to GP	21.00	0.11	2.39	
Summary of costs of laboratory tests and X-rays[2]			1.41	
Summary of costs of drugs prescribed[2]			2.70	
Total costs to GP/social services			48.20	13
Hospital costs				
Visits to out-patient clinic	78.00	0.04	3.16	
A&E visit	37.00	0.04	1.46	
Transportation to and from hospital			3.33	
Total costs to hospital			7.95	2

Table 9.2 (continued)

Items	Unit cost in £ in 1998/99		All cases $n = 81$	
	Cost vectors	Arithmetic mean	Cost	%
Direct (personal) costs to patients and carers				
Transportation costs			1.32	
Total direct costs of community case medically attended			57.47	15
Indirect costs to patients and carers				
Patient in hospital	18.85	0.00	0.00	
Patient at home in bed	88.45	1.30	114.87	
Not normal activities if carer took time off work	88.45	0.18	15.92	
Not normal activities if carer did not take time off work or no carer	18.85	8.27	155.92	
Not in bed, carer changed routine only	37.70	1.07	40.34	
Total indirect costs to patient/carer			328.37	85
Total			384.52	100

[1] Per surgery consultation lasting 9.36 min (Netten *et al.* 2000).

[2] Laboratory test unit costs and prescription costs were obtained from other research studies (Surri *et al.* 2002; Jacklin *et al.* 2003).

Cost of illness requiring hospital care

The mean duration of an admission in 1999 with an acute respiratory tract infection as the primary diagnosis using HES data was 10.3 days. The cost to the health service per admission with an acute respiratory infection in this age group was £3014 (85% of the total cost). This cost included GP costs before and after admission and out-patient attendance (Table 9.3). Indirect costs were 14% of the total costs.

Willingness to pay

Over 50% in both groups had a flu vaccination in the last year. Of those who had had an influenza-like illness, 79% said they would have a flu vaccination in the future compared with 63% who had not ($P = 0.017$).

Table 9.3 Cost per patient hospitalized with an acute respiratory illness

	Unit cost	Value	Cost per patient	
Direct costs				
Medically attended influenza in community 65+			57.5	Primary data (Table 9.1)
Cost of acute respiratory admission[1]	282.9[2]	10.3	2908	1999 HES data
Out-patient visits of those hospitalized[1]	96.6[2]	0.5	48.3	Average number of out-patient department visits, primary data from a survey of patients admitted with pneumonia[3]
Total cost to health service per hospitalization			3014	
Indirect costs to patients and carers				
Medically attended influenza 65+ (non-hospitalized)			327.1	Primary data (Table 9.1)
Patient in hospital bed[4]	18.9	10.3	194	
Informal care after discharge[5]	37.7	7.6	286	Average number of days needed for carer help post-discharge[6]
Total indirect costs of hospitalization			480	
Total costs		3494		

[1] Unit cost inflated by 15% for capital costs (personal communication Ann Netten PSSRU).

[2] From Swan et al. (1999).

[3] From Mangtani et al. (2005).

[4] Unit cost assumed leisure time lost (average daily income of a pensioner 1998/9; from Pensioners' Income Series 2001).

[5] Unit cost assumed leisure time lost to patient and carer (averate daily income of a pensioner 1998/9; from Pensioners' Income Series 2001).

[6] Plowman et al. (1999).

The question on willingness to accept compensation if there was not enough flu vaccination to go round was unanswered by most respondents; 98% responded to the WTP question.

The responses to the same WTP question of a similar sample of patients who had had pneumonia recruited at the same time as patients who had had influenza-like illness (Mangtani *et al.* 2005) are included for comparison. A total of 26 (10% of those giving a WTP value) patients responded to an open-ended question asking 'what things affect how much you would be willing to pay for it?', that their decision was influenced by the fact that the National Health Service (NHS) should pay for the vaccine or they tried to determine how much the NHS did pay for it. Since the intention was to determine the value of the vaccine to the patients, these patients were excluded from the WTP analysis.

Most patients were willing to pay up to £5 (Fig. 9.1). However, there are many patients who were not be willing to pay anything (between 8 and 19% depending on whether they had recently been ill with influenza-like illness or pneumonia) and even more who were uncertain how much to pay (9–19%). Most of the latter in response to the open-ended question gave low income as a reason; only two patients noted that they did not understand the question. Up to 21% stated that they would pay more than £5 for the vaccines.

The regression analyses showed that the biggest factor which predicted those who would pay more than £5 for vaccine was income. Even in the univariate analysis, it was clear that income is the strongest predictor (Table 9.4).

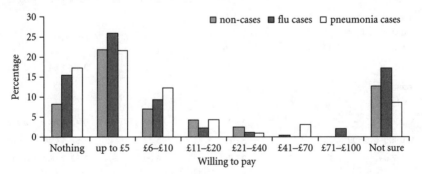

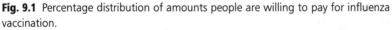

Fig. 9.1 Percentage distribution of amounts people are willing to pay for influenza vaccination.

Table 9.4 Willingness to pay more than £5 for influenza vaccine

	No.of persons in each category willing to pay >£5	% of persons in each category willing to pay >£5	Univariate analyses		
			Odds ratio	95% CI	P-value
Case					
Non-case	27	14.67	1		
Flu	13	15.29	0.76	0.34–1.66	0.487
Pneumonia	19	21.59	1.14	0.55–2.35	0.727
Age					
65–74	28	14.14	1		
Older than 75	31	19.5	1.34	0.72–2.50	0.351
Sex					
Male	35	20.11	1		
Female	24	13.11	0.69	0.37–1.28	0.239
Underlying illness according to GP					
None	28	19.05	1		
One or more	31	14.76	0.53	0.28–0.99	0.048
Underlying illness according to patient					
None	22	16.06	1		
One or more	17	12.98	0.59	0.28–1.24	0.165
Had flu vaccine in last year					
No	18	11.76	1		
Yes	40	19.9	0.86	0.43–1.70	0.662
Had pneumonia vaccine in last year					
No	40	16.26	1		
Yes	16	17.98	0.77	0.39–1.54	0.461
Income					
£0–£5199	5	10.2	1		
£5200–£10 399	19	13.01	1.23	0.41–3.69	0.715
£10 400–£15 599	19	32.2	5.32	1.62–17.44	0.006
£15 600+	10	27.03	6.00	1.52–23.67	0.011
Accommodation					
Owned	49	17.88	1		
Rented from local council	8	13.11	0.74	0.30–1.81	0.513
Rented from housing association	1	11.11	0.46	0.05–4.27	0.498

Table 9.4 (continued)

	No. of persons in each category willing to pay >£5	% of persons in each category willing to pay >£5	Univariate analyses		
			Odds ratio	95% CI	P-value
Rented privately	1	10	0.27	0.03–2.22	0.221
Live alone	19	17.92	1		
Live with spouse/partner	37	16.37	0.84	0.43–1.66	0.625
Live with children	2	15.38	1.89	0.25–14.53	0.539
Live with other relatives/friends	1	14.29	0.95	0.08–11.13	0.966
Central heating in all rooms	52	17.57	1		
Central heating in some rooms	5	12.82	0.61	0.21–1.77	0.365
No central heating	2	10.53	0.78	0.15–4.18	0.776
Townsend Disability Score					
None	27	18.12	1		
Slight or some disability	14	13.73	0.47	0.22–1.02	0.057
Appreciable or severe disability	10	17.24	0.74	0.30–1.81	0.511
SF-12					
PCS score	n/a		1.02	0.97–1.06	0.447
MCS score	n/a		1.02	0.99–1.06	0.200

In the adjusted regression model, those earning more than £15 600 were 6.16 times more likely to pay more for the flu vaccine than those in the lowest earning group ($P = 0.029$) (Table 9.5).

There was a non-significant propensity to pay more than £5 if the patient had had pneumonia but not influenza compared with people who had not experienced either illness.

Discussion

COIs from influenza-like illness incur indirect costs, i.e. costs as a consequence of the illness to patients and carers in terms of leisure or work time lost. They are, however, often overlooked in cost studies. The cost per case of influenza-like illness managed in the community by the GP was £385 at 1998/99 prices and if admitted to hospital the cost was £3494. Indirect costs of

Table 9.5 Willingness to pay more than £5 for influenza vaccine: multivariate analyses

	Odds ratio[1]	95% CI	P-value
Case			
Non-case	1		
Flu	0.69	0.26–1.81	0.449
Pneumonia	1.4	0.54–3.62	0.487
Age			
65–74	1		
Older than 75	2.12	0.94–4.78	0.069
Sex			
Male	1		
Female	0.97	0.44–2.16	0.94
Income			
£0–£5199	1		
£5200–£10399	1.18	0.34–4.11	0.789
£10400–£15599	5.35	1.38–20.73	0.015
£15600+	6.16	1.20–31.54	0.029
Townsend Disability Score			
None	1		
Slight or some disability	0.6	0.24–1.49	0.27
Appreciable or severe disability	1.03	0.34–3.13	0.965

[1] Odds after controlling for each of the other variables in the table.

medically attended influenza-like illnesses in the community amounted to 86% of the total cost and 14% of the total costs if hospitalized.

Our direct costs for a hospitalization with an acute respiratory illness were similar to those found in a study using the ingredients approach of 30 emergency admissions for the same diagnoses to a district general hospital in 1994/95 (Plowman *et al.* 2001). The mean in-patient hospital cost per case from that study was £3092 at 1998/99 prices. The HES data on length of stay we used were also similar to the mean stay of 10.6 days in the 30 patients.

The age distribution of our cases was also similar to that of the general population. The overall mean costs from the sample could be applied to the rates of influenza-like illness in people aged at least 65 years old attending general practice or requiring hospitalization to evaluate an influenza vaccination programme. For instance, from our analysis of a historical cohort, the estimated rate of hospital admissions prevented by full coverage with influenza vaccine was 39.8 per 100 000 population per year aged over 64 years averaged over 9 years (1991–1999) (Mangtani *et al.* 2004), giving the costs saved from an illness requiring hospitalization in a fully vaccinated cohort of over 64 year olds of £1.39 (3494 × 39.8 × 10^{-5}) per person. Others have calculated that 600 per 100 000 population per year consultations for influenza as well as 1600 consultations with a GP with bronchitis or otitis media per 100 000 population per year are attributable to influenza (Fleming 2000). A 58% vaccine efficacy against laboratory-confirmed influenza-like illness (Govaert *et al.* 1994) might be an optimistic estimate of protection against such consultations. However, if used, the rough cost saved by preventing such consultations would be £4.91 (384.52 × 2200 × 10^{-5} × 0.58) per person vaccinated. The cost per vaccination against influenza, including central and administration costs, was calculated at £11 per vaccine at 1998/99 prices (Mangtani *et al.* 2005). The net cost to prevent illness requiring medical attention in the community or in hospital would therefore be about £4.70 [£11 − (£1.39 + £4.91)] per person vaccinated. However, the cost savings do not take into account (i) those who remained at home and did not consult a GP [although data are limited, about 1 in 2 in this age group do not consult (Nicholson *et al.*, 1997)]; and (ii) expenses incurred by patients and those who care for them; or, include a value of lives saved. On average, the effectiveness of influenza vaccination against respiratory deaths is about 12% (Mangtani *et al.* 2004).

Would it be possible to estimate the value of lives saved using one of the measures? This result is more startling than we had anticipated!

The COIs from influenza presented here provide an idea of the distribution of the costs, e.g. within the health sector and between society and the health sector. It is therefore a useful management tool. There is, however, a need for WTP measures as it is the only method of analysing the benefits of allocating resources to a particular health care which allows people themselves to value what is important to them. Other methods of asking what should be prioritized, e.g. ranking procedures, are limited by peoples' lack of information about the other services. The more subtle welfare effects or intangible benefits to a person of an intervention are also not adequately captured by a medical assessment of health benefit. Asking people theoretically what is the maximum they would pay for a service is a simpler way of measuring how strongly they felt about the services. The WTP method is not restricted to valuing improvements in health status, e.g. pain, but can cover inconvenience, concern about worry or inconvenience to carers or family and friends, social benefit to society, reduction in their risk of infection if another person is vaccinated, the knowledge that a person is being cared for, information, reassurance and the process of treatment. The methods to place values on these benefits in the health field are still at an early stage of development.

This WTP for influenza vaccination study had a similar high response rate to that of a postal WTP question in a trial of antenatal care in Scotland (Ryan *et al.* 1997). A willing to accept question ('if there was not enough vaccine to go round so that you could not have the vaccine, how much do you think would leave you as well off as if you had had the vaccine?') was not understood by many. With a high overall response to the survey, it appears that a question on willingness to accept compensation does not work well in a population of this age and experience of health care provision free at point of use.

Though the main factor driving the amount people were willing to pay was income, the decision to receive vaccine also depended on the patients' experience of illness or disability. People with illness naturally value interventions differently from those without. It was seen here in their stated preference for flu vaccination but was not obvious when patients who had had influenza were asked about their WTP for vaccination. It is possible that uncomplicated influenza illness is not severe enough and/or the vaccine is not perceived as good enough to value it in terms of money or the categories of payment we used here, so that subjective views and prejudice about flu vaccination may have prevailed. There was a suggestion that patients who had had a more severe acute respiratory infection, pneumonia, valued influenza vaccination more than those who had not recently had an acute respiratory infection.

The value of an intervention is generally thought best to come from the community if the health care system is publicly funded. Knowledge or experience of a common illness or vulnerability may change the value of an intervention. Separate WTP values for different strata of risk should be examined. A value to those not likely to be affected could also provide a value of the positive externalities, i.e. the benefit of reduced transmission to others. A WTP value could be obtained adjusted for level of risk, as for income, using multiple regression techniques.

Although this survey of WTP for vaccine was answered by nearly all participants, of those who would have the vaccines in the future, at least 10% had difficulty replying because the scenario may not have been plausible in a health service that is paid for by taxation. They suggested that the NHS should pay for the vaccine or tried to determine the cost to the NHS. It was also not possible to exclude the potential moral hazard element of those being asked undervaluing an intervention if they thought the information might be used to guide future charges. Survey responses are sensitive to the way the questions are asked, more so when attitudes and values are ascertained. The WTP values were also sensitive to the range of values offered: there was a preference for the familiar prescription charge levied on under 65 year olds; and the starting point appeared to have been too low for a substantial proportion of people in this age group. A heavily biased summary measure of WTP, the direction of which would be difficult to assess, would result with this level of incompleteness. Ideally, comparison of the WTP value with the cost of influenza vaccination as with the COIs prevented could be examined and discussed within the limitations of some of the biases touched upon above.

The experience from this survey suggests that improvements in methods to make subjects well informed are required. Future surveys using face to face or telephone interviews, as recommended by the NOAA panel, would help reduce this information bias (improve the face validity) (Bateman *et al.* 2002), as would a formal qualitative component to decide how best to make the scenarios plausible as well as a check how health care in such scenarios is valued (Schkade and Payne 1994). Alternative avenues worth considering include a group of subjects hearing and questioning a group of experts on the benefits and costs of a policy option before asking their WTP (quoted in Schkade and Payne 1994). Work is still ongoing on which format to present the values to choose from (payment card of ordered categories, or a referendum-style bid with the range of values randomly allocated to different subjects) to give the least biased response (Ryan *et al.* 2004). Care is also needed to ensure that the values used do not exclude significant members of the population, in this example, elderly people on low incomes.

Conclusion

WTP is a relatively new technique in health economics. Its use is more accepted in transport and the environment, e.g. implementing air traffic control safety measures, rail safety or compensation for oil spills (Bateman *et al.* 2002). The advantage of transport safety is that it is easily understood because of its realism. It is not difficult to imagine choosing a car and how much extra one would pay for safety features. Many of the theoretical and practical aspects of the design of such surveys derive from the value of life lost from transport accidents to help decide investment in safety features, e.g. the Paddington rail crash.

There are a number of practical issues regarding how one sets out to obtain such WTP values for health outcomes other than accidental injuries and deaths. Methods to do so in the health field are often at the stage of testing its feasibility. Significant steps forward have, however, been made in this area (see Bhatia and Fox-Rushby Chapter 10). We have shown by this survey that there are additional difficulties in making the question plausible to a population of over 65 year olds where health care is publicly funded and largely free at point of use. The willingness to accept compensation question was, for this group, even less understandable than WTP. When estimating population-based valuations, account needs to be taken of populations more vulnerable to ill health who are likely to value health care more highly than those who are less vulnerable.

References

Arrow, K., Solow, R., Portney, P.R., Leamer, E.E., Radner, R. and Schuman, H. (1993) Report of the NOAA Panel of Contingent Valuation. *Federal Register* **58**, 4601–4614.

Bateman, I.J., Carson, R.T., Day, B., Hanemann, M., Hanley, N., Hett, T., Jones-Lee, M., Loomes, G., Mourato, S., Ozdemiroglu, E., Pearce, D.W., Sugden, R. and Swanson, J. (2002) *Economic Valuation with Stated Preference Techniques*. Edward Elgar Publishing Ltd for the Department of Transport, Cheltenham.

Birch, S., Gafni, A. and O'Brien, B. (1999) Willingness to pay and the valuation of programmes for the prevention and control of influenza. *Pharmacoeconomics* **16**, 55–61.

Bowling, A. (1997) *Measuring Health*. Open University Press, Buckingham.

Brouwer, W.B., van Exel, N.J., Koopmanschap, M.A. and Rutten, F.F. (1999) The valuation of informal care in economic appraisal. A consideration of individual choice and societal costs of time. *International Journal of Technology Assessment in Health Care* **15**, 147–160.

Clifford, R.E., Smith, J.W., Tillett, H.E. and Wherry, P.J. (1977) Excess mortality associated with influenza in England and Wales. *International Journal of Epidemiology* **6**, 115–128.

Drummond, M.F., O'Brien, B., Stoddart, G.L. and Torrance, G.W. (eds) (1997) Cost-benefit analysis. In: *Methods for the Economic Evaluation of Health Care Programmes*. Oxford University Press, Oxford, pp. 205–231.

Fleming, D.M. (2000) The contribution of influenza to combined acute respiration infections, hospital admissions and deaths in winter. *Comm Dis and Public Health* **3**, 32–8.

Govaert, T.M.E., Thijs, C.T.M.C.N., Masurel, N., Sprenger, N. and Dinant, G.J. (1994) The efficacy of influenza vaccination in elderly individuals: a randomised double-blind placebo-controlled trial. *Journal of the American Medical Association* **272**, 1661–1665.

Hassey, A., Gerrett, D. and Wilson, A. (2001) A survey of validity and utility of electronic patient records in general practice. *British Medical Journal* **322**, 1401–1405.

Hospital Episode Statistics (2001) http://www.doh.gov.uk/hes/.

Jenkinson, C., Layte, R., Jenkinson, D. *et al* (1997) A shorter form health survey: can the SF-12 replicate results from the SF-36 in longitudinal studies? *Journal of Public Health Medicine* **19**, 179–186.

Johannesson, M. (1996) The contingent valuation controversy in environmental economics and its relevance to health services research. *Journal of Health Service Research Policy* **1**, 116–117.

Kuchler, F. and Golan, E. (1999) *Assigning Values to Life: Comparing Methods for Valuing Health Risks. Agricultural Economic Report No. 784*. Food and Rural Economics Division, Economic Research Service, US Department of Agriculture, Washington, DC.

Mangtani, P., Cumberland, P., Hodgson, C.R., Roberts, J.A., Cutts, F.T. and Hall, A.J. (2004) A cohort study of the effectiveness of influenza vaccine in older people using the United Kingdom General Practice Research Database. *Journal of Infectious Diseases* **190**, 1–10.

Mangtani, P., Roberts, J.A., Hall, A.J. and Cutts, F. (2005) An economic analysis of a pneumococcal vaccine programme in people aged over 64 years in a developed country setting. *International Journal of Epidemiology* **34**, 565–574.

Mishan, E.J. (1975) *Cost Benefit Analysis: An Informal Introduction*. George Allen and Unwin Ltd, London.

Netten, A., Dennet, J. and Knight, J. (2000) *Unit Costs of Health and Social Care 2001*. Personal Social Services Research Unit, Canterbury.

Nicholson, K.G., Kent, J., Hammersley, V. and Cancio, E. (1997) Acute viral infections of the upper respiratory tract in elderly people living in the community: comparative, prospective, population based study of disease burden. *British Medical Journal* **315**, 1060–1064.

Pensioners' Income Series (2001) Pensioners' Income Series 1997/8, DSS Analytical Services Division 2000, section 2, quoted on http://www.ageconcern.org.uk accessed August 3, 2001.

Plowman, R.M., Graves, N., Griffin, M., Roberts, J.A., Swan, A., Cookson, B., and Taylor, L. (1999) The Socio-economic burden of hospital acquired infection. PHLS, London.

Plowman, R., Graves, N., Griffin, M.A., Roberts, J.A., Swan, A.V., Cookson, B. and Taylor, L. (2001) The rate and cost of hospital-acquired infections occurring in patients admitted to selected specialties of a district general hospital in England and the national burden imposed. *Journal of Hospital Infection* **47**, 198–209.

Posnett, J. and Jan, S. (1996) Indirect cost in economic evaluation: the opportunity cost of unpaid inputs. *Health Economy* **5**, 13–23.

Railway Safety (2002) *Annual Safety Performance 2001/02*. Railway Safety, London.

Ryan, M., Ratcliffe, J. and Tucker, J. (1997) Using willingness to pay to value alternative models of antenatal care. *Social Science and Medicine* **44**, 371–380.

Ryan, M., Scott, D.A. and Donaldson, C. (2004) Valuing health care using willingness to pay: a comparison of the payment card and dichotomous choice methods. *Journal of Health Economy* **23**, 237–258.

Schkade, D.A. and Payne, J.W. (1994) How people respond to contingent valuation questions: a verbal protocol analysis of willingness to pay for an environmental regulation. *Journal of Environmental Economics and Management* **26**, 88–109.

Suri, R., Grieve, R., Normand, C., Metcalfe, C., Thompson, S., Wallis, C. *et al.* (2002) Effects of hypertonic saline, alternate day and daily rhDNase on healthcare use, costs and outcomes in children with cystic fibrosis. *Thorax* **57**, 841–846.

Szucs, T.D. (1999) Influenza: the role of burden-of-illness research. *Pharmacoeconomics* **16** Supplement **1**, 27–32.

US Food and Drug Administration (1999) Labelling: trans fatty acids in nutrition labelling, nutrient size. *Federal Register* **64**, 62745–62825.

Ware, J.E., Kosinski, M. and Keller, S.D. (1994) *How to Score the SF-12 Physical and Mental Health Summary Scales*. The Health Institute, New England Medical Center, Boston, MA.

Chapter 10

Willingness to pay for insecticide-treated mosquito nets in Surat, India

Mrigesh Bhatia and Julia Fox-Rushby

Introduction

Cost-benefit analysis (CBA) is the only type of economic evaluation to put costs and benefits in monetary terms. The valuation of benefits is not restricted to health gain and can incorporate non-health benefits. Therefore, CBA can compare interventions across sectors and is the only type of economic evaluation that can question the size of resources to the health sector. However, many challenges arise in putting monetary values on benefits.

The three principal approaches used to value benefits are: the human capital approach (by measuring impact on earnings); observed preferences (by observing investment choices of decision makers or where individuals implicitly trade-off income and risk); and stated preferences (which ask individuals directly about the value they place on something). Human capital theory and observed preferences are too closely related to prices rather than value, and those that provide values may not reflect the preferences of individuals or society (Fox-Rushby and Cairns 2005). Therefore, they are not good indicators of value for use in CBA.

The two methods for eliciting stated preferences are contingent valuation and discrete choice experiments. Both methods ask individuals to make judgements in a hypothetical situation. Contingent valuation asks people directly about their maximum willingness to pay (WTP) for a good or service or the minimum they would be willing to accept (WTA) for the loss or reduction of a service contingent on a market existing (Gafni 1998). Discrete choice experiments present two (or more) scenarios to a person and ask for the preferred option. Each scenario describes a number of attributes about the option, with each option differing in the levels of each attribute. When the scenarios include a cost attribute within the choice, WTP can be estimated. Discrete choice experiments are most useful if the aim is to establish the trade-offs people are willing to make for different attributes of the choices offered, whereas WTP questions are sufficient for an overall valuation (Bateman *et al.* 2002).

Contingent valuation was originally developed in the environmental field to measure the WTP for environmental changes using survey methods (Eckerlund *et al.* 1995). In recent years, it has been applied increasingly in the health sector to obtain valuations where past preferences cannot be observed. However, as with other valuation approaches, questions have been raised about whether WTP studies really do elicit values. These concerns include: scenarios being unrealistic; values given being 'led' by WTP questions themselves; and respondents giving values that would never reflect their actual behaviour.

This chapter begins by setting out the theoretical basis for using WTP to value benefits. It moves on to present the methods used to develop a household survey designed to elicit values for insecticide-treated mosquito nets (TMNs) in Surat, India. The results section first presents descriptive statistics on who was willing to pay what amounts and then addresses whether responses were 'led' by WTP questions and whether respondents acted according to their stated values. The discussion considers how valid WTP responses appear to be and what further analysis should be conducted to address this issue.

The theory behind willingness to pay valuation

The foundation for the valuation of benefits using contingent valuation is welfare economics and the concept of consumer surplus. The aim of contingent valuation is to value the gains or losses in utility when a programme is introduced or withdrawn. This is valued using two monetary measures of change in utility: compensating and equivalent variations.

Compensating variations are evaluated prior to a policy change and aim to elicit an alternative combination of goods that a consumer considers 'as good as' the initial combination, i.e. the amount of compensation (income) that can be taken from an individual for a good that leaves their utility constant (at the same level), whilst holding real income constant. Equivalent variation is based on the expected new level of welfare once a change has taken place. In this case, it would be the amount of compensation that has to be given to the individual, in the absence of change, to make him as well off as he would be with the change (Olsen 1997).

In practice, the valuation of benefits from health care tends to adopt compensating variations. It therefore evaluates increases in health care provision or introduction of new types of care policy from the current level of utility (Donaldson 1993). In addition, there is consensus in the literature that WTP rather than WTA is the preferred approach (Olsen 1997), partly because income effects may not be small (Haneman *et al.* 1991).

Contingent valuation is consistent with utility theory and is rooted in Paretian welfare theory. This welfarist approach assumes that individuals are capable of making a rational choice between alternative bundles of goods and services in order to maximize their utility. Thus it assumes that individuals are able to reflect their preferences and that they are the best judges of their own welfare.

In a private market, for example, an individual would choose to buy a good if the marginal value of that good at least equalled the price they had to pay. Any difference between the price of a good and the amount a person is willing to pay indicates that a consumer is gaining more value than indicated by the price. Consumer surplus is the difference between the maximum that a consumer would pay to obtain a given quantity of a good and the actual amount paid.

Figure 10.1 shows a downward sloping demand curve and indicates that the area under the demand curve and above a price level equates to the amount of consumer surplus. At a lower price, consumer surplus is larger. Thus, in a private market, price is the lower bound of an individual's WTP (Bala *et al.* 1998). A demand curve is not observable in the absence of a market. However, there still exists a latent demand curve that could be 'teased out' through other means (Hanemann 1994). Figure 10.1 also indicates that if no price existed but such a latent demand was 'teased out', then any estimation of WTP is an estimation of consumer surplus.

Increments of consumer surplus are equated with increases in consumer welfare. As we know that consumption confers utility to a consumer, we accept that money confers utility indirectly as it represents a claim on consumption. Therefore, we can state that any increase in WTP represents more utility to the consumer.

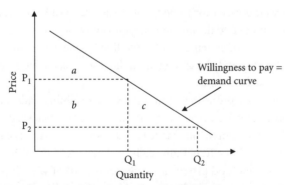

Fig. 10.1 Wilingness to pay and consumer surplus. When price = P_1, quantity demanded = Q_1 and total consumer surplus = area a. When price = P_2, quantity demanded = Q_2 and total consumer surplus = area $a+b+c$.

The cost-benefit decision rule is to choose those programmes that maximize net benefits, where benefit from a programme is defined as the sum of the maximum amounts individuals who are affected by the programme are willing to pay (Pauly 1998). CBA is directly based on the potential Pareto improvement criterion, also called the compensation test or Kaldor—Hicks criterion (Gaber *et al.* 1996), which states that 'if the amount gainers are willing to pay for a change is greater than the amount needed to compensate the losses then the change should go ahead', as this will result in Pareto improvement.

As WTP studies are conducted in settings where markets do not exist, the hypothetical nature of the studies can make them prone to various forms of bias. Thus stated, WTP has been affected by, for example, choice of elicitation method used; implied value cues and ranges of values presented (e.g. Stalhammer 1996; Whynes *et al.* 2004); perceived relevance of information presented (e.g. Brown *et al.* 1995); non-response (e.g. Miller and Smith 1983); and ordering of goods to be valued (e.g. De Ridder and De Graeve 2005) amongst others.

Various question formats for asking about WTP are set out and reviewed in a number of publications (Russell *et al.* 1995; Olsen 1997). Open-ended questions allow respondents the freedom to state the maximum amount they are willing to pay. However, its use has been discouraged in guidelines (National Oceanic Atmospheric Administration 1993) for not mimicking the market and having high rates of non-response. It is an approach that needs fairly skilled interviewers and was argued by Mitchell and Carson (1993) to be particularly prone to strategic bias, where respondents second-guess the impact of responses in setting their 'value'. Closed-ended questions ask individuals whether they will pay a specified sum. The sum is varied across respondents to generate a demand curve that approximates WTP. This format tends to have a high response rate as it is easier for respondents to answer. Whilst it is less prone to strategic bias, it is open to the bias of using quoted values (Mitchell and Carson 1993). Between the two extremes lies the bidding format, where the respondent is given a starting bid and, depending upon the response, the bid is increased or decreased by a fixed amount.

As WTP studies are prone to various biases, the reliability and validity of the stated WTP estimates are a major concern. Reliability is the level of agreement between replicate measurements made on the same subjects. It is a measure of consistency and could be tested internally and by repeatability. Validity is the extent to which a method provides a true assessment of what it purports to measure. In the absence of a 'gold standard' (criterion validity) to compare the results of the study, the majority of the studies examine the comparability of WTP estimates with indirect methods of measuring WTP; theoretical validity—to test whether the relationship between WTP responses and other variables is consistent with economic theory; and concurrent validity—to test the association of WTP estimates with estimates obtained by other measures (Harris *et al.* 1989). However, as stressed by Johannesson (1993), 'the ultimate test of validity is to compare hypothetical payments with real money transactions, and to carry out such studies is in my opinion the single most important issue in CV research'.

Methods

The aim of this study was two-fold: to estimate the WTP for insecticide-treated mosquito nets using compensating, rather than equivalent, variations, i.e. questions were framed in terms of WTP for receiving a new TMN; and to minimize and examine alternative forms of bias. [We recognize that the equivalent variation is not constrained by income and that it is possible, especially for poorer households, that income effects may not be negligible. If this were the case, we should use an income-compensated demand curve rather than a Marshallian demand curve (Coll and Holohan 1993.] This section describes where the study took place and justifies the development of the WTP questionnaire survey, including the explanatory variables, elicitation mechanism and scenario.

Context of study and study area

This study was carried out in rural villages of Surat district in Gujarat State, India. It was undertaken alongside a cluster randomized controlled trial in three different malarious zones. The three arms covered 126 villages randomized into one of the three following arms: active case detection and treatment (ACDT) as the control; ACDT plus in-house residual spraying by deltamethrin; or ACDT with mosquito nets treated with deltamethrin.

The WTP study was undertaken in 80 villages, 20 from each arm of the trial and, because we believed the trial might influence values, 20 villages were also selected from outside the trial area. Twenty out of 136 villages outside the trial area were first selected on the basis that they had an annual parasitic index of more than 2.5 and were more than 5 km from a trial village and then selected randomly from the remaining list. The 'usual care' of these village covered passive case detection and the usual government-run spraying programme.

Choice of explanatory variables

As the main aim of economic models of demand is to explain the quantity demanded of a good in terms of economic variables, we needed to consider the following: the price of the good as well as the price and use of complements (e.g insecticide) and substitutes (e.g. expenditure on alternative preventive measures) for insecticide-treated nets as well as income (including expenditure as a proxy variable) and assets (e.g. ownership of land). We also outlined a range of variables expected (see Bhatia 2000 for a review of the published literature) to represent and explain 'tastes and preferences' in the following broad categories:

+ personal characteristics of main earner and respondent (e.g. age, gender, schooling, occupation)
+ characteristics of household membership (e.g. size, number of children under six and aged 6–15, caste)
+ preferences for alternative methods of preventing mosquitoes
+ knowledge of the cause(s) of malaria
+ treatment-seeking behaviour for malaria.

Knowing which factors affect the stated WTP for TMNs would also help understand what might increase the likelihood of purchase and at what price. Both have potential policy relevance—it is important to know which variables, for example, would be under the control of policy makers other than just prices, so that the level of demand can be influenced at *all* prices.

The importance of qualitative methods in designing the questionnaire survey

Qualitative research was important in helping develop the survey questionnaire and specifically to make the bridge from theoretical models to relevant research questioning in Surat. Key informant interviews ($n = 117$) and focus group discussions (FGDs) ($n = 25$) were undertaken with community leaders, participant observers (anthropologists who were living full time in the study area), health workers, villagers from specific castes and sellers of health services (e.g. private practitioners, pharmacists, shop keepers, sellers of non-TMNs). Key informants were asked about who should be the respondents for the interview, treatment-seeking behaviour, malaria as a problem for their village, their views of affordability and level of price for TMNs, etc. FGDs were held in different groups representing the study area. The issues taken up for the FGDs to some extent were based on the outcome of the key informant interviews.

Qualitative research was immensely useful in finalizing the WTP household survey. It indicated that from the range of WTP question formats, the bidding format most closely resembled the local bargaining system. However, a suitable range of values for the bid vectors needed to be determined, such that there are minimal 'Yes' responses for the top value. We found that a bid of 100 rupees was likely to be the highest that most would accept and so, a potential highest follow-up value of 200 rupees was expected to elicit very few yes responses. In addition, qualitative research was also designed to help us with a number of practical issues such as who the respondents should be, the time when most respondents would be available and the likely acceptability of the questions (e.g. whether people were likely to be willing to pay, appropriate local language to use for malaria and WTP).

Structure of the questionnaire

The final questionnaire comprised five broad sections as outlined in Table 10.1 (see Bhatia 2000, for full questionnaire).

The sequencing of sections was designed to help respondents consider the impact that malaria had on their lives prior to answering valuation questions. Therefore, they were asked to consider their perception of the magnitude of the problem, their expenditure on prevention and treatment, and other alternatives to preventing malaria besides mosquito nets. Household income and expenditure were enquired about last in case it had an adverse impact on responses (at least all the other information would have been collected by this point of the interview).

WTP questions and the scenario for valuation

At the heart of any WTP study is the scenario for which respondents are asked to give a value. Box 10.1 gives the English translation of the scenario used. The scenario for valuation needed to give all the relevant information without

Table 10.1 Main sections of the survey questionnaire

Section	Types of questions
Household socio-economic and demographic profile	Includes household possessions, demographic and socio-economic variables
Use of preventive measures	Measures used to prevent mosquito bites, including details of mosquito net ownership, and expenditures on prevention
Treatment-seeking behaviour	Includes the history of malaria in the household, source and preferences for treatment, including expenditure on treatment
Willingness to pay	Valuation of one and multiple treated mosquito nets, their re-treatment and in-house residual spraying
Income and expenditure	Sources of household income and patterns of household expenditure

overloading the respondent with information. This is a difficult art. Careful planning and rehearsal of the verbal delivery of information by interviewers eased this. The information concerning TMNs focused on: describing the benefits, side effects, compliance and alternatives, along with a physical description of TMNs. It is important that accurate and unbiased information is given so, for example, that benefits are not overemphasized at the expense of the dis-benefits of an intervention. Each respondent was also shown a TMN and was reminded about income constraints and their expenditure commitments prior to giving values. We attempted to minimize strategic bias in the introduction of the scenario, hence statements about the balance between whether they or the government would have to pay.

A bidding format with three randomly allocated starting bids (Rs 50, Rs 75 and Rs 100) was used to elicit peoples' values. Each person was asked, for example, 'Would you be willing to buy an treated mosquito net for Rs XX?' The respondents were also offered a 'don't know' option in addition to Yes/No. This was done so as to ensure that respondents are not forced into giving a yes or no response as recommended by Harris *et al.* (1989) and National Oceanic Atmospheric Administration (1993). Those who said 'yes' to the starting bid were provided with a higher bid and similarly those who said 'no' or 'don't know' were provided with a lower bid. After a second bid, the respondents were asked for their maximum WTP as an open-ended question. The question asked, 'What is the maximum you would be willing to pay for one treated mosquito net'? Figure 10.2 provides an example of the bidding format used for the three starting bid vectors and shows that a variety of starting bids were chosen. This allowed testing of, and control for, any starting point bias.

Box 10.1 **Introduction to, and description of, the scenario all respondents were asked to give their willingness to pay for**

Introduction to the scenario

The National Malaria Eradication Programme (NMEP) Government of India (GOI) is currently looking to decide how best to control malaria. It is considering a number of options, one of which is dipping mosquito nets in insecticide. Unfortunately, this is quite expensive for the GOI and so they want to know how much people are prepared to pay, in order to judge whether this intervention will work in the future. Your responses to this

Introduction to, and description of, the scenario all respondents were asked to give their willingness to pay for (continued)

section would be used for such a policy decision. You may be required to pay according to your answer, through individual purchases.

Description of the scenario

This net that you see *[Interviewer shows net]* is not an ordinary mosquito net but treated with insecticide. By getting rid of mosquitoes and other insects (bed bugs), it will protect you and your family members from mosquitoes and other insects when inside it, thus allowing you to have a good night's sleep. In addition, it will also reduce the number of episodes of malaria in your household if your household members sleep under these each night. In some villages, use of TMNs would reduce the number of times someone in a household gets malaria from once a year to once every 2 years, thus saving time and money for the household, which would otherwise have been incurred on the treatment of that malarial episode. You know that most people suffering from malaria have severe headache and fever for about a week and are unable to work for about 4 days. In very small percentage of cases, malaria leads to complications or death.

As it has insecticide, you may experience cold-like symptoms, e.g. headache, running nose, in the first week, but thereafter there would be no symptoms. Hardly any complaints have been received from people who have used the mosquito nets. This insecticide is not harmful even to children. As the effect of the insecticide wears out with time, it needs to be treated again every year, for which you would need to bring your house-hold nets to a agreed place, e.g. the village school. Remember washing of the treated net reduces its effect. You are also aware that there are other methods to protect yourself from mosquitoes/malaria.

The mosquito nets are available in different colours and standard size of 6 × 4 ft and should last for about 5 years. Keeping the above description in mind and reminding yourself of your income; your other expenditure commitments; and your household's expenditure on treatment of malarial fever; kindly answer the following questions, which enquire about your willingness to buy treated mosquito nets.

(*Source:* Bhatia and Fox-Rushby 2002).

Reproduced with kind permission, from Bhatia, M., and Fox–Rushby, J. 'Validity of willing-ness to pay: hypothetical versus actual payment, in *Applied Economics Letters* (2003), Vol. 10, pp. 737–740. See also www.tandf.co.uk

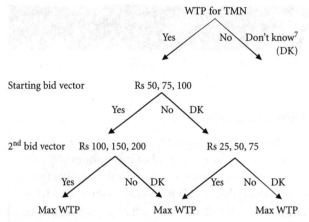

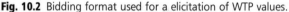

Fig. 10.2 Bidding format used for a elicitation of WTP values.

Source: Bhatia and Fox-Rushby 2002.

Reproduced with kind permission from 'Stated WTP and actual purchase of TMN accross starting bids', in Willingness to pay for treated mosquito nets in Gujarat, India, by Bhatia and Mrigresh. Health and Policy Planning Journal, Vol. 17(4), 2002, Oxford University Press. See also www.tandf.co.uk.

Quantitative data collection

Quantitative data were collected in two stages. The first stage involved a face to face interview with heads of 1200 households from a total of 80 villages using a fully structured interview schedule. The detailed methodology used has been described elsewhere (see Bhatia and Fox-Rushby 2002). The second stage involved a simulated market experiment (SME) in which 300 households from 20 villages were re-visited within 4 weeks in order to sell a TMN(s) at a fixed price of Rs 75. To the extent possible, the respondents for this SME were the same member of the household who provided the hypothetical WTP values in the first survey. This survey was undertaken to understand the impact of starting bids on actual demand for TMNs and to measure any discrepancy between the stated WTP and actual demand. The detailed methods are given elsewhere (see Bhatia and Fox-Rushby 2003).

Results

The response rate for the first survey eliciting hypothetical values was 100%, and it was 99% (with no replacement) for the follow-up survey on actual purchase. This section first describes the characteristics of the respondents and the stated values given by respondents. The second section compares responses to the hypothetical valuation and SME. The third section considers whether there was any evidence for starting point bias from the bid vectors of the hypothetical valuation exercise and whether this affected final purchase of TMNs.

Descriptive results of the first survey

Of the 1200 respondents, 87% were men and were also the main earners of the household. Almost half of the respondents did not have any formal education and only 2% had higher education (i.e. graduation and beyond). The most common occupation was manual labour (45%) followed by agriculture (23%).

The average household size was 5.1 and the mean per capita household income Rs 535. The majority of households were Hindus and fewer than 10% stated they were Christians. The Schedule Tribe was the dominant caste, with Gamits and Halpatis accounting together for more than 70% of this group. Most of the respondent's and household's characteristics varied significantly by caste (Bhatia and Fox-Rushby 2002).

The first WTP question asked respondents whether they would be willing to buy a TMN; 78.6% said they would and 21.4% said they would not. Those who said they were not willing to buy a TMN were asked if they would be willing to buy a TMN if they had the option of an instalment plan. If they said 'No', then all questions on WTP were stopped. If they said 'Yes' to the option of an instalment plan, then they were be asked the same WTP questions as all the other people who replied positively to the first question. Seventy per cent of those willing to buy TMNs ($n = 658$) said they would prefer to make a one-off payment for their TMNs, with 30% preferring to pay in instalments.

Figure 10.3 shows the histogram of all the final maximum values given. It can be seen that the distribution is not normal and that around 20% of responses were zero. There is also a clustering of values around Rs 50, Rs 75 and Rs 100. The maximum WTP for one TMN was Rs 57.4. Among those who were willing to buy a mosquito net at some price, the mean WTP was Rs 73.1 (Bhatia and Fox-Rushby 2002).

To check on the likely market demand, respondents were also asked how many nets they would be willing to buy at their stated maximum per net. On average, respondents said they would be willing to buy 1.9 nets at their maximum price. All respondents were also asked for their maximum WTP for all nets for the household. The mean total WTP was Rs 135.7. The difference reflected some inconsistencies by respondents as well as a diminishing marginal value for successive insecticide-treated nets.

There was a significant variation in responses to WTP questions between trial arms (Bhatia and Fox-Rushby 2002); 3–4 times as many people in the treated mosquito net arm stated they would not be willing to buy a mosquito net and, when they did, the mean WTP per net was around 30% lower. Much of this difference could be attributed to this trial group being given TMNs free within the trial. However, other possible explanators are differences in socio-economic and demographic characteristics. For example, respondents in the TMN group were more likely to be labourers, from the Schedule Tribe and

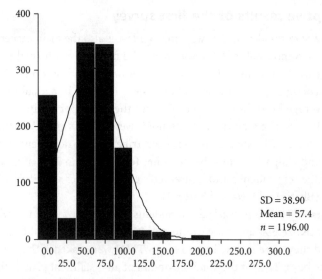

Fig. 10.3 Histogram of household's maximum WTP for one treated mosquito net[8]. Anyone stating that they were not willing to pay for a net was accorded a zero value.

Source: Bhatia and Fox-Rushby 2002.

Printed with kind permission from Bhatia, M., and Fox–Rushby, J., 'Willingness to pay for treated mosquito nets in India: The design and descriptive analysis of a household survey'. In *Health, Policy and Planning, Vol. 17(4)*, 2002, Oxford University Press.

have a house made of mud and hay, and much less likely to own any irrigated land than any other group.

Simulated market experiment to assess post-test validity

Of the 298 respondents, 48% stated they would be willing to pay at least Rs 75 for one TMN. In practice, 51% of the 298 respondents actually bought at least one TMN at this price. At the aggregate level, the null hypothesis of no difference between stated and actual WTP could not be rejected at the 95% level for one net at the price of Rs 75, suggesting that there is no discrepancy between hypothetical and observed WTP for TMNs (Bhatia and Fox-Rushby 2003).

Table 10.2 explores the behaviour below the aggregate level. It shows that, of the 142 respondents who were willing to pay Rs 75 or more for one net, only 66% actually bought a net. In addition to this, 37% of the respondents who had judged their WTP to be less than Rs 75 per net did actually buy a net. Hence a discrepancy is observed on both sides of expected behaviour. From the data in Table 10.2, various indicators to assess the performance of the WTP instrument can be computed. The sensitivity of the WTP instrument (i.e. the ability to detect households which would actually buy TMNs) is 62%

and the specificity (i.e. the ability to detect households that would not buy TMNs—the true negative values) is 67% (Bhatia and Fox-Rushby 2003).

Evidence and impact of starting point bias

Figure 10.4 compares the relationship of stated WTP and actual purchase of TMNs with starting bids. With respect to the stated WTP, Fig. 10.4 shows that the maximum WTP for one TMN varied significantly among the three starting bids. The maximum WTP was Rs 75 or more per TMN in 75% of households who were offered Rs 100 as a starting bid compared with 67 and 29% among those who were offered Rs 75 and Rs 50, respectively, as starting bids. These differences were statistically significant at the 99% level, suggesting the presence of starting point bias in this study.

Table 10.2 Comparison of hypotheticial WTP and observed demand for TMNs

	Actually bought TMN		
	Yes (%)	**No (%)**	**Total (%)**
WTP >Rs 75	94 (66.2)	48 (33.8)	142 (47.6)
WTP <Rs 75	58 (37.2)	98 (62.8)	156 (52.4)
Total	152 (51.0)	146 (49.0)	298 (100.0)
χ^2	25*		

*$P < 0.0001$.

Source: Bhatia and Fox-Rushby (2003).

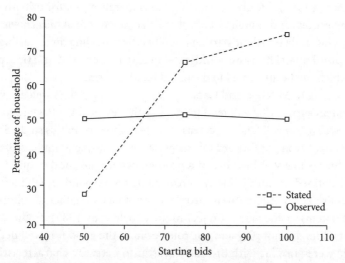

Fig. 10.4 Stated WTP and actual purchase of TMN across starting bids.

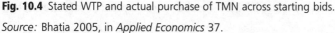

Source: Bhatia 2005, in *Applied Economics* 37.

Figure 10.4 also compares the relationship between the starting bids and the percentage of households who actually bought/did not buy nets ($n = 300$). It can be observed that irrespective of the starting bid, about 50% of the households bought TMNs. Therefore, there is no significant effect of starting bids on the actual demand for TMNs when challenged with the opportunity to buy these.

Discussion

This study had an excellent response rate. This survey showed that it was possible to undertake a WTP study with a public health good in a rural area of a developing country, in which health care has traditionally been government funded. The bidding format, which is considered to be a more complex elicitation method requiring skilled interviewers, was well received by the respondents as bargaining was commonly observed in the market place. The qualitative phase prior to the household survey proved particularly useful in setting realistic bid prices.

Descriptive analysis of the results shows that the majority of respondents were willing to buy at least one TMN. The mean stated WTP for one TMN was Rs 57 for the study population as a whole and Rs 73 for those willing to buy TMNs. The average number of TMN households willing to buy at the mean WTP was 1.92. Descriptive results indicated that perceived need for insecticide-treated nets would be important in explaining the variation in WTP values.

Starting point bias occurs when the respondent's WTP amount is influenced by a value introduced by the scenario and therefore this is a particular threat for the 'bidding game' and 'take it or leave it' elicitation techniques (Mitchell and Carson 1997). Ideally the starting bid is merely a tool for initiating the bidding process and should not affect the respondent's final bids (Boyle et al. 1985). This study tested for starting point bias by providing three starting bids to respondents. The results indicate a clear presence of starting point bias, which can be attributed to the use of bidding format.

According to Mitchell and Carson (1997), starting points well above the respondent's true WTP will tend to increase the revealed WTP while starting points well below will tend to decrease it, as was observed in this study. Several reasons have been put forward for the presence of starting point bias. Starting point bias is likely to be more of a problem where the good in question is poorly defined or not distinctly perceived by the respondent (Randall and Brookshire 1978). Alternatively, people may not be used either to valuing the specific items or the valuation technique (Boyle et al. 1985). In this study, these factors did not play a major role because: the good was well defined; people were familiar with ordinary mosquito nets; the characteristics of TMNs were explained; and a TMN was shown to respondents. However, two possible explanations raised by Stalhammar (1996) may be relevant. First, the respondents may have interpreted the initial bid as the market price and, secondly, the respondent preferences may be so unstable that they can be affected simply by being asked a direct question about them (Bhatia 2005).

One of the major limitations of contingent valuation studies is that respondents are asked hypothetical WTP questions contingent upon the existence of a market, leading to hypothetical bias. Tests of construct validity are commonly observed in the literature, which provides some confidence in WTP estimates, but there is very limited testing of criterion (post-test) validity, partly because of the lack of a criterion close to the theoretical construct (i.e. market prices). However, several researchers have stressed the need for validation of data from contingent valuation studies in health care through comparison with actual consumer choice (Diener *et al.* 1998; Johannesson, 1993). A major issue is how large the deviations from the stated WTP are from their true values.

Due to the nature of the health care good in question, it was possible to conduct an SME to assess the criterion validity. Assessment of post-test validity showed variation at the individual level, where about 35% of the sample did not act in accordance with their hypothetical preferences. However, at the aggregate level, almost the same percentage of households bought TMNs as expected. The reason for this contradictory result is that as the discrepancies occurred both ways and cancelled each other out, so the percentage willing to buy remains almost identical. Given these results, it appears that, at a population level, the results from stated WTP studies could potentially be relied upon. However, this is potentially shaky evidence for all decision makers for all aspects of health care as the results are only from one study and one country. It also raises two further issues: (i) that, like construct validity, criterion validity may only be established through a range of studies; and (ii) whether it matters that WTP results could potentially have a 100% reversal around a median value but no impact at the population level.

Researchers have argued that respondents are likely to act in an irresponsible fashion (Bohm 1972) and strategically misrepresent preferences especially if they perceive that they will not actually have to pay but want the good to be supplied (Bishop and Heberlien 1979). Alternatively, Neill *et al.* (1994) wrote that 'intentions are typically costless to express, or nearly so, which means that they may not be considered as carefully as are real consumption choices'. However, the reasons for discrepancies observed between the stated and actual WTP are not yet well documented.

A number of policy implications emerge from this study. First, it confirms that the majority of the households in rural Surat are willing to buy TMNs at a mean WTP of Rs 57 per TMN. This information, coupled with the cost of providing and distributing TMNs, could assist policy makers in taking pricing decisions and gain an idea of any subsidy required to implement this programme at different levels of coverage. Given that there are significant numbers of respondents not willing to buy TMNs, policy makers need to consider the potential role of exemption mechanisms and inducements for consumers to enter the market in the event charges are introduced for a TMN programme. Further analysis may help determine which characteristics of households could lead to the most appropriate methods of targeting exemptions and inducements.

Finally, there are number of implications for researchers from this study in terms of assessment of validity of WTP studies. First, there needs to be some debate about what the acceptable levels of sensitivity and specificity should be in WTP studies. Secondly, we doubt that criterion validity can be established by assessing discrepancies occurring at a single cut-off point. Instead we recommend that criterion validity be established over an acceptable range around the offer price over which the majority of changes are observed. However, more research needs to be undertaken to establish such an acceptable range. Finally, we will be conducting a further analysis to explain variation in values of stated and actual preferences as well as the differences between them.

Conclusion

There are number of important empirical conclusions from this study. With respect to assessing criterion validity, this study has shown that although at an individual level there are discrepancies in the stated WTP and actual purchase decision, this is nullified at the aggregate level when almost the same percentage of households bought TMNs as expected. Similarly, there is clear evidence of starting point bias in this study. By using an SME, this study has shown the absence of starting point bias in the SME, suggesting that although it is possible to influence the respondents' valuation by starting bids in hypothetical markets, this is not the case in market scenarios.

The results of this study will appeal to those both for and against taking WTP as a valid methodology. By providing evidence of the presence of starting point bias, even in a carefully designed study, and a discrepancy between hypothetical and actual behaviour, this study would satisfy those who would conclude that WTP has its limitations. On the other hand, those in favour of this methodology may draw on the knowledge that, in spite the presence of starting point bias, the mean WTP per net varied only by about Rs 1 between hypothetical and actual behaviour at a population level.

The results of this study should be considered as preliminary only and there is a need to undertake more research in this area. To increase the reliability and validity of WTP estimates, it is recommended that future studies include qualitative research methods as a part of developing an appropriate scenario as well as the overall methods. Future research on WTP studies for the same good (i.e. TMN) using different elicitation questions and in different countries, as well as WTP for different health care goods is recommended to establish the reliability and validity of WTP methodology.

Acknowledgements

This work was part of the Malaria Control and Research Project, a bilateral project between the government of the UK and the government of India funded by the Department for International Development (DfID) of the UK. However, DfID accepts no responsibility for any information provided or views expressed. We acknowledge the efforts put in by the research staff during data collection, and by data entry operators, and are extremely grateful to the people of the study villages for sharing their information with us. This chapter is based on our work published in various journals and we thank the publishers of *Health Policy and Planning*, *Applied Economics Letters* and *Applied Economics* for the copyright consent.

References

Bala, M., Wood, L., Zarkin, G., Norton, E., Gafni, A. and O'Brien, B. (1998) Valuing outcomes in health care: a comparison of willingness to pay and quality adjusted life years. *Clinical Epidemiology* **51**, 667–676.

Bateman, I.J. *et al.* (2002) *Economic Valuation with Stated Preferences Techniques: A Manual.* Edward Elgar Publishing, Cheltenham.

Bhatia, M. (2000) Economic Evaluation of Malaria Control Interventions in Surat, India. PhD Thesis, University of London.

Bhatia, M. (2005) From evidence to calibration for starting point bias: willingness to pay for treated mosquito nets in Gujarat, India. *Applied Economics* **37**, 1–7.

Bhatia, M. and Fox-Rushby, J. (2002) Willingness to pay for treated mosquito nets in Surat, India: the design and descriptive analysis of a household survey. *Health Policy and Planning* **17**, 402–411.

Bhatia, M. and Fox-Rushby, J. (2003) Validity of willingness to pay: hypothetical versus actual payment. *Applied Economics Letters* **10**, 737–740.

Bishop, R.C. and Heberlein, T.A. (1979) Measuring value of extra market goods: are indirect measures biased? *American Journal of Agricultural Economics* **61**, 926–930.

Bohm, P. (1972). Estimating demand for public goods: an experiment. *European Economic Review*, **3**, 111–130.

Boyle, K.J., Bishop, R.C. and Welsh, M.P. (1985) Starting point bias in contingent valuation bidding games. *Land Economics* **61**, 188–194.

Brown, T., Barro, S., Manfredo, M. and Paterson, G. (1995) Does better information about the good avoid the embedding effect? *Journal of Environment Management* **44**, 1–10.

Coll and Hollahan (1993) *Microeconomics Text Book*. 2nd edn, Chapter 4.

De Ridder, A. and De Graeve, D. (2005) Order bias in estimates of willingness to pay for drugs to treat attention-deficit/hyperactivity disorder. *European Journal of Health Economics* article published online 10 February 2005.

Diener, A., O'Brien, B. and Gafni, A. (1998) Contingent valuation studies in the health care literature: a review and classification. *Health Economics* 7, 313–326.

Donaldson, C. (1993) *Theory and Practice of Willingness to Pay for Health Care*. HERU Discussion Paper, University of Aberdeen.

Eckerlund, I., Johannesson, M., Johansson, Tambour, M. and Zethraeus, N. (1995) A contingent valuation study of the optimal size of the Swedish health care budget. *Health Policy* 34, 135–143.

Fox-Rushby, J.A. and Cairns, J.A. (2005) Monetary valuation of health and non-health consequences. In: Fox-Rushby, J.A. and Cairns, J.A. (eds), *Economic Evaluation: An Introductory Guide to Practice*. McGraw Hill, New York.

Gabber, A.M., Weinstein, M.C., Torrance, G.W. and Kamlet, M.S. (1996) Theoretical foundations of cost-effectiveness analysis. In: Gold, M.R., Siegel, J.E., Russel, L.B. and Weinstein, M.C. (eds), *Cost-effectiveness in Health and Medicine*. Oxford University Press, New York.

Gafni, A. (1998) Willingness to pay: what's in a name? *Pharmacoeconomics* 14, 465–470.

Hanemann, W.M. (1994) Valuing the environment through contingent valuation *Journal of Economic Perspectives* 8, 19–43.

Hanemann, M., Loomis, J. and Kanninen, B. (1991) Statistical efficiency of double-bounded dichotomous choice through contingent valuation. *American Agricultural Economic Association* 73, 1225–1263.

Harris, C., Driver, B.L. and McLaughlin, W.J. (1989) Improving the contingent valuation method: a psychological perspective. *Journal of Environmental Economics and Management* 17, 213–229.

Johannesson, M. (1993) The contingent valuation method—appraising the appraisers. *Health Economics* 2, 357–359.

Miller, L.E. and Smith, K.L. (1983) Handling non-response issues. *Journal of Extension* [on-line], 21(5), 45–50. Available at: http://www.joe.org/joe/1983september/83-5-a7.pdf (PDF)

Mitchell, R. and Carson. R. (1993) *Using Surveys to Value Public Goods: The Contingent Valuation Method*. Resources for the Future, Washington, DC.

Mitchell, R. and Carson, R. (1997) *Using Surveys to Value Public Goods: The Contingent Valuation Method*. Resources for the Future, Washington, DC.

National Oceanic Atmospheric Administration (1993) Report of the NOAA Panel on Contingent Valuation. *Federal Register* 58, 4601–4614.

Neill, H.R., Cummings, R.G., Ganderton, P.T., Harrison, G.W. and McGuckin, T. (1994) Hypothetical surveys and real economic commitments. *Land Economics* 70, 145–154.

Olsen, J.A. (1997) Aiding priority setting in health care: is there a role for the contingent valuation method? *Health Economics* 6, 603–612.

Pauly, M.V. (1998) Valuing health care benefits in money terms. In: Sloan, F.A. (ed.), *Valuing Health Care: Costs, Benefits and Effectiveness of Pharmaceuticals and Other Medical Technologies*. Cambridge University Press, Cambridge.

Randall, A. and Brookshire, D.S. (1978) *Public policy, public goods and contingent valuation mechanisms*. Paper presented at the Western Economic Association Meeting, Honolulu, HI.

Russell, S., Fox-Rushby, J. and Arhin, D. (1995) Willingness and ability to pay for health care: a selection of methods and issues. *Health Policy and Planning* **10**, 94–101.

Stalhammer, N.O. (1996) An empirical note on willingness to pay and starting-point bias. *Medical Decision Making* **16**, 242–247.

Whynes, D., Wolstenholme, J. and Frew, E. (2004) Evidence of range bias in contingent valuation payment scales. *Health Economics* **13**, 183–190.

Chapter 11

Disentangling value: assessing the benefits of containing antimicrobial resistance

Joanna Coast, Richard Smith and
Michael Millar

Introduction

Resistance to antimicrobials is increasing rapidly, undermining the ability to
treat many infectious diseases successfully (Cox *et al.* 1995; Davey *et al.* 1996).
Concern about resistance has led to the evaluation of interventions designed
to tackle the problem, but conceptual difficulties associated with valuing
benefits have received little attention. A 'standard evaluation', in which an
epidemiological assessment of the likely impact on health of avoiding the
development or transmission of resistance is followed by asking individuals to
value these different health impacts, may considerably undervalue the full
benefits associated with its control as it concentrates only upon use value. For
most commodities, use value predominates given that value in consumption is
the main benefit. For preventing the emergence or transmission of antimicrobial resistance, use value and externality value (health benefits conferred on
others) cannot be disentangled and, together, will be equivalent to the value of
the health gained as a result of the policy. In practice, this is difficult to assess
because of the problem of measuring the differential impact on health of
resistant organisms compared with susceptible organisms. Option value is
a potentially important source of benefit as individuals may attach value to
the existence of antimicrobial treatments in addition to the expected value in
consumption, because it provides the option to consume the commodity in
the future. Estimating option value may be difficult because of the potential
interaction between time preference and option value. The importance of
these different sources of value is largely unknown, and this chapter discusses
the conceptual problems in identifying and measuring these aspects of value,
considering the use of both quantitative and qualitative methods.

Background

Antimicrobial resistance is a global problem, although it arguably has greater potential for harm in the developing world, where many of the second- and third-line therapies for drug-resistant infections are unavailable, and many of the narrow spectrum antimicrobials available in the developed world are not affordable (Fasehun 1999; Smith 1999). The containment of antimicrobial resistance has received increasing attention from governments and international agencies (Standing Medical Advisory Committee Sub-Group on Antimicrobial Resistance, 1998; World Health Organization 2001), health professionals (Amyes 2000) and the media (Hunt 1996), and is undoubtedly one of the major challenges facing public health. Economists too have begun to respond to this challenge, conceptualizing antimicrobial resistance as a negative externality—an impact that occurs unintentionally when a choice is made to consume antimicrobial treatments (Evans 1984; Brown and Layton 1996; Coast et al. 1996, 1998)—and beginning to consider appropriate policy responses, based largely on the applications of economics to the environmental field (Coast et al. 1998; Smith and Coast 2002; Laxminarayan 2003)

There are numerous policies which may have as a primary aim the containment of resistance. These can be broadly divided into those policies which aim to reduce the emergence of resistance and those which aim to reduce its transmission. The former includes policies where the intermediate purpose is to reduce usage of antimicrobials [e.g. education policies such as the recent initiative by the UK Government (Communicable Diseases Branch 2002), the regulation of antimicrobials in countries where their use is currently unregulated, the development of substitutes such as vaccinations and the use of taxation or permit systems (Coast et al. 1998; Smith and Coast 1998)] and those where the intermediate purpose is to ensure that antimicrobial therapy is used optimally (e.g. influencing the choice of agent, its method of administration, the magnitude of the dose, the frequency of administration, the duration of therapy and the use of combinations, and patient adherence (Standing Medical Advisory Committee Sub-Group on Antimicrobial Resistance 1998). Policies where the aim is to reduce transmission include hand washing, patient isolation, patient and environmental decontamination, and surveillance of resistant infection.

Information about the effectiveness and efficiency of different policies is vital for policy makers at all levels in making decisions about the optimal set of policies to pursue. Efforts to evaluate the effectiveness and efficiency of these different policies are hampered, however, by the uncertainty and complexity that surround the phenomenon of antimicrobial resistance. Although the effects of antimicrobial resistance are documented in both developed and developing nations, uncertainties range from the basic scientific and epidemiological information about the development and spread of resistance, through to evidence about the costs and effectiveness of strategies which may prevent the emergence of antimicrobial resistance or limit its transmission.

One important difficulty in evaluating different policies is in the assessment of the value of these interventions, which is the topic of this chapter. We first examine the notion of value and the elements it comprises. Secondly, we consider what evidence there is about the existence and extent of these different elements of value. In the third section, there is a discussion of how, empirically, evidence about these values can be obtained and how the different elements of value can be disentangled. The final section concludes with a discussion of the implications for future research and policy development.

What is value?

'Value' can be defined as the level of utility that a person is prepared to forgo to obtain the utility from the good or service in question. It is essentially the level of worth, benefit or importance placed on a good or service. There are a number of elements of value associated with the containment of antimicrobial resistance, termed here use value, externality value and option value. Interacting with all of these is the value of time. Each aspect of value is discussed in greater detail below, and this classification is used throughout the remainder of the chapter for the examination of existing empirical evidence and of methods for obtaining further empirical evidence. Prior to discussing each element in detail, however, it is helpful to consider the question of 'value to whom?'

Economists do not generally confine their interest in the costs and benefits of an action to particular individuals or sectors of the economy, but rather to society as a whole. In relation to antimicrobial resistance, it is important to question who this 'society as a whole' comprises. This is because interventions to contain resistance confer benefits across geographical and temporal boundaries (Smith and Coast 2001). Standard techniques of economic evaluation (based on the market price method) take into account the costs and benefits to future generations only insofar as they are valued by current generations. Broome considers this to be 'a major weakness in the method' (Broome 1994, p. 137) noting that it '. . . is only the disenfranchisement of future generations that gives us the share of the world's resources that we have' (Broome 1994, p. 152). At a conceptual level, this paper steps outside the usual economic convention and explicitly concerns itself with all value generated by interventions which aim to contain antimicrobial resistance, whether that value accrues to this generation or future generations, and wherever, geographically, that value results.

Use value

For most commodities, the major source of benefit is 'use value'. Use value refers to the change in utility of the person directly consuming the good (which may or may not be the person who purchased the good). Thus, for example, the main source of value from food, shoes and Internet access is that attributable to the person directly consuming these commodities.

In relation to the containment of resistance, however, it is likely that use value does not predominate, at least not in all situations. For example, where the containment strategy being pursued is hand washing, benefits may accrue to those individuals who are treated by health professionals who have just washed their hands, and thus who are not infected by transmitted resistant infections. Where, however, the containment strategy is an educational intervention to doctors, which reduces 'inappropriate' prescribing, the particular patient who does not receive treatment will obtain little use value from that decision—indeed, the use value is likely to be negative in that the patient will forgo that benefit which they would have obtained through consuming an antimicrobial (note here, that value may relate to the patient's 'wants' as well as their 'needs', e.g. a patient may lose benefit if they wanted a prescription for an antibiotic to validate time off work, even if that prescription was not needed in the sense of improving their health status). In this case, it is difficult to imagine how any direct use value could be assigned, causing a problem for standard (economic) evaluation techniques.

Externality value

In both the examples described above, there is value which occurs to those other than the individual directly consuming the good. This is termed 'externality value', and can be defined as the value which accrues to those other than the person directly consuming the commodity. It is likely that, in relation to antimicrobial resistance containment strategies, a very large proportion of the value obtained accrues to those in society other than the person directly consuming these 'commodities'. In the second example quoted above, of the educational intervention designed to reduce antimicrobial usage, it is likely that almost all the value obtained from improved health care is due to externality, rather than use, value. It is clear that some, possibly large, elements of externality value will also accrue to future generations rather than the current generation.

Use and externality value combined: 'health' value?

In practice, it is likely to be extremely difficult, and perhaps not worthwhile, assessing separately the elements of use and externality value that accrue from interventions where the aim is to contain antimicrobial resistance. Instead, these two elements can be thought of in combination as the value of the 'health' benefits that accrue from a particular action. Almost certainly the total 'health' value arising from any action will be affected by interactions with other, different, containment strategies. The form and importance of such interactions is unknown but may involve some form of threshold (as, for example, with the notion of herd immunity linked to vaccination).

Option value

Option value is the value of maintaining access to a commodity so that it may be consumed in the future. Thus, although in the future individuals may not choose/need to use an antimicrobial, they may '. . . be willing to pay something for the option to consume the commodity in the future' (Weisbrod 1964, p. 472). Option value is, potentially, an important source of benefit relating to anti-microbials, particularly given the way in which antimicrobial resistance develops. This relationship generally follows a sigmoid distribution (Austin and Anderson 1999) with a lag phase before resistance appears, then a relatively rapid increase in the proportion of resistant organisms, followed by a third phase in which this proportion has reached an equilibrium. In the first phase, the option to use antimicrobials remains, but by the third phase this option is (in some cases totally) diminished. People may attach value (i.e. be willing to 'pay' for) to the existence of the option to use antimicrobials in the future, even if they do not in the event use them. In this case, there may be a value attached to maintaining the option to benefit from antimicrobials in the future which would not be captured by valuations of the health impacts of different policies alone.

Value of time

It has already been stated that this chapter is explicitly concerned with value across generations. There are, however, two important and distinct questions in relation to the value of time. The first is the extent to which the current generation values the present more highly than the future in the context of the development and transmission of antimicrobial resistance. The second is whether future generations should have less weight than current generations. The first question is empirically concerned with the preferences of the current generation, whilst the second question may be related to preferences of the current generation but may also be dealt with by ethicists or philosophers.

The importance of the impact of the value of time on the assessment of total value should be noted. Discounting of costs and benefits that occur in the future is standard practice in economic evaluation, with the result that even large absolute costs/effects occurring only a few decades into the future are insignificant in current terms. For example, discounting at 3.5% (the current treasury discount rate used as standard in the UK) would result in costs occurring in 25 years time being valued in the present day at only 42% of their non-discounted value, and costs incurred in 50 years time being valued at only 18% of their non-discounted value.

Option value and the value of time combined?

Unlike the combination of use and externality value discussed above, formally combining option value and the value of time would be inappropriate because a time preference rate which does not include option value needs to be applied to each of the different aspects of value. During the rest of the chapter, they are, however, discussed in combination because, in practice, it may be difficult to separate the interactions between the two.

Evidence about values

'Health' value: use value and externality value

In a previous paper (Coast *et al.* 2002), the authors noted a tendency towards larger numbers of evaluations of strategies to contain transmission [e.g. containment strategies such as hand washing (Larson 1988; Hedin and Hambraeus 1993), decontamination (Quinio *et al.* 1996; Verwaest *et al.* 1997), surveillance (Haley *et al.* 1985) and isolation policies (Rao *et al.* 1988; Chaix *et al.* 1999)] and smaller numbers of evaluations of strategies to contain emergence. This may be explained by the larger and more obvious elements of use value that result from transmission containment strategies than emergence reduction strategies as those affected by the strategy are more likely to be identifiable. Although use value is not always easy to disentangle from other treatment impacts, it is at least easier to identify than externality value where even the person(s) ultimately affected by a containment strategy is unlikely to be obvious. These studies, however, also often ignore any externality value. For example, one study examining hospital control policies for endemic methicillin-resistant *Staphylococcus aureus* (MRSA) concentrated on the direct effects of the control policy, but was unable to value other potential benefits such as avoiding the further development of resistance (Chaix *et al.* 1999).

It is also notable that these studies have all assessed cost-effectiveness, and have not made any attempt to place a value upon the use benefits that have been found. Values associated with death from antimicrobial resistance could be inferred from other areas, such as those used in transport and environmental economics (Jones-Lee 1989; Johansson 1995) (although such values have diverged widely according to context and measurement techniques). Values associated with the non-fatal health consequences of antimicrobial resistant infections are, however, less easy to infer without dedicated empirical studies.

Option value and the value of time

Whether option value exists among members of society for the availability of antimicrobial treatments is currently unknown. In practice, it is likely to be difficult to disentangle any option value from time preference given the temporal nature of both, although there is also no empirical evidence about the current generation's time preference in the context of the containment of antimicrobial resistance.

There is, however, some evidence that may illuminate, to some extent, issues surrounding the value of time. A number of studies have estimated time preference rates in health care. These have used person trade-off methods (Cairns 1994), discrete choice experiments (Van der Pol and Cairns 2001) and the trading of benefit units (Olsen 1993), and have tended to find very high time preference rates suggesting that the future benefits of reduced resistance would have very low present values. Mean rates of between 15 and 25% for short time horizons such as 5 years and lower mean rates of between 7 and 16% for longer time horizons such as 20 years have been found (Olsen 1993; Cairns 1994; Ganiats *et al.* 2000), with even higher rates in developing countries (Poulos and Whittington 2000). Surveys have, however, tended to be postal, thus allowing little opportunity to determine respondents' understanding of the questions or the information upon which they base their answers. This latter point may be particularly important given that it has also been noted that discount rates are specific not only to the length of time involved, but also to the particular context in which the decision is to be made (Olsen 1993). It is also important to note that studies have not tended to use time horizons which can be clearly linked to future generations, e.g. time horizons of 50 or 100 years.

In examining the question of how the benefits to current generations should be weighted vis-à-vis those of future generations, there is some literature related to the discounting of environmental problems. For example, the problem of global warming is not dissimilar to that of antimicrobial resistance, in that its worst effects can be expected to be incurred by future generations. Broome (1992) argues for a zero discount rate in this instance, concluding that current generations are not justified in applying a positive discount rate to major harms imposed on future generations.

Obtaining evidence and disentangling values

It is clear from the above discussion that current evidence about the value obtained from containing antimicrobial resistance is extremely limited. The current evidence specific to antimicrobial resistance concentrates almost exclusively on use value, yet use value may be only a small proportion of the total value available from containing resistance. For the purposes of estimating the costs and benefits of particular interventions, it will be important to have estimates of those aspects of value that have so far been ignored. Of course, obtaining such estimates will be difficult, but this chapter continues by exploring some of the options available. Throughout, this section will concentrate on the estimation of monetary benefits rather than health-related utility values for one main reason: not all the elements of value described above can be converted into health-related utility. In particular, option value is not an element of health-related utility, and to concentrate on the 'QALY (quality-adjusted life years) currency' would imply its disregard.

Use and externality value combined: 'health' value

Although estimates have been made of use benefits during particular studies, the value of these use benefits has not generally been estimated, in terms of either utility or money. Although this is a disappointment generally for the evaluation of such interventions, it is of more concern here because it means that the benefit of the interventions has been externally imposed; changes in some clinical or narrow health-related parameter to those directly receiving the intervention. Thus, the 'externality' value to others who may be affected, and thus avoid catching a resistant bug, is not captured. It is therefore recommended that estimates of 'use value', i.e. the value of improved health for those patients identified as part of evlutions of interventions, should therefore be obtained in monetary terms from future studies.

Uncertainty will inevitably surround estimates of the combined use and externality value associated with any policy. This uncertainty will, in some aspects, be great. There will be uncertainty about the relationships between use of antimicrobials and the development of resistance, about the likely spread of resistance once it has emerged and about the likelihood of new antimicrobials being developed. These uncertainties need to be acknowledged rather than ignored. Modelling is the most obvious way of dealing with these uncertainties, and of estimating not just the use value associated with an intervention but the externality value as well. Further, such modelling could, at least in theory, deal with the potential for interaction between different containment strategies.

This is an easy conclusion to state; the reality is that even modelling the use and externality values associated with particular interventions will be complex. Issues which will need to be dealt with include the following. What is the appropriate form of the model? What parameters (disease-specific, context-specific and external) must be incorporated into the model? Over what time period will the model be constructed? What are the mathematical relationships between these parameters? Once constructed, any model will need to be tested for its applicability and usefulness in a specific situation.

Option value and the value of time

Whereas use and externality value are, ultimately, concerned with the value of their health to individuals, option value and the value of time are societal preferences. The appropriate group from which to obtain evidence about these values is, then, not patients but citizens. The need is to, first, obtain monetary estimates (to enable combination with the use and externality values proposed above) of option value from citizens, and second, obtain information about the extent to which the current generation values the present more highly than the future in the context of the development and transmission of antimicrobial resistance. For the first aim, a willingness to pay method (Johannesson 1996; Diener *et al.* 1998; Olsen and Smith 2001) would be appropriate, whilst the second could be achieved using person trade-off methods (Cairns 1994). Willingness to pay questions would need to ask informants to estimate their willingness to pay to: (i) retain the option of effective antibiotic treatment in the future, with current levels unaffected; (ii) retain effective antibiotic treatment in the future, with current levels reduced; and (iii) retain effective antibiotic treatment now, with future levels reduced. Person trade-off questions would ask informants to trade directly between numbers of lives saved in the current time period compared with numbers of lives saved in the future using both relatively short time periods such as 10 years, and much longer time periods that imply intergenerational issues such as 50 and 100 years.

These are likely to be difficult questions for members of the public to answer unless they are provided with information about resistance and its implications (e.g. covering health care prior to the discovery of antibiotics, the development of antibiotics and their influence on health care, the development of resistance and its current and potential influence on health care; and future scenarios (Standing Medical Advisory Committee Sub-Group on Antimicrobial Resistance 1998; World Health Organization 2000) and given the opportunity to discuss and reflect upon this information (Dolan *et al.* 1999).

Further, whilst quantitative methods will be able to provide some estimate of the current generation's time preference, these methods may be less successful in tapping the second value of time issue (whether future generations should have less weight than current generations) given its essentially philosophical nature. For this reason, a combination of qualitative and quantitative methods is most likely to provide both reasoned numerical estimates of option value and the value of time, and some understanding of the judgements used by citizens which will inform the intergenerational question (Glaser and Strauss 1968; Strauss and Corbin 1990). By obtaining quantitative estimates before and after the provision of information and opportunities for discussion, 'uninformed' and 'informed' estimates would be able to be compared.

An important empirical issue, however, is the potential for interaction between each informant's time preference and option value relating to resistance. The assessment of willingness to pay over different time periods could be used to attempt to isolate a 'pure' time preference effect from option value. The time preference rate estimated in this manner could also be compared with that estimated from the person trade-off analysis to establish systematic relationships between these two rates. Qualitative data, particularly if obtained during interviews, could also assist in the estimation of the relative importance of time preference and option value. From these sources of information, the magnitude, and relative robustness, of the rates of 'pure' time preference and option value could be estimated.

Discussion

This chapter has outlined the main elements of value, indicated the paucity of evidence that exists for each and has suggested methods for obtaining further evidence. It is clear that, both conceptually and empirically, it can be difficult to disentangle these different elements of value. It is our contention that, even if the empirical assessment of value combines these different elements, conceptual clarity is vital in ensuring, first, that there is not double-counting of different elements of value and, second, that no elements of value have been missed.

This chapter has essentially recommended three empirical methods for assessing the value of interventions aimed at combating the emergence and transmission of antimicrobial resistance: (i) to obtain monetary values for health benefits in ongoing assessments of use value; (ii) to model the impacts of resistance to incorporate both use and externality values; and (iii) to obtain, using quantitative (willingness to pay and person trade-off) and qualitative methods, information about option value and the value of time. There are some caveats to these recommendations. The first concerns the use of modelling exercises. One danger in the use of modelling is the tendency to take the 'best estimate' as the basis for policy. Given the apparent irreversibility of resistance, this may not be appropriate. The 'worst case' scenario may be a better basis for policy given that irreversibility suggests the loss of future options (Arrow and Fisher 1974). The second concerns the interaction between externality value and the value of time, which has not so far been dealt with. Essentially, the extent to which a future externality needs to be estimated is dependent upon the value of time both within and across generations, given that high discount rates ensure that values quickly tend towards zero. The third difficulty is that the evidence that can be obtained can only ever be acquired through the current generation. Whatever the efforts to incorporate the values of future genera-tions, it is inevitable that those values will be coloured by the perspective from which they are taken. This problem cannot, of course, be readily solved.

Elements of value which were not discussed were the wider externality values arising from two sources. The first is the wider externality value that arises from poor health and death in terms of the economic and social impact on society. Such impacts include the impact on national incomes and the impact on families, particularly dependent children and older people, that may result from a widespread increase in untreatable infections. They may be quantitatively and qualitatively important—witness the effect of acquired immune deficiency syndrome (AIDS) on some developing nations. The second is the negative value that may accrue to health care providers, including pharmaceutical companies, particularly if efforts to curtail antimicrobial use result in greater unemploy-ment among some groups. Both these elements of value are even more uncer-tain than those that have already been discussed, and they are often ignored in the partial analysis that is economic evaluation. Nevertheless, such factors could be incorporated by extending the scope of modelling exercises.

This chapter concentrates upon the provision of information for use in pol-icy decisions, rather than how those decisions should be implemented. Thus the chapter does not deal with the sorts of problem—noted in an earlier paper (Coast *et al.* 1996)—of how to ensure that the optimal policy or set of policies is pursued. Within particular organizations, e.g. a hospital, there may be the incentive to emphasize short-term gains, such as the control of outbreaks or improvements in patient care associated with introduction of a new and effec-tive antibiotic, leaving medium- and long-term issues overshadowed. Here, there has been a concentration upon the estimation of benefits from a societal and intergenerational viewpoint but, just because the collection of such informa-tion is advocated for policy development, it does not ensure that it will be used (although of course, once quantified, these longer term externality aspects of the problem are more difficult to ignore). The development of incentives in relation to antimicrobial resistance is covered to some extent elsewhere (Coast *et al.* 1998; Smith and Coast 1998), although undoubtedly further work is needed in this area.

The evaluation of policies whose aim is to reduce transmission is likely to be less difficult than the evaluation of policies whose aim is to reduce the emergence of resistant microorganisms, yet in relation to long-term policy development, the latter policies are likely to be of greater benefit. One of the main reasons for this problem relates to the difficulty in assessing the value of these particular policies. An important role for economists is to provide conceptual clarity about these issues and to assist in the acquisition of empirical evidence. We hope that the current chapter moves one step closer to achieving these aims.

References

Arrow, K.J. and Fisher, A.C. (1974) Environmental preservation, uncertainty and irreversibility. *Quarterly Journal of Economics* **88**, 312–319.

Amyes, S.G.B. (2000) The rise in bacterial resistance. *British Medical Journal* **320**, 199–200.

Austin, D.J. and Anderson, R.M. (1999) Studies of antibiotic resistance within the patient, hospitals and the community using simple mathematical models. *Philosophical Transactions of the Royal Society of London* **354**, 721–738.

Broome, J. (1992) *Counting the Cost of Global Warming.* White Horse Press, Cambridge.

Broome, J. (1994) Discounting the future. *Philosophy and Public Affairs* **23**, 128–156.

Brown, G. and Layton, D.F. (1996) Resistance economics: social cost and the evolution of antibiotic resistance. *Environment and Development Economics* **1**, 349–355.

Cairns, J. (1994) Valuing future benefits. *Health Economics* **3**, 221–229.

Chaix, C., Durand-Zaleski, I., Alberti, C. and Brun-Buisson, C. (1999) Control of endemic methicillin-resistant *Staphylococcus aureus*. A cost-benefit analysis in an intensive care unit. *Journal of the American Medical Association* **282**, 1745–1751.

Coast, J., Smith, R.D. and Millar, M.R. (1996) Superbugs: should antimicrobial resistance be included as a cost in economic evaluation? *Health Economics* **5**, 217–226.

Coast, J., Smith, R.D. and Millar, M.R. (1998) An economic perspective on policy to reduce antimicrobial resistance. *Social Science and Medicine* **46**, 29–38.

Coast, J., Smith, R.D., Wilton, P., Karcher, A.M. and Millar, M.R. (2002) Superbugs II: how should economic evaluation be conducted for interventions which aim to reduce antimicrobial resistance? *Health Economics* **11**(7):

Communicable Diseases Branch (2002) *Public Education Campaign on Antimicrobial Resistance* (letter). Department of Health, London.

Cox, R.A., Conquest, C., Mallaghan, C. and Marples, R.R. (1995) A major outbreak of methicillin-resistant *Staphylococcus aureus* caused be a new phage-type (EMRSA-16). *Journal of Hospital Infection* **29**, 87–106.

Davey, P.G., Bax, R.P., Newey, J. *et al.* (1996) Growth in the use of antibiotics in the community in England and Scotland in 1993. *British Medical Journal* **312**, 613.

Diener, A., O'Brien, B. and Gafni, A. (1998) Health care contingent valuation studies: a review and classification of the literature. *Health Economics* **7**, 313–326.

Dolan, P., Cookson, R. and Ferguson, B. (1999) Effect of discussion and deliberation on the public's views of priority setting in health care: focus group study. *British Medical Journal* **318**, 916–919.

Evans, R.G. (1984) *Strained Mercy: The Economics of Canadian Health Care*. Butterworths, Toronto.

Fasehun, F. (1999) The antibacterial paradox: essential drugs, effectiveness and cost. *Bulletin of the World Health Organization* **77**, 211–216.

Ganiats, T.G., Carson, R.T. and Hamm, R.M. (2000) Population-based time preferences for future health outcomes. *Medical Decision Making* **20**, 263–270.

Glaser, B.G. and Strauss, A.L. (1968) *The Discovery of Grounded Theory: Strategies for Qualitative Research*. Weidenfeld and Nicolson, London.

Haley, R.W., Culver, D.H., White, J.W. *et al.* (1985) The efficacy of infection surveillance and control programs in preventing nosocomial infections in US hospitals. *American Journal of Epidemiology* **121**, 182–205.

Hedin, G. and Hambraeus, A. (1993) Daily scrub with chlorhexidine reduces skin colonization by antibiotic-resistant *Staphylococcus*. *Journal of Hospital Infection* **24**, 47–61.

Hunt, L. (1996) Perfect culture for a 'superbug'. *The Independent* 27 February, part 2:7.

Johannesson, M. (1996) *Theory and Methods of Economic Evaluation of Health Care*. Kluwer Academic Publishers, Dordrecht.

Johansson, P.O. (1995) *Evaluating Health Risks: An Economic Approach*. Cambridge University Press, Cambridge.

Jones-Lee, M. (1989) *The Economics of Safety and Physical Risk*. Basil Blackwell, Oxford.

Laxminarayan (2003) *Battling Resistance to Antibiotics and Pesticides. An Economic Approach*. Resources for the Future, Washington, DC.

Larson, E.L. (1988) A causal link between handwashing and risk of infection? Examination of the evidence. *Infection Control* **9**, 28–36.

Olsen, J.A. (1993) Time preferences for health gains: an empirical investigation. *Health Economics* **2**, 257–265.

Olsen, J.A. and Smith, R.D. (2001) Theory versus practice: a review of 'willingness-to-pay' in health and health care. *Health Economics* **10**, 39–52.

Poulos, C. and Whittington, D. (2000) Time preferences for life-saving programs: evidence from six less developed countries. *Environmental Science and Technology* **34**, 1445–1455.

Quinio, B., Albanese, J., Bues-Charbitt, M., Viviand, X. and Martin, C. (1996) Selective decontamination of the digestive tract in multiple trauma patients. A prospective double-blind, randomized, placebo-controlled study. *Chest* **109**, 765–772.

Rao, N., Jacobs, S. and Joyce, L. (1988) Cost-effective eradication of an outbreak of methicillin-resistant *Staphylococcus aureus* in a community teaching hospital. *Infection Control and Hospital Epidemiology* **89**, 255–260.

Smith, R.D. (1999) Antimicrobial resistance: the importance of developing long-term policy. *Bulletin of the World Health Organization* **77**, 862.

Smith, R.D. and Coast, J. (1998) Controlling antimicrobial resistance: a proposed transferable permit market. *Health Policy* **43**, 219–232.

Smith, R.D. and Coast, J. (2001) Antimicrobial resistance and global public goods for health. In: Woodward, D., Smith, R.D., Beaglehole, R. and Drager, N. (eds), *Global Public Goods for Health*. World Health Organisation, Geneva.

Smith, R.D. and Coast, J. (2002) Antimicrobial resistance: a global response. *Bulletin of the World Health Organization* **80**, 126–133.

Standing Medical Advisory Committee Sub-Group on Antimicrobial Resistance (1998) *The Path of Least Resistance.* Department of Health, London.

Strauss, A. and Corbin, J. (1990) *Basics of Qualitative Research. Grounded Theory Procedures and Techniques.* Sage, London.

Van der Pol, M. and Cairns, J. (2001) Estimating time preferences for health using discrete choice experiments. *Social Science and Medicine* **52**, 1459–1470.

Verwaest, C., Verhaegen, J., Ferdinande, P. *et al.* (1997) Randomized, controlled trial of selective digestive decontamination in 600 mechanically ventilated patients in a multidisciplinary intensive care unit. *Critical Care Medicine* **25**, 63–71.

Weisbrod, B.A. (1964) Collective-consumption services of individual-consumption goods. *Quarterly Journal of Economics* **78**, 471–477.

World Health Organization (2000) *Overcoming Antimicrobial Resistance.* WHO/CDS/2000.2. WHO, Geneva.

World Health Organization (2001) *Global Strategy for the Containment of Antimicrobial Resistance.* WHO/CDS/CSR/DRS/2001.2. WHO, Geneva.

Chapter 12

Economics of animal health: implications for public health

Ana Riviere-Cinnamond

Introduction

The past decade has witnessed an increase in emerging and re-emerging disease incidence. Bovine spongiform encephalopathy (BSE), severe acute respiratory syndrome (SARS), avian influenza (AI) and others have made the headlines of many newspapers. The population is therefore increasingly aware of the links and risks existing between animals and humans.

Two main (and highly intertwined) factors are influencing the change in patterns of diseases spread. These are (i) the trends in livestock production and (ii) the pathogens' evolutionary response to changing environment (also referred to as 'ecological factors').

First, the International Food Policy Research Institute (IFPRI) has recently pointed out that 'Since the early 1980s, total meat and milk consumption grew at 5 and 3% per year respectively through the developing world. In East and South-East Asia, where income grew at 4–8% per year, population at 2–3% per year and urbanisation at 4–6% per year, meat consumption increased between 4 and 8% per year. Between 1983 and 1993, the share of the world's meat consumed in developing countries rose from 37% to 47%, and the share of the world's milk rose from 34 to 41%' (Delgado *et al.* 2000). IFPRI's calculations demonstrate that by 2020 developing countries will be producing 38% more meat and 62% more milk per capita than in the early 1990s (Delgado *et al.* 1999). Such production trends are, unlike the 'Green Revolution' in crop production, demand driven. The international scientific arena has labelled these livestock production trends as the 'Livestock Revolution'. The associated implications of the 'Livestock Revolution' have already been debated extensively by Delgado *et al.* (1999) These are namely (i) nutrition, food security and poverty alleviation; (ii) environmental sustainability; (iii) world trade and food prices; and (iv) public health. The latter relates to the expected increase in animal–human contact due to livestock production increase (Delgado *et al.* 1999). As part of this process, it is therefore expected that there will be an increase in human–animal contact.

Secondly, such livestock production increases the effect on the environment where pathogens exist. Changes in agricultural practices and production systems associated with an increase in urbanization have affected the way in which pathogens adapt to new hosts, as well as their development and spread amongst the new host population. For example, recent studies regarding the AI outbreak in Southeast Asia (e.g. Vietnam) show that the risk of disease spread is not amongst highly intensive poultry productions, but amongst small production systems. Public health hazards were therefore concentrating in rural areas.

The combination of these two factors therefore points out the increase in public health risks associated with emerging and zoonotic disease occurrence. It seems logical that an increase in livestock production will lead to an increased demand for animal health care services. These services play a key role in the prevention of animal-related public health risks. At the same time, it needs to be highlighted that for most of the rural population in low- and middle-income countries (as in the case of the aforementioned AI case), live-stock represent the main source of income and act as a safety net. Thus, the compulsory culling of their animals might force them into poverty. Public health and animal health policies aim, therefore, at minimizing the risks arising from animal production, while limiting the loss of livelihood for, in particular, small producers. Leaving animal health policies outside the public health policy and research arena might therefore have important repercussions at economic and public health levels.

Justification

Animal diseases are not only a public health threat, but they might cause important economic losses at a national and regional level (a ban on exports for example) in the event of outbreak occurrence [e.g. foot-and-mouth dis-ease (FMD) in the UK]. Additionally, a country's animal health disease status might affect its accession and competitiveness in international markets (i.e. World Trade Organization and Sanitary and Phyto-sanitary Standards). Despite the consequences that derive from each these three levels, it is interest-ing to see that economic and policy analysis in the animal health care sector has scarcely been given attention.

Furthermore, in the last decade, most developing countries have undergone structural adjustments and have seen their national budgets heavily reduced. This process has also affected animal health services (AHS), which were previ-ously publicly financed and provided (Leonard 2000). Guidelines on how to privatize AHS were therefore launched by the World Bank in 1991–1992 (deHaan and Bekure 1991; Umali-Deininger *et al.* 1992). Such guidelines were based on the classification of goods and services following their 'rivalry' and 'excludability' characteristics. Thus, all goods falling into the *private* category would necessarily be left to the market, whereas those classified as *public* would remain a state duty.

Although the process was aimed at increasing effectiveness and efficiency of AHS, the results were not as expected. The privatization process disrupted the previously frail AHS structure and especially its provision in rural areas. Consequently, a widening gap has been growing between high and low potential areas (in production terms) (Dorward *et al.* 1998). The process has left producers in rural areas that derive their livelihood from livestock more vulnerable to epidemic disease spread among the livestock population. Additionally, such virtual lack of services associated with increased small-holder production leaves rural areas at high risk of potential public health hazards.

Objectives

This chapter therefore aims to:

1. Identify components and actors involved in the animal health sector.
2. Investigate the usefulness of different economic perspectives in the analysis of animal health care systems.
3. Point out the possible factors that influenced the outcomes of the privatization of AHS.
4. Highlight the public health implications of the lack of economic analysis in the animal health field.

Methodology and materials

In order to explore the aforementioned objectives, the subject was analysed following (i) a comparison with human health care systems; (ii) a review of key authors in economic theory; (iii) a review of the health economics literature; and finally (iv) using the scarce examples existing in animal health economics.

Although innovative, the idea of analysing AHS structures following the comparison with the human health counterpart has already been applied by Leonard (2000). He stated that 'the two professions [human and animal medicine] are close enough that [their] differences help each to look at its own structures and operations in new and illuminating ways'. He based his approach on the similarities existing between the two sectors. Hence, similarities at the scientific level were put forward when mentioning that 'the biological science that undergirds human and veterinary medicine is the same; in fact a great deal of medical research on which the treatment of humans depends is actually veterinary research, for it is conducted on an array of animals. Although the various species of mammals do have important differences in their responses to disease and treatment, there are significant physiological parallels and many diseases—and cures—pass back and forth across the human/animal divide' (Leonard 2000). Additionally, further similarities may be highlighted in terms of training and hierarchical organization given that 'physicians and veterinarians receive similar training, work in professions that are structured much like one another, and oversee analogous hierarchies of paraprofessionals and auxiliaries', and therefore enjoy an information advantage over their clients (Leonard 2000). The theoretical frameworks used for analysing human health care markets can be then used to illustrate the mechanisms underlying the animal health care market.

Structure of the chapter

The chapter is divided into six sections. In the introduction, the background and justification of the chapter are mentioned. The next section aims at putting into context the existing linkages between public health risks and categories of producers. This is followed by an extensive analysis of AHS, including its components and key players. The following section introduces the rationale for the economic perspective taken in the analysis of AHS, which is extensively debated in the penultimate section. Finally, the main conclusions are exposed.

Public health relevance

A recent study done by the IFPRI under the umbrella of agricultural economics attempts to analyse the linkages between agricultural markets and the rural poor (Orden *et al.* 2004). Its usefulness in the context of this study lies in the typology of farmers. Three groups are therefore identified. The first relates to those smallholders generally in peri-urban areas which have good linkages with markets and are globally competitive (denoted as rural world 1). The second group refers to smallholders engaged in domestic production and eventually accessing international markets (rural world 2). Finally, the third category focuses on the marginalized smallholders whose primary production is for self-subsistence (rural world 3).

When overlapping this categorization of smallholder with emerging disease spread patterns such as AI, strikingly it is the smallholders categorized as rural world 2 that are most at risk. There may be several reasons to explain this phenomenon, but the rapid trends in production intensification have been widening the gap between those small producers which reach competitiveness and those who do not and therefore are pushed to marginalization (to rural world 3 where, due to the remoteness and low animal density, risks of rapid spread of disease outbreak are improbable) (J Slindenberg, personal communication). These trends are highly related to the above-mentioned 'Livestock Revolution'. Additionally, over the same period, AHS have seen their efficiency and effectiveness decrease, partly due to existing budgetary constraints in most developing countries and partly to the aforesaid privatization guidelines.

Small producers in rural world 2 are those most at risk of emerging or zoonotic disease outbreaks. Given the public health and economic risks associated with such disease spread, this category needs to be a target group for increased provision of effective and efficient AHS. However, as resources are scarce, a rationale needs to be found in order to elucidate the methods of funding and provision of these services.

Before entering into applied economic theory, the next section will introduce the concept of AHS, stating the boundaries, components and actors.

Structure and boundaries of animal health services

In the animal health literature, several authors have attempted to draw up the boundaries of AHS (deHaan and Bekure 1991; Umali-Deininger *et al*. 1992; Holden 1999; Ahuja *et al*. 2000). Some components are systematically taken into account (such as clinical services). However, there is less concordance when referring to other sections, such as, for example, public health and extension.

Previous sections highlight dichotomous, and sometimes contradictory, purposes of AHS. On one hand, it seeks to improve animal production and productivity (hence improving human nutrition and welfare), while on the other hand it aims at protecting human health. This links with Murray and Frenk's definition of human health care systems which follows the concept of 'health action' (Murray and Frenck 2000). The latter is defined by any activity 'whose primary intent is to *improve* or *maintain* [human] health' (Murray and Frenck 2000) (emphasis added by author). Thus, AHS would deal with: (i) preventing disease occurrence (from food or animal origin) in humans, thus helping to 'maintain [human] health'; and (ii) increasing animal production, therefore improving human nutrition and welfare, which links with the health action concept in that it helps in 'improving [human] health'.

These activities put forward the logic for eligibility of AHS as a crucial player in the broader definition of human health systems stemming from the 'health action' concept. The dual nature of AHS (increasing production, i.e. economic, and human health protection, i.e. public health) poses difficulties in analysing the subsector in a systematic and methodological way, especially in relation to economics and financial resource generation mechanisms.

Components

AHS have generally been divided into three main categories, namely curative services; preventive services and regulatory bans; and pharmaceutical supply (Umali-Deininger *et al.* 1992; Ahuja *et al.* 2000). However, as mentioned in the previous section, this study will include other aspects such as public health, education/extension and research and development, all of which are closely entangled (see Fig. 12.1).

First, curative services refer mainly to animal disease diagnosis and treatment. Secondly, preventive services aim at limiting the occurrence of new animal diseases. The activities included under this heading will encompass vaccination campaigns, vector and/or carrier control or eradication, and measures such as segregation. Practically, these activities include dipping, quarantine, slaughter of at-risk animals, movement restrictions, import and export control of livestock and livestock products, inspection and control of animal products, etc. The third component refers to pharmaceutical supply for both preventive and curative activities. This component therefore covers the production of veterinary pharmaceuticals, and their quality control, marketing and distribution. Fourth is the public health component. This includes the control of food-borne and zoonotic diseases, food hygiene and feed safety, as well as environmental health aspects related to animal production. Part of vector control strategies might also fall into this category, such as the water-borne

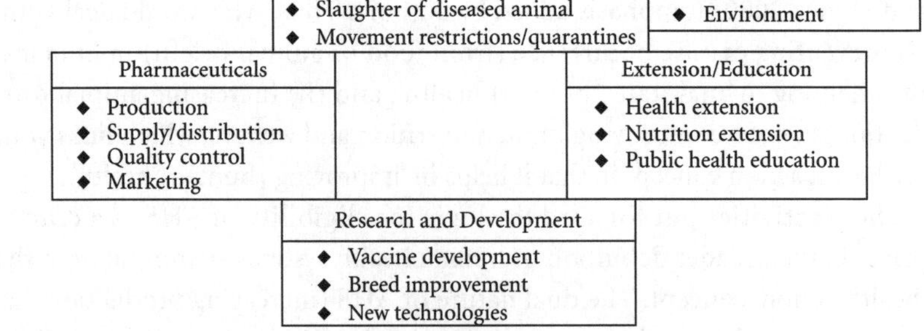

Fig. 12.1 Components of animal health services.

vector control strategies which might help in controlling vector-borne human diseases as well as animal diseases (e.g. malaria). Other examples will include water contamination due to mismanagement of animal waste in different types of production systems. Fifth comes extension in animal health and nutrition and public health education. Finally, the last component includes research and development and encompasses several strata varying from laboratory-based research to policy and economics.

A common point between the above components are the actors involved in the animal health system. Their characteristics will help in defining their roles and interactions.

Actors involved

Following the comparison with the human health sector, the actors in AHS will be analysed using the 'health care triangle' framework (Reinhardt 1990; Mossialos *et al.* 2002).

The actors may therefore be grouped into three categories (see Fig. 12.2), namely: (i) consumers of the service (or first party) which will include stock owners and the society (considered here due to externalities arising from certain goods and services in the animal health field); (ii) providers of the service (or second party) encompassing veterinarians and related paraprofessionals (such as animal health assistants, community-based animal health workers, etc.); and (iii) a third party insurer or purchaser which might be of public or private nature [e.g. national governments, donors, non-governmental organizations (NGOs), private entrepreneurs, etc.].

Thus, livestock owners, whether small or large scale, sedentary (mixed farming) or nomad (i.e. pastoralists), are considered the direct consumers of the services (Leonard 1990). They might produce individually or be organized

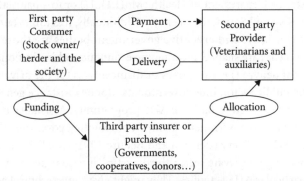

Fig. 12.2 The triangle (adapted from Mossialos *et al.* 2002)

Reproduced with kind permission, from Mossialos, E.A. Dixon, *et al.*, Funding Health Care: Options for Europe. Open University Press, 2002.

into cooperatives or producers' associations (which would therefore play the role of third party). Following Umali *et al.*(1992), society is also considered a direct consumer of AHS due to several externalities arising from livestock, livestock-derived products and livestock production methods or systems. Hazards stemming from these externalities are a threat to human health, and thus are of public health concern.

Key players in AHS delivery are therefore veterinarians and paraprofessionals, which might deliver through public and/or private channels. For example, in India, where privatization has recently started, government veterinarians are allowed to practise privatively. As a consequence, clients are generally referred to private practice hours in order to receive a timely and higher quality service. This is perceived by those working exclusively in the private sector as 'unfair competition'. The latter are of special importance in rural and remote areas as in some countries there is a lack of veterinarians and/or they are not willing to work in rural (and especially remote) areas. Paraprofessionals supplement and expand the areas that might be covered by veterinarians (Sidibe 2003), increasing the number of stock owners reached (Umali-Deininger. 1992).

The third actor in the animal health care triangle refers to insurers or purchasers. As previously mentioned, they might be public or private. When dealing with the public sector, it is generally the role of the Ministry of Finance (MoF) to allocate some budget to the Ministry of Agriculture (MoA). The latter determines the internal budget allocation to the Department of Veterinary Services (DVS). Thus, competition arises not only at a ministerial level (i.e. between the MoA and other ministries), but also within the MoA (i.e. allocation to other departments). However, and especially in developed countries, some competences and activities of AHS have been transferred to the Ministry or Department of Health (MoH/DoH) or to a parastatal agency (e.g. the UK's Food Standards Agency). Additionally, it is important to highlight that legislative and executive government bodies are those in which domestic policies are shaped, creating the economic and institutional context for AHS manoeuvre (i.e. incentives or disincentives for the private sector). Within the public sector, intergovernmental donor assistance generally provides funding targeted to national AHS programmes. Assistance is generally channelled through government channels, pinpointing government's influential role in AHS delivery (deHaan and Bekure 1991; Umali-Deininger *et al.* 1992). Focusing on private sector third parties, it is common to find NGOs funding particular AHS activities. They might give some technical advice, but they generally focus on livestock development programmes. However, as previously mentioned, private entrepreneurs are increasing in the animal health sector although, as expected due to market forces, not in an equal manner within a country (i.e. they concentrate in high production potential areas and specific commodities such as dairy or poultry). Such private initiatives (cooperatives, etc.) may offer a wide variety of services ranging from curative to preventive services, and in some cases production and distribution of veterinary supplies (Umali-Deininger *et al.* 1992).

The characteristics of these actors have been pointed out. It is, however, important to analyse their behaviour in the context of the animal health market.

Economics of agency in the animal health sector

The human health economics literature has extensively debated the principal/agent theory (Arrow 1985; Pratt and Zeckhauser 1985; Evans 1998). In the animal health field, some authors have attempted to apply such theory, notably Leonard (2000). Following his perspective, the study attempts to adapt the transaction model of Mossialos *et al.* (2002) to the animal health care sector.

Thus, as exemplified in Fig. 12.2, the simplest form of transaction between actors would be direct payment from consumer to provider, i.e. from farmer to veterinarian (and/or auxiliary), in exchange for animal health care resources. However, given the relatively unpredictable nature of illness (whether in humans or animals), it is difficult to forecast the future consumption of AHS. It might be argued that some prognoses might be feasible in relation to certain chronic conditions. Thus, in that case, losses might be, to some extent, calculated in economic terms. However, in most cases, future animal health status remains uncertain and thus consumption of AHS unplanned. As a consequence of this situation, an unregulated market would react, developing some insurance mechanism whereby one or more of the stock owners would make a payment to a risk-pooling agency (which might differ in the degree of risk sharing) to ascertain some financial economic compensation in case of animal ill health [or death or slaughter in some instances, as for example in some EU countries; see van Asseldonk *et al.* (2003) for further details of private livestock insurance]. However, in some developing countries, the third party or insurer falls in the public sector domain [examples of compulsory national livestock insurance may be found in some Asian countries such as India, Nepal and Thailand; for further details, see Mathema and Joshi (2000)]. Thus farmers insure themselves against the financial burden of their animals falling ill (and arguably against the event of zoonotic disease occurrence). The concept of 'livestock insurance', whether private (PLI) or public (NLI), therefore encompasses the wider notion of income maintenance through interpersonal redistribution (between stock owners and to some extent between farmers and the society).

Having examined the components, actors and, to some extent, their agency relationship in the animal health care market, the next section provides an innovative perspective to the economic analysis of the AH sector.

Taking a public choice approach

It has been highlighted by authors such as Buchanan (1975) that the methodologies used in the analysis of public expenditure, and the nature and structure of collective decisions, have important implications in the approach traditional public finance has taken. Government behaviour theory therefore points out two ways in which government's role may be analysed (Cullis and Jones 1998). These are the public interest approach and the public choice school.

It has been argued that the first approach looks at markets in an idealized way. Through this viewpoint, it is assumed that public interventions are shaped to *eliminate* inefficiencies arising from market failure [for further discussion about market failures in the animal health care market see Riviere-Cinnamond (2004)]. This is the approach that has mainly been taken in the analysis of AHS. Such an approach focuses primarily on outcome efficiency which refers to the Pareto optimality principle (also known as top-level economic efficiency). This traditional outcome approach has been emphasized in the economic literature by authors such as Musgrave (1959) and Musgrave and Musgrave (1989). Its aim is to point out economically correct choices for the public sector. It therefore takes a normative perspective. It is this standpoint that was first taken in economic analysis of the animal health sector (i.e. privatization guidelines) by authors such as Umali, de Haan, Feder and Bekure. Such an approach to animal health economics was innovative in the 1990s. However, the privatization process has not reached its aims of increased efficiency and effectiveness of AHS while limiting public expenditure (see Dorward *et al.* 1998). Such consequences point out that reconsidering the original economic perspective taken in the analysis of AHS might shed light on the weaknesses of previous analysis.

Hence, the present analysis takes the *public choice school* perspective. This school considers, in contrast to the previous approach, that public interventions may add inefficiencies to existing regulations. The underlying reasoning focuses on the assumption that governments are not free in making their choices. Rather, powerful interest groups are likely to interfere in decision-making processes. This is a crucial point given the existing context and political interests in the agricultural sector (in both developed and developing countries). Hence, policy makers' choices should not be separated from the decisions taken. Following this reasoning, Wiseman (1980) pointed out an economic perspective known as *process* efficiency (as opposed to the previous one, outcome efficiency). His perspective identifies existing weaknesses in the marginal equivalence principle and that such principle should not divert attention from efficiency in techniques of prioritization of resource allocation.

Thus the public choice school see the government as an added source of inefficiencies to the decision-making process in a given market. Hence, attention should be drawn to the procedures of decision making (therefore not exclusively focusing on outcomes) (Wiseman 1980). The rationale is therefore to find if another decision-making process would have resulted in a 'closer to optimal' outcome (Cullis and Jones 1998). In the animal health context, this is the most recent perspective taken by authors such as Leonard and Ahuja.

Still under the public choice perspective, it is worth highlighting that some authors, notably Stigler (1971), started the debate over regulation. He pointed out that regulation is the result of financial and political support of special interests groups in return for favourable legislation. The agricultural sector provides an interesting list of examples, varying from the Kenyan Veterinary Board's reluctance to accept legislation in favour of official recognition of community-based animal health workers (CAHWs) in Kenya, to international trade (dis)agreements in relation to livestock and livestock products under the World Trade Organization (WTO). Interestingly, Laffont and Tirole (1993) analysed the regulatory environment following the public choice approach. They searched to find out the nature of constraints preventing regulators from implementing preferred policies. As a result, three key constraints were put forward, namely (i) information gaps; (ii) transaction costs; and (iii) administrative and political constraints. Propper (1995) analysed the process of *regulatory capture* in the interface between agriculture and public health in relation to the BSE outbreak in the UK. The *capture* process refers to the close association existing between the regulating agency and the regulatee. Hence, it is prompted that the regulatee 'captures' or controls the regulator, thus guiding the regulatory process towards their interest. This might explain certain chain effects originated during the BSE outbreak as the Ministry of Agriculture, Fisheries and Food (MAFF, currently known as Department of Environment, Food and Rural Affairs; DEFRA) was 'captured' by interest groups in the industrial sector, hindering the government's responsiveness. These mechanisms may well apply to more recent events highlighting the public health and agriculture interface relevance, such as the AI outbreak in Asia.

The agricultural sector (and especially the animal health subsector) is subject to a highly politicized environment. This fact sheds light on the usefulness of moving from a traditional approach to a public choice perspective especially in the animal health sector. Following this perspective, the next section compares different ways in which animal health goods and services may be classified and the implications derived.

Defining public goods: taxonomic types

Although economic theory has been used in the analysis of several types of markets and neoclassical economics in the human health care sector developed during the 1960s and 1970s, its application in the animal health field only started a decade ago. The main triggering event was the widespread public financial crisis in several developing countries [especially, the 'Great African Depression' (Leonard 2000)]. Consequently, animal health care services were classified following the previously debated *outcome* approach. Under this perspective, governments were advised on service categorization following the rather dichotomous criteria of 'public' versus 'private' goods (Umali-Deininger *et al.* 1992).

Historically, goods were classified following Samuelson's rivalry and excludability principles (Samuelson 1954). However, several economic theorists have especially debated his definition of a 'public good'. They argue about the difficulty of finding public goods in the purest sense. Hence, examples such as law and order, or the classical one on lighthouses, were debated by authors such as Margolis (1955), Sandler (1977) and Coase (1974). It has been argued that the debate about goods should not focus on the two extremes (*pure* private and *pure* public goods), but rather on their degree of 'publicness' (Cullis and Jones 1998) (also referred to as *impure* public goods). The way in which goods are classified will determine an alternative rationale for governments to take decisions on adequate ways of financing and/or provision of services.

Cullis and Jones (1998) devised three ways in which goods and services may be classified. The first one relates to Head (1962) and Peston's (1972) classification following Samuelson's principles. The second, which is supported by Musgrave (1969) and to some extent by Weisbrod (1988), focuses on assessing the mix of benefits stemming from the provision of a good. This approach is referred to as 'mixed goods or quasi-public goods'. The rationale of the third approach is associated mainly with Buchanan (1965). His categorization is based on the relationship between the degree of indivisibility and the number of people consuming the good.

It is important to mention that in the animal health sector, it is mostly the first approach that has been applied (Umali-Deininger *et al.* 1992). Few other authors have attempted to take the second perspective (Leonard 2000). Each of these approaches will be analysed in the animal health context.

Excludability and rivalry

As previously mentioned, this has been the approach most commonly taken in animal health economics. Although Umali *et al.* (Umali-Deininger *et al.* 1992, 1994; Holden *et al.* 1996) pioneered such analysis, the most extensive interpretation comes from Holden (1999). Given the aforementioned controversy over *pure* public goods, in her analysis she purposely uses the criteria of high and low rivalry and excludability. It is interesting to see that in her analysis she associates a funding mechanisms with each of these categories (see Table 12.1).

Table 12.1 Classification of goods following the rivalry and excludability principles

		Excludability	
		High	**Low**
	High	**Private goods**	**Common pool goods**
		Endemic disease control and prevention *(a)*	Tsetse control on communal land using traps, targets or aerial spraying *(j)*
		Sales of drugs and vaccines *(b)*	
		Some extension *(c)*	
		Some research *(d)*	
		Clinical services *(e)*	
Rivalry		**PRIVATE FINANCE** **A**	**PUBLIC FUNDING** **B**
	Low	**Toll goods**	**Public goods**
		Vaccine production *(f)*	Epidemic or zoonotic disease control (surveillance, movement control, quarantine services) *(k)*
		Diagnostic services *(g)*	Some extension
		Veterinary clinics *(h)*	Some research
		Dips *(i)*	Control of food borne diseases *(l)*
		PRIVATE FINANCE **C**	**PUBLIC FINANCE** **D**

Adapted from Holden (1999).

Reproduced with kind permission, from Holden, S., 'The Economics of Delivery of Veterinary Services', in *Revue Scientifique et Technique 18(2)*, pp. 425–439.

Even if the list depicted in Table 12.1 is not exhaustive, the taxonomy of some of the examples is highly debatable, as well as the associated funding source. Elements (a–l) have been extensively debated elsewhere (Riviere-Cinnamond 2004), but some of the examples of public health relevance are mentioned here.

For goods falling into category A, there is theoretically a strong incentive for the private buyer or consumer to pay for the good. Typical examples included by Holden are clinical services, vaccines and pharmaceuticals, and prevention and control of endemic diseases. However, some concerns arise as some of the items might have positive spillovers [especially (a)] to other herders (e.g. in the case of common grazing). When focusing on item (a), Holden argues that such services should be privately funded given that 'private benefits of vaccination against endemic (livestock) diseases usually outweigh the benefits to other' (Holden 1999). While this holds true, it is also applicable in the case of epidemic diseases.

Of special concern to the public choice approach would be items (e) and (b). Following Samuelson's rationale, these items are highly excludable and rival. One might argue that their funding may fall exclusively on end-consumers. Although the rationale is accepted, the underlying reason for delivering private goods is the need for enough aggregated demand for these goods or services, as well as sufficient suppliers so as to ascertain adequate market competition. The guidelines given for privatizing AHS did not take into account either the physical or the institutional context of rural and remote areas. In some of these areas, it could be argued that market failure is complete. Although farmers or livestock keepers may have the willingness to pay (WTP) for services, depending on the targeted population, they might not have the ability to pay (ATP), especially in the case of 'rural world 3'. In these situations, and of course depending on the poverty reduction goals at a governmental level, a certain degree of public intervention would be needed. Similarly, in 'rural world 2' where ATP might be higher, concerns may be highlighted over potential public health hazards arising in this category (as mentioned in previous sections). Thus, even if market failure is not complete, there would be a need for a certain degree of public intervention under the public health umbrella. It can therefore be argued that not all highly rival and excludable goods find their funding source in the private sector.

When focusing on toll *goods* [category C, items (f–i)], economic theory generally suggests that end-users should pay for the services. Although they are characterized by low rivalry (as several animals might be treated or samples processed), services are excludable for non-paying users. However, the inclusion of veterinary clinics as a toll good might be argued against given that services are paid in relation to the (individual) animals treated. Thus, they will fall under the 'private good' category. Most of the services included in category C are found in high production areas (i.e. 'rural world 1'), relatively near to urban settings. In these settings, aggregated demand, access to markets and competition among suppliers tend to be high enough to leave these items to market forces. However, the same situation as for items in category A would be found for toll goods in the rural and remote settings, therefore indicating the need for government intervention.

Of special interest in these high potential areas is the pressure exerted by (in developing countries) a recent trend in growth of supermarkets, especially in Asia and certain parts of Africa (Orden *et al.* 2004). Increased consumer demand for standard quality products has put pressure on transformers and producers. The latter need to ascertain adequate quality levels (specified for each commodity of livestock-derived product) in order for their product to enter the transforming industry. Consumers will force the transforming industry to meet these levels. At the same time, the latter will force producers to increase the quality of raw products. Hence, goods that have a certain degree of public good characteristics (included in category B and D) might be privately funded and provided due to market pressures (e.g. food-borne disease control), provided there is the adequate legislative framework for enforcement. Examples of such movements include Australia's National Animal Health Authority. Although being a parastatal agency financed through compulsory contributions, such contributions come mainly from producers' associations, the system is enabled by legislation. Interestingly, the creation of this authority came from a proposal from the industry sector in order to enable them to be competitive in the national, but, most importantly, in the international market (Animal-Health-Australia 2003).

In other less developed settings, examples such as trypanosomosis (try-panosomosis is a zoonotic disease known in humans as sleeping sickness) control illustrate the changing nature of goods (and their funding source) due to technological innovations. Trypanososmosis control on communal land through traps, target or aerial spraying may fall into the category of common pool goods (B) as non-paying users cannot be prevented from using the good or service, while increased consumption of the good diminishes supply for others. As non-paying users cannot be prevented access, there is no incentive for the consumer to pay for the service. Hence, people tend to 'free-ride'. However, trypanosomosis control may have positive externalities not only related to decreasing cattle mortality rates but also by lowering the occurrence of (human) sleeping sickness. Therefore, trypanosomosis control may have characteristics not only of a common pool good but also of a public good if its zoonotic disease aspects are considered. However, new technologies have allowed the creation of pour-on insecticides, therefore increasing the service's excludability and thus changing its nature.

Not only might the nature of the good change over time, but the economic consequences of an animal disease outbreak (i.e. externalities as it affects national economy and international market competitiveness), which may not necessarily be of a zoonotic nature, may cause a re-evaluation of the nature of the good or service. Hence, animal diseases with high national socio-economic and/or public health repercussions might be of particular relevance in developing countries due to the contribution of livestock to wealth generation and employment. In addition, in the case of public health hazards associated with animal disease spread, the state would benefit from its control as this might lower national health care costs (Holden 1999).

However, when assessing the nature of a good in this study's context, one might think of who is the end beneficiary of AHS. Is it the society as a whole, the farmer population or the national state government? The question is relevant as outbreaks of highly contagious animal diseases but with rather low mortality rates might have different effects at different levels. For example, in the event of FMD spread, a meat-exporting country will be banned from the international market. As a consequence, beef prices and the prices of derived products are likely to fall, thus benefiting the poorest consumers in the nation. However, given the closure of export markets, beef producers as well as governments will see their economic benefits from trade heavily diminished (i.e. lower prices in beef products in the case of farmers and less revenue from export duties for the state).

This case may exemplify the aforementioned 'capture' process and influence of powerful interest groups over decision-making processes. Given that economic theory defines a good as 'public' when it relates to the whole society, the negative effects of an FMD outbreak at a societal level remain debatable and will vary in relation to the political standpoint of governments. Thus, control measures against epidemic diseases may provide a 'public' good only to a subset of the society (although it requires government legislation and enforcement control measures). This example links to the third method for classifying goods and services (i.e. consumption sharing), especially with Buchanan's 'theory of clubs' (Buchanan 1965), which will be debated later.

Hence, it has been pointed out that, even in the AHS, one good may fall into different categories when conditions vary. This point was highlighted by Peston (1972). However innovative this technique was at the beginning of animal health economic analysis, its current validity may be contested. At this level, two points have been raised that shed light on the possible reasons for the privatization of AHS failure. These relate first to the targeted population (i.e. for whom is the service public) and, secondly, to the context (physical and institutional) in which goods and services are delivered. These issues are debated in the next section.

Mixed goods/quasi-public goods

The quasi-public goods approach was first taken by Musgrave (1969). In the context of AHS, it has been adopted by authors such as Leonard (2000) and to a certain extent Ahuja (2004). Koma's research in Uganda (Koma 2000) has highlighted that this approach towards animal health goods and services is preferable to the previous one mainly because evaluating through the externalities lens 'leads one to do a better job in evaluating the adequacy of private demand, because it quantifies rather than categorizes both internal and external benefits' (Leonard 2000).

Services such as research (d) and extension (c) show the difficulty the public–private categorization of goods might pose. For example, the outcomes of research might have private good characteristics (i.e. patent on a vaccine), but at the same time it might increase knowledge on, for example, animal disease prevention and treatment. The latter may profit not only the farmer population but also the society as a whole, depending on the nature of the disease. Similarly, education or extension directed towards livestock owners or producers is expected to help increase their production and consequently the income earned. Simultaneously, extension messages may prevent or limit the extent of disease outbreaks, thus not only affecting nearby farmers' production but, in relation to the specificities of the disease, avoiding important losses at a national level. At the same time, extension and education are likely to increase future generation's knowledge on production management and facilitate basic research, thus creating non-rival and non-excludable knowledge and information benefiting others (however distant these examples might seem from the initial education or extension message).

A concrete example of the mixed good perspective may well be a herder vaccinating his herd against CBPP (contagious bovine pleuro-pneumonia). While he benefits from the vaccination of his herd, he creates an external benefit as the chance of infection of neighbouring producers' herds diminishes. It becomes clear that the external effect of consumption of a private good (the vaccine) bears to some extent characteristics of public good. Thus the mixed goods approach recognizes that goods may have private benefits as well as external effects.

The importance of the approach of Musgrave (1969) in dealing with the blend of privateness and publicness of goods lies in its usefulness in policy making. If costs and benefits of introducing a new policy could be evaluated, it would be possible to prioritize activities in the policy agenda. However, operationalizing this approach is not exempt from technical constraints. Private benefits should be weighted against spillover benefits. However, measuring the effect of spillover at different levels, and especially in the animal health—public health interface, might prove to be difficult as it encompasses human, animal and environmental levels. One attempt has been through cost-benefit analysis (CBA); however, such a method is not exempt from criticisms. For an extensive debate between private and social CBAs, see Stiglitz (2000).

As previously mentioned, CBAs could be a useful tool for allocation of public resources. However, these analyses were established on the assumption that governments seek 'benevolently to maximise social welfare' (Cullis and Jones 1998). It is a framework to assess different elements in the desirability of a project but does not convey the idea of it being a perfect method. In that context, mainly two criticisms have been made. First, problems arise when trying to determine social benefits arising from a precise animal health intervention. In that area, several authors have attempted to make the case for further use of CBA techniques in relation to AHS (Marsh 1999; Morris 1999; Rushton *et al.* 1999). However, most of the existing studies lack carefully documented analysis (Ramsay *et al.* 1999) and/or lack disaggregated and reliable data (Coleman 2002), especially in the case of zoonotic diseases. Secondly, it needs to be highlighted that CBAs are not exempt from political interference and influence from interest groups. Hence, a public choice approach would focus on *how* the investment was *chosen*, which has more to do with political costs and benefits than the normative approach of *which* investment should be chosen (Cullis and Jones 1998). Cullis and Jones mention that 'the fact that government departments invest time and effort when undertaking cost-benefit analysis does not preclude the possibility that they are motivated far more by political factors than by welfare economics', highlighting the susceptibility to regulatory capture from powerful industries.

Thus, the main difference between the private–public good and the 'quasi-public good' approach lies in that the latter tries to evaluate the public–private mix of benefits stemming from a policy intervention. Hence, physical and institutional contexts, as well as the 'blend of publicness' of consequences are taken into account in the evaluation.

This analysis therefore may be a powerful tool for decision making in the animal health care sector. However, the arrangements relating to the optimization of resource allocation at a service provision level are not taken into consideration. It is the next section that provides a conceptual framework for the classification of goods in relation to their degree of consumption sharing among a certain population.

Consumption sharing

Essentially, what Buchanan's theory explores is the relationship between the degree of indivisibility of a good or service and the number of people consuming that service. Thus it analyses the degree to which consumption sharing is possible among a given population (see Fig. 12.3).

Applying his conceptual framework to the animal health setting would point out that services or goods in (1) in Fig. 12.3 would mainly have private characteristics and be fully divisible between a few individuals (in that case farmers or producers). Examples would include clinical services or diagnostic tests used for one given producer/farmer. Such services, it is argued, 'should' be left to market provision. At the opposite end, services falling into (5) would be public goods completely indivisible among a large farmer population. For example, AI or FMD control in a given district may be considered in this category for slightly different reasons: AI for its public health risks as well as its associated production and economic losses, and FMD exclusively under an economic rationale. The control of such diseases is fully indivisible between producers, and all the farmer population (as well as the general population in the case of AI) of the district will profit. Items in (3) may apply for less highly infectious diseases (e.g. CBPP), whose control could profit nearby producers.

Items in (2) are those which are shared within a small group, but are relatively indivisible. Extension services at a community level may be taken as an example as they are shared amongst a small number of community members. Buchanan suggests that the provision of these services is left to voluntary arrangements between the individual members of the small group concerned. Finally, those services included under item (4) refer to Buchanan's 'clubs' and would necessarily be highly indivisible among a small group of individuals. Cooperatives may serve as an example, where dipping facilities could be used

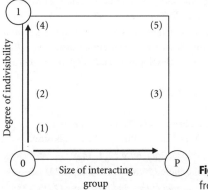

Fig. 12.3 Consumption sharing (adapted from Cullis and Jones, 1998).

by all members having paid a premium fee. The provision of the service will continue as long as the number of members is not excessive. It could be argued that the effectiveness of the dipping product diminished with use, thus incurring some level of rivalry.

Buchanan states that such services or goods are arrangements in the private sector where the service is excludable (through a membership fee or premium) but not private below capacity levels (thus non-rival). The interest of such an approach lies in the optimization of efficiency conditions in the provision of these services.

Conclusions

The novelty of these approaches in the economic analysis of AHS lies in that they call into question the appropriate role for the public sector. Hence, those goods that are not perfectly public might well be better supplied through the market, whereas under certain conditions it might be more appropriate for governments to provide private goods.

When linking this economic analysis of AHS to IFPRI's categorization of smallholders, it seems obvious that the virtual lack of AHS in some areas, and especially in rural world 2, may have helped trigger the spread of highly infectious disease outbreaks such as AI or SARS. Given the trends in animal production, not only will the gap between those farmers in rural world 1 and 3 be widening (thus increasing inequality within countries), but the increase in human–animal contact will provide the ecological conditions for potential outbreaks of emerging and zoonotic disease spread.

AHS need therefore to be viewed as a key preventive measure when assessing public health risks.

References

Ahuja, V. (2004) The economic rationale of public and private sector roles in the provision of animal health services. *Revue Scientifique et Technique* 23, 33–45.

Ahuja, V., George, S. *et al.* (2000) *Agricultural Services and the Poor: Case of Livestock Health and Breeding Services in India*. Indian Institute of Management, Ahmedabad, India, the World Bank, Washington, DC, Swiss Agency for Development and Cooperation. Bern, Switzerland.

Animal-Health-Australia (2003) Animal Health Australia, http://www.aahc.com.au/about/what.htm.

Arrow, K.J. (1985) The economics of agency. In: Pratt, J. and Zeckhauser, R. (eds), *Principals and Agents. The Structure of Business*. Harvard Business School, Boston.

Buchanan, J.M. (1965) An economic theory of clubs. *Economica* 32, 1–14.

Buchanan, J.M. (1975) Public finance and public choice. *National Tax Journal* 28, 383–394.

Coase, R. (1974) The lighthouse in economics. *Journal of Law and Economics* 17, 357–376.

Coleman, P. (2002) Zoonotic disease and their impact on the poor (Annex 9). In: Perry, B.D., Randolph, T.F., McDermott, J.J., Sones, K.R. and Thornton, P.K. (eds), *Investing in Animal Health Research to Alleviate Poverty*. International Livestock Research Institute, Nairobi.

Cullis, J. and Jones, P. (1998) *Public Finance and Public Choice*. Oxford University Press, Oxford.

deHaan, C. and Bekure, S. (1991) *Animal Health Services in Sub-Saharan Africa. Initial Experiences with Alternative Approaches*. The World Bank, Washington, DC.

Delgado, C.L., Rosegrant, M.W. *et al.* (1999) *Livestock 2020. The Next Food Revolution*. International Food Policy Research Institute, Washington, DC/United Nations Food and Agriculture Organization, Rome/International Livestock Research Institute, Nairobi.

Delgado, C.L., Rosegrant, M.W. *et al.* (2000) *The Coming Livestock Revolution*. Background paper no. 6, Department of Economic and Social Affairs, Commission of Sustainable Development, Eighth Session, Food and Agriculture Organisation, New York.

Dorward, A., Kydd, J. *et al.* (1998) *Smallholder Cash Crop Production Under Market Liberalization: A New Institutional Economics Perspective*. CAB International, Wallingford, UK.

Evans, R.G. (1998) Going for gold: the redistributive agenda behind market based health care reform. In: Chinitz, D., Cohen, J. and Doron, C. (eds), *Governments and Health Systems: Implications of Differing Involvements*. Wiley, Chichester.

Head, J.G. (1962) Public goods and public policy. *Public Finances/Finances Publiques* 17, 197–219.

Holden, S. (1999) The economics of delivery of veterinary services. *Revue Scientifique et Technique* 18, 425–439.

Holden, S., Ashley, S. *et al.* (1996) *Delivery of Animal Health Services: Synthesis of Research Needs*. Livestock in Development, Crewkerne, Somerset, 33.

Koma, M.P.K. (2000) Can private veterinarians survive in Uganda? In: Leonard, D.K. (ed.), *Africa's Changing Market for Health and Veterinary Services. The New Institutional Issues*. MacMillan Press, London.

Laffont, J.-J. and Tirole, J. (1993) *A Theory of Incentives in Procurement and Regulation*. MIT Press. Cambridge, MA.

Leonard, D.K. (1990) Draft research proposal on the organisation of animal health services in Africa presented at the International Livestock Centre for Africa. Umali, L.D., Feder, G. and de Haan, C. (eds), *The Balance Between Public and Private Sector Activities in the Delivery of Livestock Services (1992)*. World Bank Discussion Paper 163, The World Bank, Washington, DC.

Leonard, D.K. (2000) *Africa's Changing Market for Health and Veterinary Services. The New Institutional Issues*. MacMillan Press, London.

Margolis, J.A. (1955) Comment on the pure theory of public expenditure. *Review of Economics and Statistics* 37, 347–349.

Marsh, W. (1999) The economics of animal health in farmed livestock at the herd level. *Revue Scientifique et Technique* 18, 357–366.

Mathema, V.R. and Joshi, D.D. (2000) *Livestock and Livestock Insurance in Nepal*. Padma Mathema and Ram Narayan Kunj Publishers, Kathmandu, Nepal.

Morris, R.S. (1999) The application of economics in animal health programmes: a practical guide. *Revue Scientifique et Technique* 18, 305–314.

Mossialos, E., Dixon, A. *et al.* (2002) *Funding Health Care: Options for Europe.* Open University Press, Buckingham.

Murray, J.L. and Frenck, J. (2000) A framework for assessing the performance of health systems. *Bulletin of the World Health Organization* **78**, 717–731.

Musgrave, R.A. (1969) Provision for social goods. In: Margolis J. and Guitton, M. (eds), *Public Economics.* St Martin's Press, New York.

Musgrave, R.A. and Musgrave, P.B. (1989) *Public Finance in Theory and Practice.* McGraw-Hill, New York.

Orden, D., Torero, M. *et al.* (2004) *Agricultural Markets and the Rural Poor (preliminary draft).* IFPRI, Washington, DC.

Peston, M. (1972) *Public Goods and the Public Sector.* Macmillan, London.

Pratt, J. and Zeckhauser, R. (1985) *Principals and Agents. The Structure of Business.* Harvard Business School, Boston.

Propper, C. (1995) Agency and incentives in the NHS internal market. *Social Science and Medicine* **40**, 1683–1690.

Ramsay, G.C., Philip, P. *et al.* (1999) The economic implications of animal diseases and disease control at the national level. *Revue Scientifique et Technique* **18**, 343–356.

Reinhardt, U.E. (1990) *Economic Relationships in Health Care, in OECD Health Care Systems in Transition: The Search for Efficiency.* Organisation for Economic Co-operation and Development, Paris,

Riviere-Cinnamond, A. (2004) A public choice approach to the analysis of animal healthcare systems. *FAO-Pro Poor Livestock Policy Initiative Working Paper* **11**.

Rushton, J., Thornton, P.K. *et al.* (1999) Methods of economic impact assessment. *Revue Scientifique et Technique* **18**, 315–342.

Samuelson, P.A. (1954) The pure theory of public expenditure. *Review of Economics and Statistics* **36**, 387–389.

Sandler, T. (1977) Impurity of defence: an application to the economics of alliances. *Kyklos* **30**, 443–460.

Sidibe, A.S. (2003) Organisation actuelle et future des services veterinaires en Afrique. *Revue Scientifique et Technique* **22**, 473–484.

Stigler, G.J. (1971) The theory of economic regulation. *Bell Journal of Economics and Management Sciences* **2**, 137–146.

Stiglitz, J.E. (2000) *Economics of the Public Sector.* W.W. Norton and Company, London/New York.

Umali-Deininger, D., Feder, G. *et al.* (1992) *The Balance Between Public and Private Sector Activities in the Delivery of Livestock Services.* World Bank Discussion Paper **163**, 114.

Umali-Deininger, D., Narrod, C. *et al.* (1994) *Private Sector Development in Agriculture: Constraints, Opportunities and New Approaches.* Private Sector Development Department, World Bank, Washington, DC.

Van Asseldonk, M.A.P.M., Meuwissen, M.P.M. *et al.* (2003) European public and private schemes indemnifying epidemic livestock losses: a review. *Livestock Insurance Products.*

Weisbrod, B.A. (1988) *The Nonprofit Economy.* Harvard University Press, Cambridge, MA.

Wiseman, J. (1980) The choice of optimal social expenditures. In: Roskamp, K. (ed.), *Public Choice and Public Finance.* Editions Cujas, Paris.

Chapter 13

Risk assessment models, economic analysis and food safety policy

Tanya Roberts[1]

Introduction

Risk assessment models are important tools in economic analysis of infectious disease. Risk assessment is the science of identifying and understanding hazards (unwanted events), of estimating the likelihood of these events occurring and of estimating the consequences if they do occur. Disease outcome tree models can organize medical data to estimate the probability of lifetime outcomes due to food-borne pathogens. Economists can then estimate public health costs for these outcomes. If the damage to society is significant, a cost-benefit analysis of public and private control options can be conducted. After the options for controlling pathogens in food production and distribution are determined, scenario models can be combined with probabilistic risk assessment (PRA) models to estimate quantitatively the impact of alternative risk-reducing options. Both individual companies seeking to control pathogens better and the public regulators setting priorities among food-borne hazards can use these risk assessment models. The 'market failure', due to limited information about the presence of pathogens in food, has a strong impact on economic incentives. Some remedies to the information problems are suggested. How economic incentives affect investment in both short- and long-term control options is also discussed. The various risk assessment models presented here are applicable to economic analysis of any infectious disease.

Disease outcome tree models

Most food-borne illnesses are 'acute' and usually self-limiting. The gastrointestinal problems, generally of short duration, range from mild to severe. While deaths from acute food-borne illness are rare, they are more likely to occur in the elderly,

[1] The views expressed here are those of the author, and may not be attributed to the Economic Research Service or the U.S. Department of Agriculture or the Food and Drug Administration.

Table 13.1 Chronic complications associated with food-borne pathogens

Bacterial and parasitic infections transmitted by foods	Complications/sequelae
Bacterial infections	
Aeromonas hydrophila enteritis	Bronchopneumonia, cholecystitis
Brucellosis	Aortitis, epididymo-orchitis, meningitis, pericarditis, spondylitis
Campylobacteriosis	Arthritis, carditis, cholecystitis, colitis, endocarditis, erythema nodosum, Guillain–Barré syndrome, haemolytic–uraemic syndrome, meningitis, pancreatitis, septicaemia
Escherichia coli (EHEC-types) enteritis	Erythema nodosum, haemolytic–uraemic syndrome, seronegative arthropathy, thrombotic thrombocytopenic purpura
Q-fever	Endocarditis, granulomatous hepatitis
Salmonellosis	Aortitis, cholecystitis, colitis, endocarditis, epididymo-orchitis, meningitis, myocarditis, osteomyelitis, pancreatitis, Reiter's disease, rheumatoid syndromes, septicaemia, splenic abscesses, thyroiditis, septic arthritis (sickle-cell anaemic persons)
Shigellosis	Erythema nodosum, haemolytic–uraemic syndrome, peripheral neuropathy, pneumonia, Reiter's disease, septicaemia, splenic abscesses, synovitis
Vibrio parahaemolyticus enteritis	Septicaemia
Yersiniosis	Arthritis, cholangitis, erythema nodosum, liver and splenic abscesses, lymphadenitis, pneumonia, pyomyositis, Reiter's disease, septicaemia, spondylitis, Still's disease
Parasitic infections	
Cryptosporidiosis[1]	Severe diarrhoea, prolonged and sometimes fatal
Giardiasis[2]	Cholangitis, dystrophy, joint symptoms, lymphoidal hyperplasia
Taeniasis	Arthritis, cysticercosis (*T.solium*)
Toxoplasmosis	Encephalitis and other central nervous system diseases, pancarditis, polymyositis
Trichinosis	Cardiac dysfunction, neurological sequelae

[1] Suspected to be food-borne or water-borne.

[2] Water-borne.

Source: Council for Agricultural Science and Technology (CAST) (1994).

children (including the fetus) or others with compromised immune systems [such as those suffering from acquired immune deficiency syndrome (AIDS) and cancer, taking medication to prevent rejection of a transplanted organ, etc.].

Complications of food-borne illness, called chronic sequelae, can occur in any part of the body including the joints, nervous system, kidneys or heart. These chronic illnesses may afflict the patients for a short time or for the remainder of their lives, or cause premature death. Most food-borne pathogens have a variety of chronic sequelae that occur in a small, but often unknown, percentage of persons with acute illness (Table 13.1). For example, *Campylobacter* infections are estimated to be responsible for 20–40% of Guillain–Barré syndrome (GBS) cases (a major cause of paralysis unrelated to trauma) in the USA (Buzby *et al.* 1997).

About 1.5% of *Escherichia coli* O157:H7 disease patients develop haemolytic–uraemic syndrome (HUS), which usually involves red blood cell destruction, kidney failure and neurological complications, such as seizures and strokes. In Fig. 13.1, a disease outcome tree model, showing the full range of acute

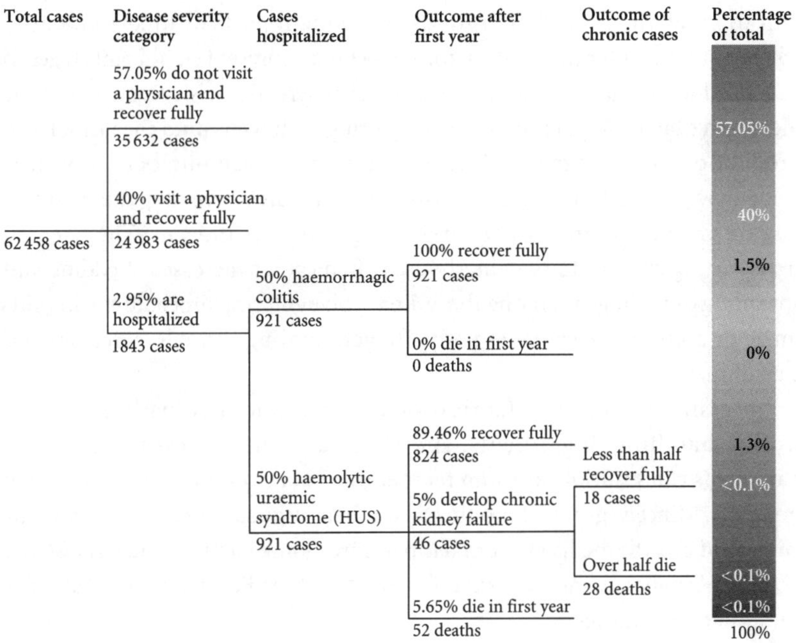

Fig. 13.1 Distribution of estimated US food-borne *Escherichia coli* O157:H7 disease cases and outcome. Percentages and number of cases may be rounded. Prepared by the Economic Research Service, USDA.

and chronic disease outcomes, is illustrated for *E.coli* O157:H7 cases in the USA. The model is a useful tool for organizing medical data. Economists can then estimate the medical costs, productivity losses, premature deaths and other consequences associated with each node of the disease outcome tree model (Roberts *et al.* 1998).

Identifying control options

Food-borne disease risks can either be prevented from entering the farm-to-fork food chain, or removed/controlled once they are present. For example, pathogens that sneak into the food chain may be controlled by killing them in food production and processing (e.g. canning foods or sterilizing food contact surfaces); by limiting their growth with careful temperature control, monitoring and other procedures; and/or by product formulations that discourage growth. Most food companies use prevention as well as several control procedures to control pathogens—called the 'multiple hurdle' strategy in the trade.

The rest of this section identifies where food-borne disease risks could enter the food chain for beef (for further details, see Roberts *et al.* 1995). It is important to break the food chain into its component parts or links to identify where risks can enter the food chain. These links represent significant stages in beef production, handling and consumption where high-risk practices may be identified (Table 13.2). Farm inputs may bring pathogens onto the farm. Farm production practices may reduce or amplify pathogen numbers, as well as bring new pathogens into contact with food animals where they cause animal disease or cause animals to be carriers for human pathogens. The stress of transporting animals to slaughterhouses often causes increased shedding and spreading of pathogens among the animals. Slaughtering procedures can minimize or amplify the spreading of pathogens among animals, carcasses and cuts of meat.

Processing and product fabrication can introduce new pathogens from worker handling, ingredients, and water used in processing. Bacterial pathogens can multiply at room temperature in or on nutrient-rich animal products. Minced (ground) products with their large surface areas are particularly good growth media at room temperature. Some bacteria, such as *Listeria, Yersinia, Aeromonas* and *Clostridium botulinum* type E, can also grow at refrigeration temperatures.

Transporting meat products to wholesale/retail operations may permit pathogen growth, cross-contamination of products or introduction of new pathogens. How foods are stored and displayed affects pathogen growth through temperature control, possibilities for cross-contamination and length of shelf-life. How food is handled in the kitchen affects the probability that

Table 13.2 Variables of potential concern in estimating food-borne disease risks in beef production, handling and consumption.
Copyright (2006) from Interdisciplinary Food Safety Research, edited by Neal H Hooker and Elsa A Murano. Reproduced with kind permission by Routledge/Taylor & Francis Group, LLC

Farm input use	Farm production practices	Animal transportation
Production animal: Animal breeds (e.g., Holstein, Hereford), animal purpose (dairy, beef, veal), gender, age. **Type of housing:** Open range, feeding shed, group pens, individual calf housing, enclosed barn for all animals (concrete/wood/dirt floor), etc. **Feed inputs:** ♦ Use of colostrum (fresh or frozen) fed to newborns and protective effect against pathogens (amount fed, timing of feeding). ♦ Calf feed type (udder or pail milk, formula, milk replacer). ♦ Other types of feed (pelleted feed, roughage, additives, silage, etc.) and treatment of feed (irradiated, steam sterilization, medicated). ♦ Use of pasture, rotation and manure . management on pasture. **Water sources and access:** Well water, municipal water supply (chlorinated, filtered, etc.), on-farm pond, irrigation water, manure lagoon.	**Type of operation:** Product (e.g., dairy, veal calf, grow-out, finishing, feedlot, range-fed beef), vertical integration (owned, contract, independent) and purchased and/or farm-produced feed. **Herd management systems:** Calving management, calf rearing management (e.g. weaning practices), breeding practices, replacement strategies, barn cleaning practices. **Feed handling:** Delivery system (bulk feeding at-will, computer-programmed rations), types of rations/roughage, additives (rumensin, vitamins, antibiotics, idophones) and cleaning of system. **Animal health practices:** Herd health monitoring, use of veterinarian services, source of drugs and drug use patterns **Pathogen testing:** Use of pathogen test information from the individual/herd in farm management and to support probability modelling; quality of test information (sensitivity/	**Transport type:** Independent trucker, company truck, and/or railroad car, ship, plane. **Travel:** Length (local/regional/national/ international), timing season. **Feeding system:** Feed and water practices during transit. **Manure handling:** Loading procedures, stanchions in transportation, number of layers of animals. **System cleaning:** Type of cleaning, location and timing of cleaning of transportation vehicles. **Identification:** Maintenance of animal identification.

Table 13.2 (continued)

Farm input use	Farm production practices	Animal transportation
Wildlife access to farm: Rodents, birds or other animal access to farm ponds, food animals and pathways to contamination (aerosols, urine, feces; ingestion of vermin). **Geographic factors:** Local climate and pathogen survival, local wildlife vectors, and trade patterns/impact on replacement stock and pathogen probability. **Pathogen testing:** Testing farm inputs and the environment to identify pathogens (test sensitivity, sampling design, and frequency and breadth of pathogen testing).	specificity, sampling design, frequency/breadth). **Water delivery:** Delivery system (pipes, troughs, etc.), testing for pathogens and cleaning of system. **Manure handling practices:** Type of system (open pit, other liquid, dry, free range), disposal and cleaning of system; animal exposure to manure. **Wildlife control:** Pest surveillance and control (e.g. traps, poison); presence or absence of cats. **Control of visitors/trucks:** Restrictions on truck/human entry. **Animal identification system:** Maintenance of animal identification.	

Animal slaughter system	Beef processing system	Product transportation system
Type of operation: Integrated with processing or farm operation, single/multiple types of animals slaughtered, single/multiple slaughter lines. **Antemortem treatment:** Live animal inspection, hide wash, dry manure removal from animal. **Carcass preparation:** Hide removal, opening of abdominal cavity, tying off digestive tract, and	**Type of operation:** Integrated with slaughter or retail operation, single/multiple types of products/ animal species processed, single/multiple processing lines. **Cross-contamination control:** Physical separation of incoming trucks/personnel that may be contaminated from plant workers and product; equipment cleaning programme, knife sterilization, worker glove use/hand	**Transport type:** Independent trucker, company truck, and/or railroad car, ship, plane. **Length of trip:** Local, regional, national or international movement of raw or cooked product. **Temperature control:** Refrigeration practices during transit, temperature monitoring, use of temperature indicators.

other procedures to minimize manure contamination of meat.

Cross-contamination control:
Plant air ventilation system; physical separation of product/workers from beginning to end of line; equipment cleaning and/or sterilization between carcasses (e.g. knives); worker glove use/hand washing; and refraining from handling food when ill.

Digestive tract removal:
Minimizing spillage on meal, organoleptic examination of organs.

Carcass treatment:
Removal of fecal contamination and minimization of cross-contamination among carcasses and from workers. Carcass cooling and temperature maintenance.

Plant sanitation programme:
Weekly/daily/shift/lot schedule for cleaning building, drains and equipment.

Pathogen testing:
Testing animals, equipment, the environment, workers and meat for pathogen occurrence.

Identification:
Maintaining farm/carcass/lot identification linkages.

washing, and refraining from handling food when ill; air ventilation system; separation of raw from cooked products; special control procedures for ground (comminuted) products.

Meat cutting/trimming:
Removal of fecal contamination; minimization of cross-contamination along the processing line and from workers to product.

Meat temperature control:
Control of meat temperature during fabrication, cooling of processed products, and temperature maintenance after processing.

Inventory control:
Special date control programmes for ground (comminuted) products and for cooked products, and coordination with lot identification system for products.

Plant sanitation programme:
Weekly/daily/shift/lot schedule for cleaning building, drains, conveyor belts, grinders, and the like.

Pathogen testing:
Testing raw meat, finished product, equipment, workers and the environment for pathogens

Identification:
Maintaining slaughterhouse/lot identification linkages.

Cross-contamination:
Requirements for driver's hygiene; sanitary handling practices.

Cleaning system:
Type of cleaning, location and timing of vehicle cleaning.

Pathogen testing:
Testing vehicles, raw product, processed product and environment for pathogens.

Identification:
Maintaining lot and company identification.

Table 13.2 (continued)

Meat wholesale/retail system	Kitchen handling/consumption	Food link to human health
Type of operation: Degree of integration with processing and food preparation activities. **Cross-contamination:** Physical separation of plant workers and product from incoming trucks/personnel that may be contaminated: equipment cleaning programme; knife sterilization; worker glove use/hand washing; air ventilation system; separation of raw from cooked products. **Product fabrication:** Minimization of cross-contamination from raw to cooked product, among products, and from workers to product. Risk level may vary depending upon fabrication practices (origins of meat used in ground product, age of pieces, location of grinding, number of regrindings) and reworking practices. **Temperature control:** Control of meat temperature during fabrication, cooling of fabricated products, and temperature maintenance after processing.	**Type of kitchen:** Home, restaurant, fast food chain, schools, group homes/elder care, military, detention facilities and the like. **Cross-contamination:** Kitchen sanitation (washing utensils, counters); glove use/hand washing; separation of raw from cooked products; refraining from handling food when ill. **Temperature control:** Rapid refrigeration after purchase and maintenance at low temperature. Cook raw animal protein products well-done. **Inventory control:** Use of raw product within a few days, especially ground meats. **Pathogen testing:** Testing raw meat, finished product, equipment, workers and the environment for pathogens. **Consumption:** Avoid ordering undercooked beef, sending restaurant food back for more cooking if not well done.	**Surveillance and monitoring:** Food-borne association is variable depending on the pathogen/food combination and whether the illness is caused by cells or their toxins. Improved monitoring and surveillance combined with epidemiological investigations using new tests can link disease outbreaks to causative pathogens/food. **Acute illness:** Variable incidence for various chronic illnesses and variable severity distribution, depending on the pathogen and food combination. **Chronic illness:** Human-to-human transmission is variable, depending on the pathogen and food combination. **High-risk individuals:** Increased risk of acute illness, more severe illness and chronic illness in immunocompromised and other individuals. Variable, depending on the pathogen and food combination.

Inventory control:
Special date control programmes for ground (comminuted) products and for cooked products, and coordination with lot identification system for products.

Sanitation programme:
Weekly/daily/shift/lot schedule for cleaning knives, grinders, display cases, drains and the like.

Pathogen testing:
Testing raw meat, finished product, equipment, workers and the environment for pathogens.

Identification:
Maintaining lot/company identification linkages.

Identification:
Source of product.

Secondary cases:
Variable, depending on the pathogen and food combination.

Outrage factors:
Variable, depending on who is at high risk, the pathogen/food combination, the ability to control the pathogen using a variety of risk-reducing techniques and the like.

Anticipating the future:
Improved knowledge about evolving food-borne pathogens and human illness, especially linkages to chronic disease.

From Roberts *et al.* (1995).

pathogens multiply, cross-contaminate other products or are killed thorough cooking. Consumer food consumption choices (rare burgers versus well done) and behaviour in storing and handling food at home is the last link in the chain (Ralston et al. 2002).

The complexities of the food safety chain are exacerbated by such natural events as the appearance of new pathogens and changes to existing ones. Zoonotic agents may be pathogenic for humans but not for their animal hosts; therefore, assessing the health of the live animal may not indicate if it is carrying human pathogens. Human activities also add to the complexity. Consumers seek novelty in foods, which leads to the development of new food processes. This may result in foods with new pathogen profiles. Proper procedures in cooking and handling food in the kitchen at home are not well understood. Food preparation jobs in institutions are often low paid, which leads to rapid turnover, further complicating the proper training of food service workers.

Models to analyse control options can either be developed for a specific company (or even just one plant) or the models may try to capture practices in the whole industry. There are pros and cons for each approach. If data are available, plant-specific models are easier to construct, since only a small set of personnel, management, equipment and input variables are included. To construct a nationwide estimate of risk representing all plants processing a particular food, all the processes, procedures, worker training and management systems that vary greatly among the US plants would need to be accounted for in the model.

Probabilistic risk assessment (PRA) models

The first use of modern probabilistic modelling as a research tool stems from work on the atomic bomb. In the 1950s, Hermann Kahn of RAND Corporation used 'what if' scenarios to evaluate the probabilities of nuclear proliferation. By 1960, PRA models were used for financial analysis, engineering applications and general economic evaluations. The method has been well tried, and proved useful in many fields, including plant and animal health. It is an excellent tool for estimating the probability of an unwanted event occurring, such as contamination of food with pathogens (Roberts et al. 1995).

PRA models can be built for the whole farm-to-fork food production and processing chain. Alternatively, several models could be built for segments of the food chain and then linked together. Usually such models are tackled by a team—composed of decision scientists (including economists), modellers and subject matter experts (veterinarians, meat inspectors and plant operators). The team attempts to capture the scenarios that can lead to significant levels of contamination in the model. Here a scenario model illustrates the events that are likely to play a significant role in contamination or decontamination of beef carcasses in a slaughterhouse (Fig. 13.2).

The first node on the far left shows cattle entering the slaughterhouse. The (+) indicates an animal's contamination with pathogens that can lead to human illness, either on their hide or in their gastrointestinal (GI) tract. The contaminated (+) cattle are the top branch of the node, while clean (−) cattle are the lower branch. The second node depicts cattle stunning and bleeding (killing), shackling hocks (feet) to an overhead rail, and hide removal. The upper node indicates whether a slaughtered animal that entered with contamination on its hide or GI tract (+) has its normally sterile carcass contaminated (+) during

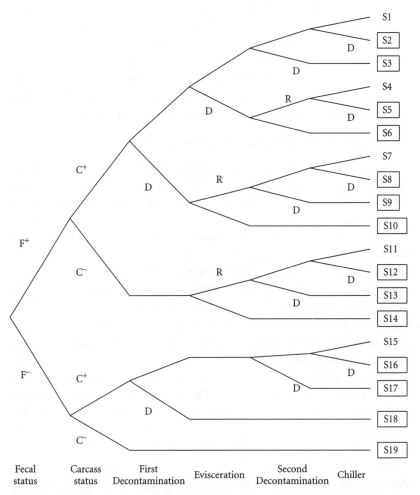

Fig. 13.2 Event tree and possible outcomes in a slaughterhouse. □—clean carcass status. Adapted from Roberts *et al.* (2001).

hide removal, or whether the carcass remains free of contamination ($-$) after hide removal. The lower node indicates whether a ($-$) animal has its carcass contaminated ($+$) with human pathogens in the air, on hands/knives, or contact with a ($+$) hide being removed from an adjacent carcass. The lower node ($-$) indicates that the carcass remains uncontaminated ($-$) during hide removal. The carcasses then proceed through subsequent steps of decontamination (steam vacuum and carcass washes), evisceration (removal of the GI tract) which can cause contamination, another decontamination step (perhaps steam pasteurization of the carcass or a carcass rinse) and the final step of carcass chilling for 18–48 h.

The final column in the figure shows 14 scenarios, identified by the boxes, that result in clean carcasses coming out of the chiller. The other five scenarios show contamination. For all these scenarios, evidence is collected and a PRA model is built to estimate the distribution of carcasses likely to be contaminated, and the area and level of contamination. Monte Carlo simulations can then be run to estimate a probabilistic distribution for carcasses leaving the chiller being contaminated and the level and area of contamination.

PRA model of statistical process control

To illustrate the impact of plant practices on process control and contamination with generic E.coli, Roberts et al. (1999) modelled a series of beef slaughter scenarios. The output of the model is the $\log_{10}$ colony-forming units (c.f.u.) of generic E.coli in quarter pound raw hamburgers. The model is a simplified version of the slaughter procedures described above. The four steps in the model for pathogen reduction or increase are:

$$X = h + s + c + f$$

where, X = average number of generic E.coli per quarter pound raw hamburger (expressed as $\log_{10}$ c.f.u.); h = hide removal from the carcass; s = steam pasteurization of the carcass at the end of the slaughter line; c = carcass chilling overnight; f = fabrication where the carcass is cut into steaks and trim for hamburger.

The values used in the model for plants with 'normal' and 'improved' process control are summarized in Table 13.3. The computation begins by assigning a level of generic E.coli in $\log_{10}$ c.f.u.s reported by Gill (1999) on the hindquarters of beef carcasses after normal hide removal. Improved skinning practices can prevent the hide from touching/contaminating the carcass and can reduce the cross-contamination that can occur. Gill found a 99% reduction in contamination when the plants studied earlier improved their practices.

The second step, s, models the effectiveness in killing generic E.coli on carcasses by applying steam or hot water to the carcass before it goes into the

Table 13.3 Slaughter plant model variables and ranges

Process	Distribution[1]	
	Normal procedures	**Improved procedures**
Hide removal (h)	Normal (2.47, 0.5)	Normal (0.23, 0.5)
Steam on carcass[2] (s)	Triangle (−1, 0, 0)	Triangle (−2, −2, −1)
Carcass chilling[2] (c)	Triangle (0, 1, 1)	Triangle (−1, −1, 0)
Fabrication[2] (f)	Normal (1, 0.5)[3]	Normal (0, 0.5)[3]

[1] Values are given as $\log_{10}$ c.f.u. of generic *E.coli*/cm² of carcass surface. The triangle distribution parameters are minimum, most likely and maximum values, and the normal distribution parameters are mean and SD for changes in $\log_{10}$ c.f.u./generic *E. coli*/cm².

[2] Change in $\log_{10}$ c.f.u. of generic *E.coli*/cm² of carcass surface. References for these values are cited in the text.

[3] Truncated at zero.

Adapted from Roberts *et al.* (1999).

chiller. There is considerable variability in the systems used, with water and acid washes generally less effective than steam. There is also variability in how steam systems are operated, depending on the time and temperature of the steam. Normal practices can reduce contamination up to 90%, while improved practices can reduce contamination up to 99% (Gill and Bryant 1997; Gill 1998).

The third step, c, is chilling the carcasses for 18–48 h. Studies of plants have found great variability in their ability to control their chilling operations (Gill and Bryant 1997). Normal plants can increase contamination by cross-contamination between carcasses and temperatures that permit bacterial growth. The normal case is modelled as up to a 90% increase in contamination. The improved situation is modelled as up to a 90% reduction in contamination because the low chill temperature kills some pathogens.

The final step, f, in this model is fabrication, where the trim from steaks and much of the older, tougher cows/bulls are placed in combo bins and will be ground into hamburgers. Using a conservative interpretation of Gill's data (1999), normal fabrication processes cause a 90% increase in contamination. Improved processes have a very slight increase, on average.

Model results show that the distribution of generic *E.coli* contamination in raw quarter pound hamburgers from slaughterhouses with normal process control was significantly greater than in plants with improved process control. Monte Carlo simulations were used to compute the distribution of contamination levels per quarter pound raw hamburger. There are two kinds of cattle slaughter plants: steer/heifer plants that produce mostly steaks and roasts with the trimmings going into hamburgers, and cow plants where the majority of the meat is trimming going into hamburgers (although some of the roasts are salvaged). We ran the model for 10 000 iterations for both types of plants and got similar results. Table 13.4 shows the results for the cow plant model. In each of the 16 scenarios, the results range from a 0.2% contamination rate to 99.9% for the cow plants with a different mix of 'normal' and 'improved' practices. Normal hide removal practices produced the eight scenarios with the highest levels of generic *E.coli*—illustrating the importance of careful hide removal to prevent contamination occurring. The impact of improving hide removal can be seen in Table 13.4 by comparing the 0.2% contamination rate that occurs when all four improved practices are used with the 62.7% contamination rate that occurs when normal hide removal is used along with the other three improved practices. The net difference is the benefit of improved hide removal, or 62.7 – 0.2% = 62.5% of the raw hamburgers are no longer contaminated above the threshold. Normal practices in the fabrication room

Table 13.4 Effect of cow slaughter plant practices

Process control practice				$P(N>4)$[1]
Hide removal	**Steam on carcass**	**Chilling carcass**	**Fabrication**	
Normal	Normal	Normal	Normal	99.9%
Normal	Normal	Normal	Improved	99.4%
Normal	Normal	Improved	Normal	98.8%
Normal	Improved	Normal	Normal	98.7%
Normal	Improved	Improved	Normal	90.9%
Normal	Normal	Improved	Improved	90.9%
Normal	Improved	Normal	Improved	90.9%
Normal	Improved	Improved	Improved	62.7%
Improved	Normal	Normal	Normal	55.5%
Improved	Normal	Improved	Normal	24.2%
Improved	Improved	Normal	Normal	23.7%
Improved	Normal	Normal	Improved	14.9%
Improved	Improved	Improved	Normal	5.7%
Improved	Improved	Normal	Improved	2.5%
Improved	Normal	Improved	Improved	2.4%
Improved	Improved	Improved	Improved	0.2%

[1] $P(N>4)$ means the raw quarter pound hamburgers are contaminated with more than 4 $\log_{10}$ c.f.u. of generic *E.coli*. We arbitrarily chose 4 $\log_{10}$ c.f.u. (10 000 c.f.u.) as a rough indicator of an adequate process control. Adapted from Roberts *et al.* (1999).

resulted in a 5.5% increase in hamburgers contaminated compared with a plant with all 'improved' practices. Normal practices in chilling and steam pasteurization contributed to a 2.5% increase or less of quarter pound hamburgers above the threshold of more than 4 $\log_{10}$ c.f.u of generic *E.coli*.

Roberts *et al.* (1999) arbitrarily chose 4 $\log_{10}$ c.f.u. (10 000 c.f.u.) as a threshold to indicate adequate process control. Slaughter plants with good process control were very effective in producing low levels of contamination in raw hamburgers. Only 0.2% of quarter pound raw hamburgers were contaminated above 4 $\log_{10}$ c.f.u. of generic *E.coli* in improved process control cow plants (Table 13.4).

Each hamburger plant will set its own threshold, higher or lower, depending on which market it is serving. For example, is the company one of Porter's (1985) first movers in a niche market providing the highest level of food safety? Or is the company selling hamburger patties to the local supermarket where most of the population is healthy? Is the company producing for a fast food chain with specific microbial testing requirements? Or is the company selling to nursing homes or day care centres where the populations are more vulnerable? As the Supreme Beef case in the USA shows, some companies are willing to produce hamburgers with contamination levels that do not meet minimum regulatory standards (United States Department of Agriculture, Food Safety and Inspection Services 2001). Alternatively, a company could do its own cost-benefit analysis of producing hamburgers for these different markets to discover where its comparative advantage lies.

This model is an illustration only, to show the power of the PRA technique. It is important that any model use distributions, such as the log normal distribution used here, that have a long right-hand tail to reflect that a few carcasses are likely to be highly contaminated. Data of Sofos *et al.* (1999a) show that beef carcasses can have up to 6 logs of contamination. The beauty of this PRA model is that it can show a slaughter plant the risk trade-offs associated with various interventions in the plant. Once the risk trade-offs have been estimated, economic data can be added to estimate the benefits and costs of alternative options. One such model was presented by Clare Narrod at the American Agricultural Economics Association meeting (Narrod *et al.* 1999) and has been published (Malcolm *et al.* 2004).

The data in the model for a particular slaughter plant will, of course, have to be modified to fit the plant's actual operations. For example, small plants may have a comparative advantage in preventing contamination in the first place. Small slaughter plants with low employee turnover and low line speeds might maximally reduce contamination with improved employee training programmes that focus on more sanitary hide removal that prevents the mostly sterile carcass from being contaminated. They can sterilize knives in between short cuts, use a dual knife system to ensure sterilization of the knives, minimize air-borne particles coming off the hide, ensure that tail/hide do not touch the carcass, minimize hand contact, etc. Plants with fast line speeds and larger throughputs may find their comparative advantage in investing in more automated processes and larger equipment to kill pathogens, such as carcass steam pasteurizers or irradiation equipment.

Cost-benefit analysis of HACCP

To encourage the private sector to produce safer meat and poultry, the United States Department of Agriculture's (USDA) Food Safety and Inspection Service (FSIS) issued the Pathogen Reduction/Hazard Analysis and Critical Control Point systems (HACCP) rule, which took effect in stages starting in 1997. Federally regulated meat and poultry slaughter and processing establishments are required to:

+ develop a HACCP plan to identify and control pathogens in their products
+ meet targets for microbial pathogen reduction
+ conduct microbial testing to determine compliance with the targets
+ establish and follow written sanitary standard operating procedures.

The HACCP regulations for meat and poultry slaughter and processing are designed to control or prevent food contamination by four pathogens: *Campylobacter*, *E.coli* O157:H7, *Listeria monocytogenes* and *Salmonella*. Food-borne disease for the first two pathogens is thought to be associated with raw meat and poultry 75% of the time. Food-borne disease for the second two pathogens is thought to be associated with raw meat and poultry at least 50% of the time.

Benefits of HACCP

The public health protection benefits come from preventing food-borne diseases caused by these four pathogens. The economic benefits reflect the improved Centers for Disease Control and Prevention's (CDC) food-borne disease estimates (Mead *et al.* 1999). The benefits of preventing non-fatal illnesses are avoidance of medical costs and productivity losses. When illnesses result in death, the Economic Research Service (ERS) measures the economic losses by using an age-adjusted value of statistical life based on Viscusi's review of the risk premium labour markets (higher wages paid for risky jobs). Because the likely reduction in human disease is unknown, the analysis used different assumptions of a 20% reduction in pathogens (in raw meat and poultry) and in human disease, a 50% reduction and a 90% percent reduction. The analysis also uses two interest rates, 3 and 7%, to evaluate the lifetime consequences of exposure to these pathogens and the stream of industry costs. In its analysis, ERS assumed that the benefits of pathogen reduction begin in 2000 (when the rule is fully implemented) and extend for 20 years (see Buzby *et al.* Chapter 16 for a discussion of alternative methods to estimate public health protection benefits).

Costs of HACCP

Meat and poultry plants are required to develop and implement HACCP plans, follow sanitation standard operating procedures, meet *Salmonella* standards and conduct *E.coli* generic tests. Plant costs include assessing and developing control procedures, antimicrobial treatments, record keeping, employee training and microbial testing. For this analysis, ERS used costs estimated by FSIS.

Estimated net benefits

HACCP benefits outweigh costs, even for the lowest range of benefits, in combating food-borne diseases caused by four pathogens (Table 13.5). With the most conservative assumptions, ERS found that HACCP provided net benefits of US$7 billion or more over a 20 year time horizon. When the

Table 13.5 Four HACCP/PR[1] scenarios illustrate the range of net benefits

Scenarios	Pathogen control	Interest rate	Present value[2] evaluated over 20 years [US$ billion (2000)]		
	%	%	Industry costs	Public health benefits	Annual net benefits
Low-range benefits estimate	20	7	1.3–1.5	8.5	6.8–7.2
Mid-range benefits estimate I	50	7	1.3–1.5	21.2	19.7–19.9
Mid-range benefits estimate II	50	3	1.7–2.1	24.3	22.2–22.6
High-range benefits estimate	90	3	1.7–2.1	43.8	41.7–42.1

[1] Hazard analysis and critical control point/pathogen reduction rule.

[2] The present value is the discounted value of either the stream of costs of the programme or the benefits of the programme over the 20 year time horizon. This is reported in year 2000 dollars.

Source: http://www.ers.usda.gov/briefing/FoodSafetyPolicy/features.htm

For more detail on the calculation methodology, see ERS report: Crutchfield *et al.* (1997).

analysis assumed higher rates of pathogen control and lower interest rates, the present value of the net benefits provided by HACCP were US$42 billion.

Future HACCP research

As PRA models for individual pathogens are developed, future models could elegantly estimate the likely risk reduction for the four pathogens HACCP is designed to control (rather than arbitrarily assume a 20, 50 or 90% reduction in illness due to the four pathogens in this cost-benefit analysis). The USDA and the US Department of Health and Human Services have built PRA models for several food-borne pathogens. For the latest details, see the models on the web pages of these departments or the Risk Assessment Consortium (RAC) http://www.foodrisk.org/index.efm.

Another consideration is the short-term versus long-term costs of implementing superior pathogen control options. Testing for pathogens is continuing to be cheaper, faster, more sensitive and more reliable. Pathogen test data from various locations in the plant and in the product can be combined with new data on the performance of existing HACCP programmes. This will allow identification of problem locations, continual evaluation of current operating systems and management programmes, and evaluation of the success of new improvements to solving pathogen problem areas. In addition, research and development efforts are looking for and evaluating new solutions to improve pathogen control in the slaughterhouse (such as steam pasteurization of carcasses) as well on the farm, in transporting animals, in transporting meat, case-ready products, etc.

Ranking food-borne disease risks

Setting priorities among the competing hazards (pathogens, pesticides, hormones, etc.) is critical for both public policy officials and companies who have scarce resources to allocate. The importance of estimating actual risks of food-borne illness, and not perceived risks, is often not appreciated. Both the precautionary principle and risk assessments using 'safety factors' (e.g. the US Environmental Protection Agency's estimates for pesticide and dioxin risks) are designed to overestimate risks. This makes comparisons across all food-borne hazards difficult for a private company or government regulators. To compare food-borne risks across pathogens, pesticides, hormones and other hazards, it is important to calculate 'best estimates' of risk for each hazard. To include the scientific uncertainty, confidence intervals can also be calculated around the 'best estimate', be it a point estimate of the mean or a probability distribution of all possible outcomes.

Economic incentives

In an efficient market, prices reflect the economic value of a good or service (see Golan *et al*. 2005 for a more complete discussion of the economic concepts in this paragraph). However, we do not observe different prices for products with reduced microbial contamination in the US marketplace. (Although irradiated hamburger is starting to be sold.) Thus, food safety is often a credence attribute—where consumers cannot usually discern before purchase, or even after consumption, whether a food was produced with the best or worst safety procedures, or whether a food poses a health risk. The fact that food safety attributes are difficult for consumers to detect means that firms producing high-risk food could charge low-risk prices and, because of their safety cost cutting, have greater profits than low-risk producers. As a result, producers may have an incentive to provide lower quality, higher risk food. Of course, if a firm is linked to an outbreak of food-borne illness, the loss in reputation and sales could outweigh the benefits of any food safety cost cutting. Though the threat of bad publicity may curtail incentives to cut safety corners, difficulty identifying the contaminated food responsible for an illness lessens both this threat and the threat of litigation. Complex diets, long incubation periods, incomplete laboratory analyses and the fact that the food evidence is usually destroyed (eaten) all reduce the chances of successful litigation (Buzby *et al*. 2001).

The ERS estimate of US$6.9 billion lost annually in medical costs, productivity losses and premature death for five US pathogens suggests an undersupply of food safety (http://www.ers.usda.gov/Emphases/SafeFood/features.htm#start). Because of the information problems associated with detecting hazards, companies have an incentive to underspend on food safety. This may suggest that the government should step in and put things right. The UK's problems with bovine spongioform encephalopathy (BSE) illustrates imperfect actions by government agents charged with ensuring food safety. USDA's FSIS has no ability to levy fines for non-compliance, limiting costs of non-compliance to companies cutting food safety corners (Buzby *et al*. 2001).

One regulatory option is improving food safety information to buyers in the marketplace. Approaches to address the lack of information directly (and minimize the market failure causing an undersupply of food safety) include the following.

1. Government or industry web sites posting data on each food company: its policy toward controlling pathogens, monitoring/testing data on the level of various pathogens found in the firm's testing programmes (for inputs, plant environment and products), and the company's actions taken after

each test result indicating contamination. This could be an expanded version of the UK programme that posts Hygiene Assessment Scores for all UK meat plants, accessible to both the food industry and consumers (Spriggs and Isaac 2001, p. 178).

2. Consumer labels that identify foods produced under a superior pathogen control programme, such as a 'gold star for safety'. This can be either a government or an industry programme. The Underwriters Laboratory rating for electricial products sold in the USA is a private programme with a good reputation for accuracy. ISO certification 9000 or 22000: 2005 could be examined, if a well-defined minimum level of safety was clearly defined for all companies meeting the standard.

3. Improved government surveillance systems could be set up to estimate more accurately the current level of food-borne disease in a country overall and from specific pathogens, foods and companies.

4. Improved information on food-borne pathogens and risk factors could be made available. For example, electronic databases could be built for use by consumers, industry and researchers that include the following information: the incidence of acute illness and complications from food-borne pathogens; identification of who the high-risk demographic groups are; quantification of which foods (including brand names) are associated with specific food-borne pathogens; and identification of which risky behaviours by consumers are associated with food-borne pathogens. One strategy to encourage better self-reporting of food-borne disease would be printing on the bottom of all menus and posting in all supermarkets, both a phone number (1-800-BAD-FOOD is a hypothetical phone number) and an Internet address at a national location where a form could be filled out.

An economic analysis could evaluate the short- and long-term impact of various options for increasing information on microbial food safety. In the long run, how does each option increase the economic incentives for developing new processes and technologies to provide safer food? What are the most efficient mechanisms for reducing information and transaction costs in the market for food safety?

By enacting a 'due diligence' clause in the 1990 Food Safety Act, the UK increased the private economic incentives for food safety. Supermarkets became legally liable for purchasing contaminated inputs and this empowered them to require suppliers for their private brand foods to exert more control over pathogens. The marketplace has responded, and new businesses have been created to certify the food safety efforts by UK food suppliers. Other countries could follow the UK's lead and enact stricter legal liability systems for all foods. Viscusi (1989), however, cautions that the legal liability system cannot address all market failure issues when safety is involved.

Spriggs and Isaac (2001) criticize the US HACCP regulations and *Salmonella* performance standards—they prefer a specific HACCP system identifying critical control points for *all* firms. The *Salmonella* (or other pathogen) performance standards, however, provide strong incentives for innovation. Each company has an incentive to invest in research and development and implement their innovations to meet the standard. Each company can determine if they have a comparative advantage in preventing contamination versus removing/killing contaminants on meat products, and choosing the mix of equipment and management systems that best achieve the level of microbial control required by the standard. (Note the *Salmonella* performance standard was challenged in the US courts and industry won. In response, USDA integrated the *Salmonella* test results more explicitly into HACCP regulatory and enforcement procedures.)

Discussion

The next decade will show vast changes in our ability to detect pathogens (Unnevehr *et al.* 2005), to develop risk assessment models for food-borne pathogens, to better identify and quantify the impact of improved control techniques on food-borne risks and to better understand the role economic cost-benefit analysis and economic incentives can play in improving food safety systems. Both the public and private sectors will be in a better position to control food-borne pathogens in the future. Unnevehr and Roberts (2002) discuss how food safety incentives are changing, even today, in the world food system: 'Food safety is becoming more important in food markets due to several structural changes in the world food system. These changes include advancements in the science of public health, changes in how consumers obtain and prepare food, and increased international trade in food products. These changes, which are apparent in both industrialized and developing nations, are creating enhanced market incentives for producers to improve food safety and enhanced political incentives for public intervention in food markets. Frequently, partnerships between the public and private sectors are needed to respond to the incentives for improved safety' (p. 73).

Spriggs and Isaac (2001) identify outbreaks of food-borne illness, domestically and abroad, as the major driver for change in national and international regulations and markets. As the world moves toward international markets, even for fresh beef, the responsibility for food safety is shifting among private and public agents. International arrangements, such as the Codex and the World Trade Organization (WTO), are gaining more oversight over food safety. For example, the WTO's Agreement on Sanitary and Phyto-sanitary Standards requires scientific proof of risks, transparency in the regulations, and basing national standards on Codex food safety standards.

Also the issue of how to develop international Food Safety Objectives, pathogen performance standards and/or Statistical Process Control will be long debated (Bisaillon *et al.* 1997; Sofos *et al.* 1999b, c; Powell *et al.* 2001; Spriggs and Isaac 2001).

Acknowledgements

The author appreciates the insightful review comments by Elise Golan, Helen Jensen and Jean Buzby.

References

Bisaillon, J.-R., Charlebois, R., Feltmate, T. and Labbe, Y. (1997) HACCP, statistical process control applied to post-mortem inspection and risk analysis in Canadian abbatoirs. *Dairy, Food, and Envirnmental Sanitation* **17**, 150–155.

Buzby, J., Robertsm T. and Allos, B.M. (1997) Estimated annual costs of *Campylobacter*-associated Guillain–Barre syndrome, USDA/ERS Agricultural Economics Report No. 756. On ERS website: http://www.ers.usda.gov/publications/aer756/.

Buzby, J.C., Frenzen, P.D. and Rasco, B. (2001) Product liability and microbial foodborne illness. ERS Agricultural Economic Report No. 799. On ERS website: http://www.ers.usda.gov/Publications/aer799/.

Council for Agricultural Science and Technology (CAST) (1994) *Foodborne Pathogens: Risks and Consequences*. CAST, Ames, IA.

Crutchfield, S.R., Buzby, J.C., Roberts, T., Ollinger, M. and Lin, C.-T.J. (1997) Economic assessment of food safety regulations: the new approach to meat and poultry inspection, Economic Research Service, USDA, Agricultural Economics Report No. 755. On ERS website: http://www.ers.usda.gov/publications/aer755/index.htm

Gill, C.O. (1998) *Apparatus for Pasteurizing Red Meat Carcasses*. Technical Bulletin 1998-5E, Agriculture and Agri-Food Canada, Lacombe, Alberta.

Gill, C.O. (1999) HACCP: by guesswork or by the numbers? *Food Quality* **6**, 28–32.

Gill, C.O. and Bryant, J. (1997) Assessment of the hygienic performances of two beef carcass cooling processes from product temperature history data or enumeration of bacteria on carcass surfaces. *Food Microbiology* **14**, 593–602.

Golan, E., Buzby, J., Crutchfield, C., Frenzen, P., Kuchler, F., Ralston, K. and Roberts, T. (2005) The value to consumers of reducing foodborne risks. In: Hoffman, S.A. and Taylor, M.R. (eds), *Toward Safer Food: Perspectives on Risk and Priority Setting*. Resources for the Future, Washington, DC, pp. 129–158.

Malcolm, S., Narrod, C., Roberts, T. and Ollinger, M. (2004) Evaluating the economic effectiveness of pathogen reduction technology in beef slaughter plants. *Agribusiness: An International Journal* **20**, 109–123.

Mead, P.S., Slutsker, L., Dietz, V., McCaig, L.F., Bresee, J.S., Shapiro, C., Griffin, P.M. and Tauxe, R.V. (1999) Food-related illness and death in the United States. *Emerging Infectious Diseases* **5**, 607–625.

Narrod, C.A., Malcolm, S.A., Ollinger, M. and Roberts, T. (1999) Pathogen reduction options in slaughterhouses and methods for evaluating their economic effectiveness. American Agricultural Economics Association meeting selected paper. http://agecon.lib.umn.edu/cgi-bin/pdf_view.pl?paperid=1786&ftype=.pdf

Porter, M. (1985) *Competitive Advantage: Creating and Sustaining Superior Performance.* Free Press, Simon and Schuster, New York.

Powell, M.R., Ebel, E.D., Hogue, A.T. and Schlosser, W.D. (2001) The promise and challenge of food safety performance standards. *Dairy, Food, and Environmental Sanitation* 21, 582–590.

Ralston, K., Brent, C.P., Starke, Y., Riggins, T. and Lin, C.T.J. (2002) Consumer food safety behavior: a case study in hamburger cooking and ordering. ERS, Agricultural Economic Report No. (AER804). On ERS website: http://www.ers.usda.gov/Publications/aer804/

Roberts, T., Ahl, A. and McDowell, R. (1995) Risk assessment for foodborne microbial hazards. In: Roberts, T., Jensen, H. and Unnevehr, L. (eds), *Tracking Foodborne Pathogens from Farm to Table: Data Needs To Evaluate Control Options.* US. Department of Agriculture, Economic Research Service, Miscellaneous Publication No. 1532, pp. 95–115. On ERS website: http://www.ers.usda.gov/publications/MP1532/mp1532.pdf

Roberts, T., Buzby, J., Lin, J., Nummery, P., Mead, P. and Tarr, P.I. (1998) New & resurgent infections: prediction, detection and management of tomorrow's epidemics. In: Greenwood, B. and De Cock, K. (eds), *London School of Hygiene & Tropical Medicine's Seventh Annual Public Health Forum.* John Wiley & Sons, Chichester, UK, pp. 155–172.

Roberts, T., Malcolm, S.A. and Narrod, C.A. (1999) Probabilistic risk assessment and slaughterhouse practices: modelling contamination process control in beef destined for hamburger. In: Modarres, M. (ed.), *Probabilistic Safety Assessment PSA '99: Risk-Informed Performance-based Regulation in the New Millennium.* American Nuclear Society, La Grange Park, IL, pp. 809–815. On ERS website: http://www.ers.usda.gov/briefing/IndustryFoodSafety/pdfs/psa9.pdf

Roberts, T., Narrod, C., Marcolm, S. and Modarres, M. (2001) An interdisciplinary approach to developing a probabilistic risk analysis model: application to a beef slaughterhouse. In: Hooker, H.N. and Murano, E.A. (eds), *Interdisciplinary Food Safety Research.* CRC Press, Boca Raton, FL, pp. 1–23.

Sofos, J.N., Kochevar, S.L., Bellinger, G.R., Buege, D.R., Hancock, D.D., Ingham, S.C., Morgan, J.B., Reagan, J.O. and Smith, G.C. (1999a) Sources and extent of microbiological contamination of beef carcasses in seven United States slaughtering plants. *Journal of Food Protection* 62, 140–145.

Sofos, J.N., Kochevar, S.L., Reagan, J.O. and Smith, G.C. (1999b) Extent of beef carcass contamination with *Escherichia coli* and probabilities of passing U.S. regulatory criteria. *Journal of Food Protection* 62, 234–238.

Sofos, J.N., Kochevar, S.L., Reagan, J.O. and Smith, G.C. (1999c) Incidence of *Salmonella* on beef carcasses relating to the U.S. meat and poultry inspection regulations. *Journal of Food Protection* 62, 467–473.

Spriggs, J. and Isaac, G. (2001) *Food Safety and International Competitiveness: The Case of Beef.* CABI Publishing, Wallingford, UK.

US Department of Agriculture, Food Safety and Inspection Service (2001) Inaccuracies in news articles concerning the decision by the U.S. Court of Appeals for the Fifth Circuit. In *Supreme Beef Processors, Inc. v. USDA* On USDA website: http://www.fsis.usda.gov/oa/news/2001/supremem&f.htm>

Unnevehr, L. and Roberts, T. (2002) Editorial: food safety incentives in a changing world food system. *Food Control* **13**, 73–76.

Unnevehr, L., Roberts, T. and Custer, C. (2005) New pathogen testing technologies and the market for food safety information. *AgBioForum* **7**, 212–218. Available online at www.agbioforum.org.

Viscusi, W.K. (1989) Toward a diminished role for tort liability: social insurance, government regulation, and contemporary risks to health and society. *Yale Journal on Regulation* **6**, 203–220.

Chapter 14

Transaction cost economics and principal–agent theory: insights into investigations of outbreaks of infectious diseases

Azarmeen Jamasji-Pavri

Introduction

Outbreaks of infectious disease occur when the incidence rises above the normal endemic level (Barker and Rose 1990) or when there are two or more linked cases of the same disease. The purpose of investigating these outbreaks is to identify the cause of the outbreak so that control measures can be implemented. Systematic, routine procedures exist for the investigation process. The plethora of instructional literature regarding these procedures (Goodman *et al.* 1990; Palmer 1990; Palmer 1995; Mackenzie and Goodman 1996; Reingold 1998) indicates their acceptance by the public health community. Despite the existence of technical literature on the subject, the situation-specific nature of outbreaks makes it impossible for a 'gold standard' to exist.

Investigations comprise epidemiological, microbiological and environmental components, each of which is composed of various steps (Table 14.1), not all of which are needed in every investigation. It is more important that the investigation be conducted in an organized and coordinated fashion, such that information from one step feeds into another and data from one component provide the basis for action in another. Considering that knowledge and expertise in various disciplines is required during investigations, it is recommended that investigations be conducted by teams of experts.

These experts are employed in public sector organizations and therefore are agents whose operations are affected by the bureaucracy of the organizations to which they belong and the external organizations with which they must cooperate. As prescriptive guidelines for the investigative process do not exist, agents representing various disciplines and different public organizations have to collaborate. In this complex web of relationships, it is difficult to ensure

Table 14.1 The steps to an outbreak investigation

Epidemiological component
Verify existence of outbreak
Confirm diagnosis
Take immediate control measures
Develop case definition
Institute case finding
Collect descriptive data in terms of time, person, place to determine common factors between cases
Develop hypotheses about the exposure responsible for the outbreak
Test hypotheses using analytical epidemiological studies
Execute control measures
Communicate findings
Microbiological component
Determine type of specimens to be collected
Collect specimens using appropriate media
Conduct tests on specimens for the appropriate pathogen as indicated by epidemiological hypotheses
Send positive specimens to reference laboratory for serotyping/phage typing
Environmental investigation
Conduct visual inspections of the environment
Take appropriate samples for testing

that investigations are conducted efficiently, expeditiously and scientifically, or to attribute weakness to any particular person or organization. It is this issue that compels one to draw on some theories of new institutional economics (NIE) to understand the implications of collaborative effort between bureaucrats on the investigative process. This class of theories proposes that the function of an organization should be studied in terms of its contracting behaviour which is a departure from the view of an organization as a production function (Williamson 1985). Figure 14.1 distinguishes between the former which is the Science of Contract and the latter that typifies the Science of Choice. The orthodox approach to economics as the study of 'human behaviour as a relationship between ends and scarce means which have alternative uses' (Robbins 1932) defines the Science of Choice.

Private ordering is split into two related branches, transaction cost economics (TCE) and incentive alignment. This chapter will consider the contribution

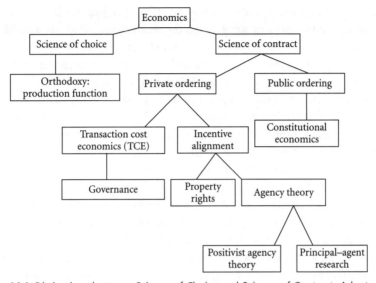

Fig. 14.1 Distinctions between Science of Choice and Science of Contract. Adapted from Williamson (2002).

of TCE and principal-agent theory to outbreak investigation practices. An overview of these theories will be presented and the rationale for using them to examine investigative practice will be explained. The theories will be applied to outbreak investigations, and the usefulness of governance solutions presented by them to control the investigative process will be considered.

This chapter draws on examples from the findings of a qualitative study that was conducted in New York State in which several investigators from various health departments participated (Jamasji 2006). The study focused on the execution of food-borne disease outbreak investigations. Data were derived from eight semi-structured interviews that were conducted with investigators in different health departments and a 9 month long case study that included participant observation, document analysis and informal interviews with various members of the Environmental Investigations Division in a health department.

The rationale for applying these theories to outbreak investigations

NIE may not immediately appear to be relevant to outbreak investigation, but as Williamson has stated any issue that can be reformulated as a contracting problem deserves to be considered through the lens of TCE (Williamson 1998). Outbreak investigations can in fact easily be conceived of as a contracting issue: a relationship in which one party agrees for a mutually agreed return to carry out some action on behalf of the other (see also Allen and Croxson Chapter 15). First, as investigators are employed in public bureaux, they are agents of the public and subordinates of managers in those organizations. These are contractual relationships that are vulnerable to the agency problems. Secondly, implicit contractual relationships exist between individuals who participate in investigations; the fact of their involvement in an investigation implies that the parties agree to be bound by the contract. Rights and obligations are exchanged; a promise or set of promises is made between agents to share relevant information and efficiently execute investigative tasks for which each agent is responsible. It should be noted that these interactions are situation specific, in that they depend on the public health infrastructure of the country in which the investigation takes place, the aetiology of the outbreak that is being investigated and the scale of the outbreak.

Figure 14.2 is a representation of some of the contractual relationships that develop within and outside an organization during the course of an investigation. This figure is derived from the findings of the New York study. Thus it describes the transactional relationships involved in the investigation of a food poisoning outbreak at a regional level using the main, local investigator as the focal point of the transactions. From the figure, it is seen that there is a core group of individuals with whom transactions occur most frequently, a secondary group within the organization which is only peripherally involved and is mostly responsible for overseeing the process, and several individuals outside the organization with whom interaction is essential. Officials from other public health organizations are usually only involved in investigations that extend beyond the local health department's jurisdiction or are so complicated that they are beyond the expertise of local investigators.

Principal–agent research

The theory

In an organization, there is a contractual relationship between the principal and the agent. The principal delegates a task, accompanied by the decision-making authority pertaining to that task, to the agent with the expectation that the task will be executed on his behalf (Jensen and Meckling 1976). If it is assumed that individuals are utility maximizers, it follows that an agent will act in his own best interests to maximize the gain from any transaction for himself. Therefore, when his interests are in conflict with the principal's, it is likely that he will choose actions that will benefit himself (Jensen and Meckling 1976). These actions can take the form of moral hazard (lack of effort on part

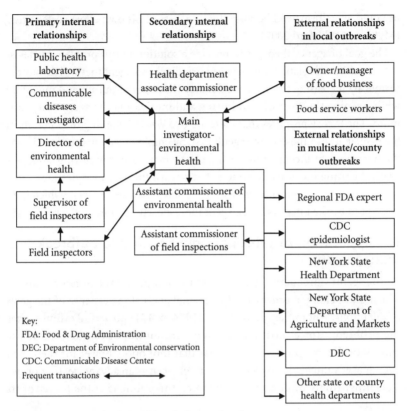

Fig. 14.2 Contractual relationships during outbreaks.

of the agent) and adverse selection (inappropriate effort that undermines the goals of the principal) (Fama and Jensen 1983). The principal is further disadvantaged because any attempts to monitor the agent and thereby check subversive behaviour are often prohibitively difficult and expensive. Consequently, an information asymmetry, that favours the agent, exists. Principals and agents may also have divergent perspectives on risk, which is a product of the fact that they occupy different levels on the rungs of the organizational ladder.

This is important because managerial decisions involve taking action in the presence of ambiguity, uncertainty and risk (Shapira 2000). Not only are principals and agents in disagreement as to the level of risk that should be assumed, they may also disagree as to who should assume that risk. Shapira (2000) argues that the greater the risk the greater is the difference in the perception between principal and agent about who should assume responsibility for that risk. As the agent is risk averse, he will supply lower effort than he could actually expend because this 'puts less of his own effort costs at risk' (Miller and Whitford 2002).

The goal of agency theory is to provide a solution to this problem by devising a contractual relationship between principal and agent that will favour the former by increasing the agent's efficiency (in terms of output and outcome) while keeping the costs of monitoring and motivating the agent to a minimum. The theory proposes that there are two ways of aligning the interests of the principal with those of the agent; first, by employing contracts that change the behaviour of the agent by raising pay or increased monitoring, and, secondly, by using incentive contracts that reward the agent for desirable outcomes by stock options or commissions (Nilakant and Rao 1994), which is an attempt to tie the interests of the agent more closely to those of the principal.

The application of principal–agent theory to outbreak management

Public sector bureaucrats are inclined to manipulate the organizations to which they belong in order to fulfil personal goals at the expense of the goals of the public, whom they serve. Savas (1974, p. 474) powerfully summarizes the problem: 'since most city agencies are monopolies, their staffs are automatically in a position to exercise that monopoly power for their own parochial advantage—and efficiency is rarely seen as an advantage. In short we have unwittingly built a system in which the public is at the mercy of its servants'.

If this is the case, it follows that the quality of an investigation will not be an investigator's primary concern. Therefore, there may be conflict between the interests of the public (the ultimate principal) and the organization and investigator (agents). The natural tendency of the investigator will be to conduct an average investigation thereby expending minimal effort. Miller and Whitford (2002) believe that the costs of attaining excellence in a public bureaucracy are so large that most agents will be unwilling to expend the additional effort that is required

This argument may be criticized for not considering the impact that intrinsic controls have in regulating the behaviour of employees, whereby the bureau, another social body and social or personal principles prevent investigators from engaging in opportunistic behaviour by inculcating conformance with the principal's goals. These intrinsic controls include professionalism, the existence of a public service ethos among investigators who believe in the moral superiority of their remit in terms of its ability to protect the public and compliance with organizational or professional norms, and perhaps even the satisfaction of resolving a problem.

However, the study in New York State (Jamasji 2006) reported that these intrinsic controls either did not exist or were superseded by agency. Investigators expended just enough effort to ensure continued employment by not arousing suspicion. They executed tasks but did not use their initiative to look into issues that arose as a result of those tasks as that would have required the expenditure of additional effort, for example they chose not to expand investigations as that would have entailed greater effort.

As his actions are not readily observable, the investigator is able to conceal his lack of effort from the public because it lacks the resources, capacity and knowledge to monitor his actions. As illustrated by Fig. 14.2, those responsible for monitoring the investigative process are not an integral part of the investigation, which reduces their ability to monitor investigations adequately. Investigators in this study demonstrated an awareness of their inefficiency and realized that their opportunism undermined the principal. However, they were comfortable doing so because as one investigator confessed 'the right hand doesn't know what the left hand does at the Health Department', which facilitates the capture of information by agents. It was also found that agents actively work towards maintaining the asymmetry as they have a vested interest in organizational malfunction.

Other asymmetries also exist between principals and agents in terms of power, perspectives and aspirations (Shapira 2000). As the principal wields greater power than the agent, he may use or abuse it. Principals can use information asymmetry to their advantage and withhold information that could demotivate agents or structure transactions in such a manner that risks are disproportionately borne by the agent. On one occasion, the main investigator (principal) instructed field inspectors (agents) to take enforcement action against a food business because she was uncomfortable doing so as she felt the action was unwarranted. Hence, she transferred the risk of taking an unnecessary action to unsuspecting agents. The asymmetries in risk perception between principals and agents could also reflect the asymmetrical aspirations of the two parties. March and Shapira (1987) contend that risk behaviour is related to an individual's resources and ambitions, and that an individual will take risk commensurate with the factor that is more important to him. They predict that those who focus on maximizing their ambitions are likely to take larger risks than those who are concerned with their financial security. Principals, being higher in the hierarchy, have greater financial security and may be less risk averse than agents. This demonstrates that conflict between principal and agent is built into the organizational structure and is therefore difficult to mitigate.

Another problem with organizational structure is that it introduces multiple principals and agents, all of whose goals conflict with each other and those of the public, the ultimate principal, for example the main investigator, being higher in the hierarchy than field inspectors, assumes the role of principal. However, as she is subordinate to others in the hierarchy, she is also their agent as well as the agent of the public. The investigation process exacerbates this problem because for the duration of the investigation additional principal-agent relationships are created between team members. Breton and Wintrobe (1982) postulated that the presence of hierarchy causes 'selective behaviour'— the behaviour of subordinates who at times are efficient (cooperative and collaborative) and at other times are inefficient in pursuing the goals of their superiors. These agency costs arise in any situation that requires cooperative effort such as the superior-subordinate relationship or between team members during an investigation. The consequence is that the investigation suffers not only because the investigator is work averse but also because other individuals who contribute to the investigation have multiple and conflicting goals. This is especially noticeable when other agencies become involved in investigations. An example of such conflict comes from the New York study in which local investigators were willing to conduct blanket screening of food service workers and untargeted sampling of food. From their perspective, any attempts to find the causative pathogen were justifiable. However, these attempts increased the burden that the laboratory had to shoulder and wasted considerable resources.

Can monitoring and incentives be used to improve outbreak investigations?

Traditional options of monitoring and offering incentives to counter the principal-agent problem cannot be successful in the context of public bureaux that undertake outbreak investigations. Several issues make monitoring investigators difficult (if not impossible). This is because outbreaks are judgment-based exercises which are non-prescriptive and do not have fixed outcome measures. The lack of pre-specified formulae to dictate the path that an investigation is supposed to take allows investigators to hide behind their decisions and makes it difficult for superiors to evaluate their performance. With the power of information asymmetry, subordinates can manipulate data, rendering the exercise of monitoring entirely meaningless. In addition, bounded rationality, which refers to behaviour that is 'intendedly rational but only limitedly so' (Simon 1957a), implies that the cognitive limitations of the principal make him incapable of perfectly monitoring an agent anyway. When monitoring is impossible, investigators have to be trusted to perform their duties; this means that conditions conducive to the development of trust have to be present.

Incentive contracts may be successful but, in order for these to operate effectively, an outcome measure that can be evaluated is needed. In the absence of such a measure for investigations, the relationship between effort and outcome remains ambiguous. Consequently, it would be futile to link employment contracts with investigative performance. Besides, in the absence of a fixed standard of investigation quality, there is bound to be disagreement between principal and agent as to what constitutes a good investigation. Even if hypothetically and unrealistically both parties agreed on this matter, the uncertainties surrounding an investigation mean that investigators do not always have full control over the quality of the investigation. These uncertainties include, but are not limited to, technical limitations, constrained resources and lack of cooperation from parties involved, including other government agencies and physicians.

So while this theory has the capacity to provide explanations for the cause of investigators' behaviour, it cannot provide an adequate solution to the agency problem in terms of outbreak investigations. Consequently, we need to turn to governance theory, which provides a more satisfactory answer to accountability problems in organizations

Transaction cost economics

The theory

According to this theory, a transaction is the basic unit of analysis and governance is the means of ensuring that order prevails during the transaction, the completion of which is always threatened by conflict because contracts by their very nature are incomplete because they are incapable of specifying all eventualities and all future events that can interfere with the transaction. As the attributes of transactions are different, they need to be aligned with appropriate governance structures which can reduce transaction costs. Transaction costs are incurred during the transformation of input to output. These costs can be *ex ante* or *ex post*. The former include measurement costs which are associated with collecting information about the attribute of a commodity or service that is the object of a contract and about the reliability and trustworthiness of the parties to the contract. *Ex post* costs are associated with the monitoring of contracts to ensure that the parties to the contract are compliant and the costs that are incurred if the parties fail to uphold their obligations. Incentive alignment attempts to reduce *ex ante* costs by building safeguards into contracts to protect against all possible contingencies. TCE focuses on *ex post* institutions of contract and makes the argument that markets and hierarchies are alternative forms of governance (Coase 1937) and that form of governance which has the lowest transaction costs will be chosen. The choice of governance structure is dependent on the attributes of a transaction and the costs and characteristics of alternative forms of governance.

According to Williamson (1985), governance is affected by the institutional environment and the individual. The former provides the 'rules of the game' and therefore any changes in this will result in changing the costs of governance, while individuals are responsible for the behavioural attributes that shape TCE theory. TCE subscribes to the view that individuals have the attributes of bounded rationality and severe self-interest. The implications of bounded rationality as a cognitive assumption are 2-fold; first, the maximizing man is replaced by the satisficing man, who is willing to accept an outcome that is 'good enough' and, secondly, the cognitive limitations of man make the creation of organizations imperative (Simon 1957b). The lesson that TCE draws from bounded rationality is that the cognitive limitations of men obviously give rise to incomplete contracts. As a result of gaps, errors and omissions, contracts are vulnerable to unforeseen disturbances. Another factor that gives rise to problems when dealing with contracts is that of opportunism.

Strategic behaviour by economic actors borne entirely out of self-interest can take supremacy over fulfilling contractual obligations faithfully. However, it should be noted that if men succumb to opportunistic behaviour in order to maximize personal gain, the theory of the satisficing man who is content 'making do' collapses. Not all economic actors are always opportunistic, but it should be acknowledged that some actors will be opportunistic at least some of the time. Hart's comments are a particularly good characterization of human nature: 'All are tempted at times to prefer their own immediate interests . . .' (Hart 1961). If such behaviour is inevitable, it is important that sanctions are available to check it. When opportunism is combined with behavioural uncertainty, it results in information impactedness. This 'exists when true underlying circumstances relevant to the transaction, or related set of transactions, are known to one or more parties but cannot be costlessly discerned by or displayed for others' (Williamson 1975).

As bounded rationality results in incomplete contracts, parties to contracts are tempted to behave opportunistically. Consequently, conflict arises and transaction costs are incurred in settling disputes. While classical contracting advocates the use of courts as a forum for addressing such disputes, TCE proposes that contractual disputes can often be settled without recourse to the courts by avoidance, self-help or mediation (Galanter 1981). In fact, courts may be less effective because they are an external party with limited knowledge of the contract and are bound to uphold legal rules which may not be entirely relevant to the disputed situation. Indeed, courts may even refuse to preside over certain types of disputes, especially intra-organizational disputes, unless there is evidence of bad faith or corruption.

Moreover, in a climate of bounded rationality and opportunism (Williamson 1975), courts become less capable of presiding over disputes effectively, and certainly the level of research required means that the costs incurred by relying on the courts become exorbitant (Williamson 2002). Therefore, it is best if courts are used as the last resort, but their very existence serves to delimit threat positions, thereby promoting private ordering.

The application of TCE to outbreak investigations

During investigations, transactions occur when information about the outbreak is converted into outcomes through transformation activities. Each step in an investigation (Table 14.1) is a transaction. Therefore, outbreak management is composed of a series of transactions. Hence transaction, as a unit of analysis, is a valid concept in terms of outbreak investigation.

The behavioural assumptions that shape TCE also hold for agents engaged in investigative activities. Bounded rationality imposes limitations on an investigator's capacity to process information perfectly. In terms of outbreak investigations, there are several interpretations of this factor. First, it means that the perfect investigation is an illusion and that the best way to minimize the impact of bounded rationality is to have a team of investigators instead of just one individual. Secondly, rather than wanting to maximize the quality of investigations, investigators are satisfied with an average product, which is 'just good enough' because they acknowledge their limitations. Therefore, they are more likely to pursue the investigation of outbreaks that are confined to clearly delineated cohorts and yield answers easily rather than outbreaks that are difficult to detect and manage as they may involve cases that are spread across a region and are not associated with a discrete event (Jamasji 2006). Thirdly, it explains investigators' tendency to focus on only that specific aspect of an investigation for which they are responsible or on the impact of the outbreak in their geographical jurisdiction without much regard to the larger picture. This translates into the pursuit of subgoals rather than an interest in obtaining answers to the investigation in general. Although agents from different agencies may be part of the investigative team, they have to abide by the organizational policies and confidentiality clauses of the agencies to which they belong. Thus transparency and coordination may be sacrificed to the detriment of the investigation.

Subgoal pursuit is complicated by the fact that individual investigators are also opportunistic. The principal-gent problem has posited that as bureaucrats, investigators have a tendency to engage in opportunistic behaviour, which arises out of self-interest. Finally, many of the actors in an investigation misrepresent or withhold information from other parties because of confidentiality rules or because they want to maintain information asymmetry.

Considering this, the transactions of outbreak investigation need to be embedded in appropriate governance structures that can minimize transaction costs. According to Milgrom and Roberts (1992), most of the characteristics of a transaction that determine the appropriate mode of governance are:

- asset specificity
- frequency of similar transactions
- complexity and uncertainty surrounding the transaction
- difficulty of measuring performance in the transaction
- reliance on other transactions involving other people.

As the specificity of the assets increases, it makes more sense for the transaction to be conducted in a hierarchical organization. In terms of an investigation, human assets are most important. The training, experience and accumulated knowledge of investigators are not easily replaceable or deployable to another use without a reduction in their productive value. The practical knowledge that investigators possess coupled with their understanding of internal bureau policies and the relationships that they have developed within and outside the bureau make their contribution to the investigative process particularly specific. Figure 14.2 has highlighted a core group of contractual relationships in which the frequency of transactions between the parties is high. Social conditioning is attained through these relationships and is responsible for developing professional and group norms which can act as intrinsic controls to reduce opportunism.

The size of the population for which the health department is responsible, the diligence and dedication of investigative agents, the ability of surveillance systems to detect outbreaks and the capacity within health departments to investigate recognized outbreaks determine the frequency with which investigations are undertaken. When investigations occur frequently, the relationship between the parties is a recurrent or ongoing one. Consequently, it makes most sense for these relationships to be contained in a single governance structure; from Fig. 14.2 it can be seen that most frequently occurring transactions during investigations take place within the local health department, i.e. within one institution of governance. However, recurrent relationships are a mixed blessing. While an ongoing relationship can discipline parties to act non-opportunistically, it can also give rise to a bilateral relationship where the creation of trust makes regulatory capture possible as vigilance against opportunism is relaxed in favour of good continuing relationships. Main investigators and inspectors work in the same division and on many investigations together. Therefore, at the case study location in New York (Jamasji 2006), in the interests of continued cooperation, the main investigator relaxes her supervisory role which allows moral hazard and shirking to prevail among inspectors.

In addition, investigations are complicated; the characteristics of outbreaks are different and the factors that facilitate or hinder investigations also vary between investigations. Consequently, as there is great uncertainty surrounding an investigation, it is difficult to gauge the kind of performance that is required by an investigator. This is compounded by the fact that there are no measurable standards of performance. These factors make it difficult to write a contract that adequately specifies the task.

Finally, as each investigation is composed of several transactions that involve various individuals, the performance during each component of an investigation (i.e. transaction) is directly affected by the performance of other individuals who control other components, for example the ability of field inspectors to gather data comprehensively and efficiently and transmit it to the main investigator expeditiously affects the ability of the main investigator to devise scientifically sound hypotheses about the cause of the outbreak, which can then be tested by the communicable diseases investigator mounting an appropriate analytical study to identify the cause of the illness epidemiologically. Therefore, transaction costs incurred during one transaction have an adverse effect on another. Thus all these factors dictate that an outbreak investigation should be performed by individuals who belong to a single bureau because in order to perform it satisfactorily there is a great need for cooperative adaptation.

Hayek's statement that 'economic problems arise always and only in the consequence of change' (Hayek 1945) indicates that the organization has to be adaptive to these changes in order to survive. Different forms of governance have different levels of adaptability. Adaptation can be autonomous or cooperative. The benefit of the price mechanism is that it can adapt autonomously to change, which is why the market form of governance does not require cooperative adaptation. Hierarchies, on the other hand, require 'that kind of cooperation among men that is conscious, deliberate, and purposeful' (Barnard 1938) and is provided by formal organization.

When conditions of bilateral dependency intrude in a contractual relationship, transaction costs can be reduced by adopting a hierarchical mode of governance because formal organization, which is a hallmark of hierarchies, is adept at dealing with unanticipated disturbances. The advantage of this mode of governance is the presence of administrative controls. On the other hand incentive intensity diminishes in hierarchies because changes in effort do not have an impact on compensation in the immediate future (Williamson 1996). Therefore, from a TCE perspective, individuals who perform investigations should ideally be governed by hierarchical organizations.

However, the type of hierarchy within which they operate is a public bureau rather than a firm as the problems of uncertainty, externality and ambiguous property rights make it difficult for infection control to be outsourced to the private sector. First, as the nature of outbreaks is variable, it is difficult to predict the scope of the outbreak, the complexity of the investigation, and the time and resources that will be required. This uncertainty makes it difficult for complete contracts to be written which would be needed if the activity was run by or contracted out to a private company. Secondly, infectious disease control is a classic externality, in that the control of infectious diseases directly affects individuals who have neither been afflicted by the disease nor are involved in any aspect of its control or prevention. Thirdly, it is difficult to assign property rights over infectious diseases because diseases do not respect organizational or geographical boundaries. In a study, Allen *et al* (2002) revealed the wrangling over responsibility for MRSA (methycillin-resistant *Staphylococcus aureus*) between different NHS Trusts. Although the public bureau is the organization form of last resort (Williamson 1998), it is most appropriate for activities related to infectious disease control.

Are instruments of governance useful during outbreak investigation?

In situations such as outbreak investigations, where cooperative adaptation is essential, hierarchies inherently have certain instruments whereby conscious, deliberate control to coordinate an organization's response to changing circumstances can be exercised. These instruments include: fiat, forbearance, and formal and informal organization.

Fiat

In order to bring about cooperative adaptation, fiat is the main instrument to which bureaux have access. There are different theories of authority; the most commonly held one is that it originates at the top of an organization and filters downwards, compelling those it encompasses to obey the rules set out by those at the top of the organization (Hobbes 1928). In Barnard's view, authority arises out of mutual consent and can only bring about cooperation if subordinates choose to accept it (Barnard 1938). This can explain why orders are routinely disobeyed because if subordinates can choose whether or not to accept authority they may choose not to. According to Barnard (1938), there is a balance between incentives and sacrifices. When the sacrifice related to an order outweighs the inducements, subordinates refuse to follow orders and in extreme circumstances they may quit, but usually resort to 'malingering and unreliability' which causes inefficiency. In the New York study (Jamasji 2006), it was found that the authority that is transmitted to officials down the hierarchical ladder was incomplete. In order to establish accountability, superiors must have adequate authority to ensure that subordinates execute the tasks assigned to them. Jaques (2005) identified the four elements that have to be present.

1. The right to veto applicants for a position whose ability falls short is not commensurate with the challenges of the job.

2. The power to assign work.

3. The power to conduct appraisals and to make decisions and not merely recommendations about raises and rewards.

4. The power to terminate employment, at least, in the division.

In public bureaux, superiors who are one hierarchical level above investigators and thus in a position of authority relative to them lack most of these essential elements. While they delegate work, assign discrete tasks and even make some attempts at appraisal, their ability to reward or punish their subordinates is limited. These are decisions that are made in the higher ranks of the ladder. The result is that the authority that direct superiors possess over their subordinates is meaningless.

The only circumstances in which individuals can be relied upon to accept authority is if the intrinsic controls of professionalism and public service ethos operate effectively or if an environment that inculcates trust between superiors and subordinates exists so that the individual is obligated to his superior to act in the latter's best interest. However, as supervisors are only peripherally involved in investigations (Fig. 14.2), the low frequency of transactions means that there is not much opportunity for trust to develop, at least during the course of investigations.

Informal organization

In his theory, Barnard made provision for formal and informal organization (which co-exist in a bureau) and claimed that the latter arose spontaneously. There are questions about the efficacy of the formal organization to govern the investigative process effectively. The official codes, rules and procedures that define hierarchies often prevent individual initiative, forbid the deletion of unnecessary or cumbersome steps, prohibit bureaucrats from changing onerous procedures and inhibit the acceptance of risk and responsibility for terminating useless operations. These restrictions effectively prevent efficiency increasing actions (Breton and Wintrobe 1982). When one considers the importance of initiative, flexibility and efficiency during the investigation of outbreaks, it becomes obvious that the strictures associated with a formal, hierarchical structure are likely to suppress these traits.

Coordination within the formal organization hinges on the presence of informal relationships which facilitate communication, organizational cohesion and personal integrity (Barnard 1938). Any formal organization provides the bedrock for informal organizations to develop which are a response to the opportunities and problems inherent in the formal structure. They offer a means of coping with the gaps in official policies and practices as well as the creation of networks of social relations (Blau and Scott 2005). While informal organizations may be a means of raising esprit de corps and bringing about conformity to group norms, they can also create problems. By using the relationships that have developed as a result of investigative team work, agents can use informal relationships to undermine the formal organization. While the hierarchy is supposed to be a tool for facilitating communication and delegating authority, bureaucrats may be able to misuse these very qualities. They can control the flow of information or commands through the hierarchy, vary the quality and quantity of information that is leaked to those who should not be privy to it and change the speed of implementing policies. All these factors cause transaction costs, yet it is impossible for a superior to chastise a bureaucrat for any of these inefficiencies because it is impossible to prove that any of the inefficiencies were deliberate. Loss and distortion of information occurs naturally in an organization, some information leakages are also inevitable, and red tape (which is a naturally occurring phenomenon) can provide an effective screen under which policies and practices can be systematically sabotaged. On the other hand, informal organizations promote cohesion among investigators by creating clans—organic associations that resemble kin networks (Durkheim, 1933). These breed a sense of community and foster professional norms which counter opportunism.

The investigative team is a form of formal organization that largely remains constant. Thus investigation as a transaction is embedded in informal relationships that develop over time due to interaction between investigators. Interactions between actors in the core group become increasingly social and thus, over the long term, trust replaces opportunism (Williamson 1996). With growing trust, transaction costs are decreased as division of labour, cooperation and information sharing become embedded in the relationships. However, when investigators who are not part of the usual team become involved on an *ad hoc* basis such as those from other agencies during multistate/county outbreaks, transaction costs may rise as there is no history of transactions between these investigators and no potential for repeated transactions. This may explain why local investigators mistrust Food and Drug Administration (FDA) investigators who are not consistently part of local investigative teams.

Forbearance law

The implicit law of forbearance presides over disputes in hierarchies (Williamson 1991). According to this, disputes are settled internally because of the existence of fiat. In public bureaux, however, forbearance may fail to operate as intended. While forbearance may be available, personnel may choose not to settle their disputes because of the negative connotations associated with this practice. Disputes can fester and resentment towards the organization and the individuals involved may build. The result can be an individual who operates at a suboptimal level and in the worst case scenario actively tries to sabotage the organization from within (Jamasji 2006).

Conclusion

These theories offer a novel interpretation of the problems inherent in investigative practice. According to this perspective, the qualities of organizations that run outbreak investigations and the bureaucratic agents who conduct them influence the performance of investigations. The conflicting goals of principal and agent caused by information and risk asymmetry allow opportunism to prevail. In investigative terms, this means that the investigator engages in moral hazard by shirking investigative tasks or executing them at a suboptimal level. However, incentive contracts and monitoring that are supposed to counter agency cannot work in this situation. Therefore, TCE and governance theory offer solutions. The most appropriate form of governance for investigations is the public sector hierarchy. While the instruments of fiat, informal organization and forbearance have the potential to reduce transaction costs during investigations, their operation within a public sector bureaucracy limits their efficacy. When investigations are viewed through the contractual lens, an important finding is that investigative networks are essential as they are a normative means of building trust and professionalism which encourage transparency and counter opportunism. The performance of investigations by teams limits bounded rationality and aligns the goals of principal and agent.

References

Allen, P., Croxson, B., Roberts, J.A., Archibald, K., Crawshaw, S. and Taylor, L. (2002) The use of contracts in the management of infectious disease related risk in the NHS internal market. *Health Policy* **59**, 257–281.

Barker, D.J.P. and Rose, G. (1990) *Epidemiology in Medical Practice*. Churchill Livingstone, New York.

Barnard, C. (1938) *The Functions of the Executive*. Harvard University Press, Cambridge, MA.

Blau, P.M. and Scott, W.R. (2005) The concept of formal organization. In: Shafritz, J.M., Ott, S. and Jang, Y.S. (eds), *Classics of Organization Theory*. Thomson-Wadsworth, Belmont, CA.

Breton, A. and Wintrobe, R. (1982) *The Logic of Bureaucratic Conduct*. Cambridge University Press, New York.

Coase, R.H. (1937) The nature of the firm. *Economica N.S.* **4**, 386–405.

Durkheim E (1933) The division of labor in society. Translated by G. Simpson. Free Press, New York.

Fama, E. and Jensen, M. (1983) Separation of ownership and control. *Journal of Law and Economics* **26**, 301–326.

Galanter, M. (1981) Justice in many rooms: courts, private ordering and indigenous law. *Journal of Legal Pluralism* **19**, 1–47.

Goodman, R.A., Buehler, J.W. and Koplan, J.P. (1990) The epidemiologic field investigation: science and judgment in public health practice. *American Journal of Epidemiology* **132**, 9–16.

Hart, H.L.A. (1961) *The Concept of Law*. Oxford University Press, Oxford.

Hayek, F. (1945) The uses of knowledge in society. *American Economic Review* **35**: 519–530.

Hobbes, T. (1928) *Leviathan, or the Matter, Form and Power of Commonwealth Ecclesiastical and Civil*. Basil Blackwell, Oxford.

Jaques, E. (2005) In praise of hierarchy. In: Shafritz, J.M., Ott, S. and Jang, Y.S. (eds), *Classics of Organization Theory*. Thomson-Wadsworth, Belmont, CA.

Jamasji, A. (2006) A Study of the Investigation of Food Poisoning Outbreaks in New York State: The Divergence of Theory and Practice. PhD thesis, University of London.

Jensen, M. and Meckling, W. (1976) The theory of the firm: managerial behaviour agency costs and ownership structure. *Journal of Financial Economics* **3**, 305–360.

Keene, W.E. (1999) Lessons from investigations of foodborne disease outbreaks. *Journal of the American Medical Association* **281**, 1845–1847.

MacKenzie and Goodman, R.A. (1996) The public health response to an outbreak. *Current Issues in Public Health* **2**, 1–4.

March, J. and Shapira, Z. (1987) Variable risk preference and focus of attention. *Psychological Review* **99**, 172–183.

Miller, G. and Whitford, A.B. (2002) Trust and incentives in principal-agent negotiations— the insurance/incentive trade-off. *Journal of Theoretical Politics* **14**, 231–267.

Milgrom, P. and Roberts, J. (1992) *Economics, Organization and Management*. Prentice-Hall, Englewood Cliffs, NJ.

Nilakant, V. and Rao, H. (1994) Agency theory and uncertainty in organizations: an evaluation. *Organization Studies* **15**, 649–672.

Palmer, S.R. (1990) Epidemiologic methods in the investigation of food poisoning outbreaks. *Letters in Applied Microbiology* 11, 109–115.

Palmer, S.R. (1995) Outbreak investigation the need for quick and clean epidemiology. *International Journal of Epidemiology* 24 (Supplement 1), S34–S38.

Reingold, A. (1998) Outbreak investigations—a perspective. *Emerging Infectious Diseases* 4 (1), 21–7. www.cdc/nc1dod/e1d/vol4No1/reingold.htm.

Robbins, L. (1932) *An Essay on the Nature and Significance of Economic Science.* New York University Press, New York.

Savas, E. (1974) Municipal monopolies versus competition in delivering urban services. In: Hawley, W. and Rogers, D. (eds), *Improving the Quality of Urban Management.* Sage, Beverly Hills, CA.

Shapira, Z. (2000) Governance in organizations: a cognitive perspective. *Journal of Management and Governance* 4, 53–67.

Simon, H. (1957a) *Administrative Behaviour.* Macmillan, New York.

Simon, H. (1957b) *Models of Man.* Wiley, New York.

Williamson, O.E. (1975) *Markets and Hierarchies: Analysis and Antitrust Implications.* Free Press New York.

Williamson, O.E. (1985) *The Economic Institutions of Capitalism.* Free Press, New York.

Williamson, O.E. (1991) Comparative economic organization: the analysis of discrete structural alternatives. *Administrative Science Quarterly* 36, 269–296.

Williamson, O.E. (1996) *The Mechanisms of Governance.* Oxford University Press, New York.

Williamson, O.E. (1998) Transaction cost economics: how it works; where it is headed. *De Economist* 146, 23–58.

Williamson, O.E. (2002) The theory of the firm as governance structure: from choice to contract. *Journal of Economic Perspectives* 16, 171–195.

Chapter 15

Governance arrangements for the control of infectious disease

Pauline Allen and Bronwyn Croxson

Introduction

This chapter is about the effect of governance structures on the ability of public health services to carry out infectious disease control. The economics of governance as developed in new institutional economics and the closely related socio-legal study of contracting will be used as analytical tools to understand how organizational structures affect infectious disease control. Data from a study of contracting for infectious disease control in the former British National Health Service (NHS) will be used to illustrate underlying principles.

The special economic characteristics of infection and infection control

Infectious disease has special characteristics which need to be taken into account when designing a governance structure. Infectious disease is difficult to predict, i.e. it is associated with uncertainty. Infections affect others both concurrently and over time: they exhibit externalities. Infection control, or the lack of it, has the characteristics of a public good: if it is provided, it is usually available to all, whether they are willing to pay or not. Some knowledge of infections and some concept of the likely implications in terms of mortality and morbidity, and cost are required by those planning and managing health services.

Agent, host and environmental factors are all important epidemiologically (Benenson 1994). The infectivity and pathogenicity of the organism, the pre-existing health or disease in the host, and the environmental features influencing geographical distribution and seasonal variation determine when and where outbreaks occur.

Hospitals are reservoirs of susceptible individuals, some predisposed to infection by virtue of their immunosupressed status and others undergoing procedures which increase their risk of acquiring infection (Plowman *et al.* 1997). Against a background prevalence of infection in hospital wards, there may, for example, be outbreaks of methicillin-resistant *Staphylococcus aureus* (MRSA). The imprudent use of some antibiotics in medical, veterinary or farming circles may encourage the development of drug resistance, so diminishing the useful armament of future drugs and in doing so jeopardizing future protection of others. Poorly organized programmes for treatment of tuberculosis (TB), for example, can result in multidrug-resistant strains of TB (MDRTB) arising, particularly affecting immunosupressed individuals (Humphreys and Duckworth 1997). What is or is not done to control infection today may influence the subsequent form and extent of future infection.

There are other 'externalities' (which are discussed in more detail below). For instance, certain infections such as hepatitis B, syphilis and human immunodeficiency virus (HIV) can be passed on to the developing fetus, and hence to subsequent generations. At the population level, some people receive preventive immunization which protects themselves and others from infection, whilst others receive medicine that, whilst not protecting themselves, might prevent them affecting others. Examples of the latter are prophylactic antibiotics for meningitis or exclusion from work of food handlers who have experienced an intestinal infection.

Hospitals have to take on the care of cases of infection that may result from failures in environmental and public health procedures. Whether these infections are directly attributable to failures of other parties or not, hospitals, in the UK NHS, will have to absorb some of the costs associated with them. These costs may or may not be adequately covered by the contracts. For example, in the case of a major outbreak of *Escherichia coli* O157 which originated in the community, the laboratory service had to absorb costs of dealing with additional diagnostic and therapeutic investigations associated with the outbreak that were far in excess of the normal work load (Roberts and Upton 2000).

If the sequelae of infection, together with externalities that arise from infection control (or the lack of it), are not taken into account by those purchasing health care and those providing it in hospitals, then infection may well have an impact on other institutions (such as nursing homes or community services), or on individuals following their discharge from hospitals.

Internal arrangements for managing budgets within a hospital may also impede the development of appropriate control procedures. Practices in hospital theatres, for example, may impose costs on surgical wards and intensive care units. Also, in the community, if adequate public and environmental health provision is not made for infections that arise, repercussions may rebound upon general practitioners and hospitals.

Moreover, infections are difficult to predict. In the community, clusters of meningococcal infections may occur (commonly in schools or colleges of higher education) against a background of sporadic cases, and influenza may outstrip its predictable winter seasonal levels in years where there is an epidemic or pandemic increase in cases (Allison 1991). Sporadic cases of *E.coli* O157 occur on a regular basis, but most districts to date have escaped the effects of a large-scale outbreak as witnessed in Scotland (Pennington Report 1997).

Major outbreaks cannot be predicted by any single hospital. Whereas major incidents are subject to 'major accident plans', infections are not usually included. This leaves hospitals exposed and sometimes unprepared to deal with such risks. For example, an outbreak of *E.coli* O157 imposed substantial burdens upon hospitals receiving cases, using up all renal dialysis facilities in a children's hospital (Roberts and Upton 2000). These exacerbations can put great strains on community and hospital resources by forcing individual organizations to incur very large, unplanned expenditures. Epidemiology of infections is collected on a population basis and, depending on the variance of such data, any particular individual or area may be much more prone to infection than others and may require additional protection, which implies the use of more resources.

Thus infectious disease and infection control are associated with uncertainty and exhibit externalities. A good infection control policy affects everyone by reducing the risk of infection. Infection control has the characteristics of a public good, i.e. if it is in place it benefits everyone regardless of whether they pay or not. This presents a number of questions for policy makers and managers. First, how much should be invested in infection control? Whose values should be used and how should they be elicited? Secondly, will the values be freely expressed or is free-riding to be expected because exclusion is not possible or efficient? Because of its public good aspects, property rights to infection control are difficult to assign.

Infections and their control present a number of problems for any system of governance.

Contract as a form of governance

Many health care systems involve the use of contracts between those purchasing the health care (such as health maintenance organizations or health insurers) and those providing it (the hospitals). The use of contracts is an example of an attempt to govern agency relationships. The principal–agent relationship can be defined as 'a contract under which one or more persons (the principal(s)) engage another person (the agent) to perform some service on their behalf which involves delegating some decision making authority to the agent' (Jensen and Meckling 1976). The principal's problem is ensuring that the agent acts in the principal's interests, overcoming any different or conflicting interests. Agency relationships are central to all complex organizations, be they private firms or public sector bureaucracies, because, in such organizations, many people are needed to carry out the aims of the organization. In circumstances of imperfect information, once any significant degree of decision making is delegated, it is possible for the agent to make decisions which will further their own ends, rather than those of the principal. The appropriate use of the contractual relationship is therefore central to the management of agency relationships.

One of the key concepts concerning such contracts is whether they are capable of being complete. Completeness means that the contractual document covers all eventualities and can specify all future events at the outset. Simple short-term contractual relationships can allow for complete contracts to be written and, in these circumstances, the principal can use the contract effectively to govern the relationship with the agent: all obligations can be specified and performance of those obligations can be fully monitored. However, it is not always the case that contracts can be complete, as will be discussed later in this chapter (see also Chapter 1).

New institutional economics and transactions costs

Contracts made for health care would be unlikely to be able to govern agency relationships by virtue of being complete. This is because health care has a number of features which mean that the transaction costs of contracts are likely to be high, and the contracts incomplete. Transaction costs result from imperfect information, either about the other party involved in the exchange (asymmetric information) or about the future (uncertainty). Imperfect information means that it is costly to enter into contracts for the exchange of rights, since the parties will have to incur the costs of searching for a suitable trading partner and then negotiate and write contracts (called *ex ante* transaction costs). It also makes it costly to monitor, enforce and renegotiate contracts (called *ex post* transaction costs). Both types of transaction costs may be high, but when there is a high level of uncertainty about relevant events there may be a trade-off between the two: the costs of making contracts may be reduced by not attempting to specify contingencies fully, leaving a contract incomplete and necessitating renegotiation (leading to *ex post* transaction costs) to accommodate events left out of the contract.

Particular transactions and environments are expected to have higher levels of asymmetric information and uncertainty, and therefore higher transaction costs. Transaction costs are expected to be higher if, all else being equal, there is less competition, exchange is less frequent, assets are dedicated to particular uses making 'hold-up' possible, cognitive capacity of individuals may be limited, and there is a greater tendency to behave opportunistically. We would expect high transaction costs in health care since it is characterized by high levels of uncertainty and asymmetric information. A number of commentators believe that the introduction of an internal market was accompanied by high transaction costs (Bartlett 1991; Croxson 1999). As will be discussed later in this chapter, there are many reasons why we might expect the transaction costs of contracts involving infectious disease to be particularly high.

Empirical work also shows that organizations economize on transaction costs by adapting to environments with high transaction costs by altering governance structures to mitigate the risk that might otherwise accompany incomplete contracts in arms-length transactions (Williamson 1975; Coase 1987; North 1990). A common response is integration, either by formally internalizing the transaction or by informally entering into networks. As will be discussed below, a number of commentators have argued that even if incomplete contracts undermine the effectiveness of complete contracts as a way of managing agency relationships, it may nonetheless be possible to use network relations and relational contracts. It is, however, important to recognize that relational contracts can be used in this way only if there are viable networks and an exchange of well-defined property rights.

Socio-legal theory of contracts

Contracts can manage agency relationships if they are complete, in other words if they specify all future matters at the outset (this is known as 'presentiation') (Macneil 1981). It would not be necessary for a fully specified contract to be open to renegotiation within the contractual period, but rather both parties would abide by the terms agreed at the outset. Such complete contracts are known as classical contracts in socio-legal theory (Macneil 1981).

Complete contracts safeguard principals' interests, whilst simultaneously giving agents an incentive to act efficiently. In the event that terms are breached, a principal can use the contractual terms to rectify matters, or use a verifiable breach of terms as grounds to exit the relationship.

There is evidence suggesting that completeness is not a true representation of many long-term commercial contractual relationships. Parties to long-term commercial contracts often do not plan and specify their contractual relationships completely (Macaualay 1963; Beale and Dugdale 1975), although many aspects of the relationship may be formally recorded. Moreover, socio-legal and economic theory suggest that this might be an efficient response when uncertainty or asymmetric information increase transaction costs, making complete contracts non-feasible. In these circumstances, relational contracts might evolve and permit efficient trade.

The theory of relational contracts was developed by Macneil (1981) to explain long-term contracts as relationships over time. In long-term contracts between separate firms, presentation is not always attempted and instead use is made of a commitment to good faith, in other words to cooperative efforts to realize their joint and several goals in the face of contingencies that arise during the course of the performance of the contract (Campbell and Harris 1983). This does not mean that parties do not have differing interests, but rather that cooperation is a way of realizing those interests. A key component of effective relational contracting is the trust between the parties. In the absence of full information about the other's performance, each party is prepared to cooperate to achieve its respective interests.

Some authors see the process of negotiating and writing the contractual documentation as part of the process of building and planning the relationship (Daintith 1986; Deakin et al. 1994).

> (By) agreeing from the start on an appropriate set of procedural rules to guide their response to unanticipated contingencies, agents can promote the kinds of mutual learning that contribute to the build-up of trust and which increase the likelihood of successful co-operation. (Lorenz 1999, pp. 313–314)

Others, in contrast, contend that the act of negotiating and writing contracts is inimical to the development of trusting, cooperative relationships between the parties (Macaulay 1963; Lyons and Mehta 1992; Sako 1992).

Relational contracts rely on the existence of personal relationships, which can sometimes be characterized as networks. The term networks can be used in either of two senses, either or both of which might be a feature of relational contracting. The first use connotes webs of informal relationships between individuals (e.g. Burt 1992). These do not exist as a means of allocating financial risk, but rather to communicate information missing from formal structures, and may also have the normative effect of constraining opportunism (Ouchi 1979). Networks may therefore be a means of regulating the behaviour of professionals, by supplying missing information both through better monitoring and through their normative role.

The second use of the term networks connotes 'virtual firms', when different organizations share risk without formally integrating (Sabel 1991). Under conditions of uncertainty, when it is not feasible fully to allocate future risk (i.e. in the absence of presentiation), risk can be managed within relational contracts by being pooled between the parties as events arise (when cooperative strategies can be developed). Personal relationships may provide the basis for this type of network, by providing the basis for cooperation between organizations.

As Granovetter (1985) and Bradach and Eccles (1991) point out, networks and contractual relationships in markets are not mutually exclusive forms of organization. Making strict distinctions between markets, integrated hierarchies and networks would overestimate the authority and coherence in hierarchies, and underestimate the networks and social relationships which exist in markets. Williamson (1985) sees relational contracting (which can be characterized as a form of network) as a way of dealing with high transaction costs in certain markets. In circumstances where complete contracts cannot be concluded, it is possible that networks will evolve to deal with deficiencies in formal contracts.

Contracting for infection control

In the case of the NHS internal market, Health Authorities were charged with using contracts to achieve their ends. In respect of infectious diseases, they had to meet three objectives: (i), they had to ensure access to appropriate treatment for those with infectious diseases; (ii) they had to ensure adequate prevention of and protection from infectious diseases, including hospital-acquired diseases; and (iii) they had to maintain the capacity of the hospitals to provide all other types of health care, despite any disruption arising from infectious diseases. It is important to note that, with respect to infectious diseases, Health Authorities were responsible both for ensuring adequate treatment for sufferers and for prevention and control of infectious diseases. To be complete in these circumstances, contracts for infectious disease control would have to be complete in respect of both the specification of what should be done by infection control personnel and the allocation of financial risk associated with infectious diseases.

Economic analysis shows that contracts for infectious disease management are likely to be incomplete. The costs of enforcing property rights and the uncertainty of contagion both raise the transaction costs of contracting for infectious diseases. Infectious diseases are often cited in health economics as a 'classic' externality because relevant property rights are often poorly defined and, if they exist, they are costly to enforce. This externality is manifested as the production or consumption of a good directly affecting people not involved in buying or selling it. The nature of contagion makes it costly to enforce rights to an infection-free environment, since infectious organisms are hard to monitor and it is often hard to assign responsibility for contagion (Crawshaw et al. 2000). Infectious disease is therefore said to be a negative externality, and a 'public bad'. Conversely, it is often costly to exclude individuals from the benefits of infection control measures, meaning that prevention may be underprovided: vaccination of one individual benefits all those with whom she/he subsequently has contact, regardless of any compensation from the latter. The transaction costs of contracting for infection-related events are also affected by uncertainty. As is the case with a number of disorders and their treatment, infection is not a certain event. The incidence of each infectious disease varies over time, and the risk of contagion varies between individuals and sites. This means that it is costly to predict and incorporate incidence rates, *ex ante*, making it likely that contracts will be incomplete. Although these problems are present in health care for other diseases, the control of infectious disease presents extreme types of problems for systems of economic governance due to the high monitoring costs.

Contracting in the NHS internal market in England

Contracting has become even more widespread in the last decade as it has been introduced into various publicly funded health systems in an attempt to improve efficiency (Organization for Economic Co-operation and Development 1992).

One example of public sector contracting is the English NHS. As the illustrations of the effect of governance structures on infection control are taken from a study of this system of contracting, a short explanation of the NHS internal market follows. The NHS was established initially in 1948 as a hierarchical public organization. By the late 1980s, an internal market was seen by the government as the best form of governance structure for the NHS. An internal market for community, secondary and tertiary health care was introduced by means of a split between the purchasers of care and its providers. The arrangement made between purchasers and providers (known as 'NHS Trusts') in the NHS internal market was referred to as a 'contract'. It was thought that purchasers (the main purchasers at the time were Health Authorities) would be in a position to undertake strategic planning of services by assessing the needs of populations and by prioritizing between groups and services. They were supposed to translate their aims for individual services, including the quality standards which those services should meet, into contractual specifications (Department of Health 1989). In this way, contracts were the crucial element in the new organizational structure.

The study of contracting for infection control in the NHS internal market reported in this chapter was funded by the British Economic and Social Research Council and was undertaken between 1997 and 2000. It explored the management and distribution of risks posed by infectious disease, and the implications of introducing contracts for infection control (see Allen *et al.* 2002 for further details of the study). The relevant data are derived from two arms of the study: an in-depth series of case studies in five sites; and a national questionnaire survey of all members of the three main professional groups with responsibility for infectious diseases in England. There are three key clinical groups with direct responsibility for infectious disease treatment or management. The first group are Consultants in Communicable Disease Control (CsCDC), whose role was created by the Acheson Report (1998). The CCDC is responsible for the surveillance, prevention and control of communicable disease throughout a Health Authority. This role incorporates membership of Hospital Infection Control Committees, District Infection Control Committees, accountability to local authorities, liaison with Public Health Laboratories and, since the introduction of the NHS internal market in 1991, responsibility for advising the Health Authority on contracts. These arrangements have now changed slightly with the setting up of the Health Protection Agency (HPA) in 2003. The two other groups, Infection Control Nurses (ICNs) and Infection Control Doctors (ICDs), are usually based in Trusts, and form part of the hospital infection control team, responsible for protecting the hospital population from the risks of infectious diseases.

The research evidence concerning governance of infection control in England

The research described above is a unique study of contracting for infection control in England. The findings of the study illustrate the principles of the economic and socio-legal theory discussed above. The contracts used to govern the control of infectious disease were not complete. In many local areas, some elements of relational contracts were present, namely the importance assigned to professional networks by the infection control professionals themselves. However, it is not clear that professional networks were able to compensate for all the missing aspects of the incomplete contracts, and thus, that effective relational contracts had evolved. In particular, there were serious problems reported in some areas concerning the burden of financial risk. These problems had not been solved either by advance allocation in contractual documents (which complete contracts would achieve) or by cooperative agreement about the allocation of such risks when they arose (which effective relational contracts would achieve). Finally, problems arose due to the externalities associated with infection control – there did seem to be the possibility of free-riding, and thus, underinvestment inside the hospitals.

Contracts and the practice of infection control

Appropriate management of infection control is central to safeguarding quality of care. As far as the practice of infection control was concerned, the contractual documents from the case study sites were incomplete. Four of the five sets of contractual documents contained no specifications of good practice in the management of infection, nor did they contain quality indicators relating directly to infection.

This finding of incompleteness is consistent with the results of the national questionnaire survey. Only a minority of each professional group reported that the contract between the acute Trust and Health Authority included clauses relating to surveillance of hospital-acquired infection (HAI). A slightly larger proportion reported that the Trust was required to meet specific standards for infection control. The descriptions of the contractual provisions by staff with knowledge of their contents suggest that the relevant clauses of the contracts were of a general nature, and, thus, the contracts were not complete. (In the absence of the documents themselves, this conclusion has been inferred.) National standards, such as those set by the Department of Health (Cooke Report 1995) and the King's Fund Accreditation Scheme, were frequently referred to by respondents.

There is positive evidence that Health Authorities were not able formally to monitor infection rates or control practices, because of high *ex post* transaction costs. One case study site had some years previously introduced specific targets for infection control, including an acceptable limit for MRSA incidence and for the rate of post-surgical infections: the 'deep infection rate' was to be less than 1%. The costs of monitoring and enforcing this rate were not incurred because they were prohibitively high. A Trust-based respondent in this site said that there was no 'infrastructure' either to deliver or to monitor this standard, and that no audits were ever conducted by the Health Authority or by the Trust.

Other interviewees suggested that transaction costs were raised by the characteristics of infectious disease: its intangibility; and the irregularity of its appearance. The monitoring costs were explained by one interviewee in the context of a particular organism, small round structured virus (SRSV), causing an acute gastrointestinal illness. This is particularly hard to monitor because it is transmitted very quickly between individuals: 'SRSV, my experience is that it's gone halfway round the ward before you get evidence and control measures up and running'. A number of Health Authority contract managers stated that they did not monitor the Trust's practice with respect to infectious diseases directly, instead they focused on its ability to deliver the contracted level of activity. They noted that they might become aware of problems with infectious disease control if it affected levels of elective activity or, connected with this, length of stay. Trusts were also aware of this: one Trust noted that although they would not report to the Health Authority an outbreak such as salmonella, it would be brought to the Health Authority's attention when they were forced to explain changes in activity levels and length of stay. The Health Authorities and Trusts themselves recognized that length of stay and activity rates were both imperfect indicators of infection, since each is affected by multiple factors. This meant that Trusts were not being monitored effectively: an increase in activity could be achieved with increasing rates HAI without any penalty being incurred. Conversely, a fall in activity could be incorrectly attributed to HAI. This, coupled with the monitoring costs, gave Trusts a financial incentive to ignore infection and focus on activity rates.

Contracts and financial risk

In each of the case study sites, responsibility for managing the financial risk normally associated with infection control was passed to Trusts by using 'sophisticated block contracts' which tied payment to activity, where activity was specified in terms of the different volumes of activity in each specialty. None of the five sites had a contract where contractual payments depended on levels of infectious disease treated in hospitals or on their efforts to control infection. The allocation of financial risk in the event that an outbreak of HAI disrupted normal activity was not dealt with at all in three of the contracts. In two sites, *force majeure* clauses allowed renegotiation of the contract in the event of a 'major outbreak'. These clauses did not attempt to specify what would constitute a 'major outbreak'. Thus, the contracts imply that, in all but exceptional circumstances for two of the sites, financial risk was passed to the provider. On a strict reading of the contracts, the silence concerning the allocation of the normal financial risk of infection implies that it was intended to be passed to the providers. This is confirmed by the interviews conducted at the case study sites, which suggested that the costs of managing or controlling HAI were viewed by Health Authority and Trust management staff as overheads, as a 'risk that the Trust bears'. Interviewees at three sites, based in both Health Authorities and Trusts, likened managing the risk of infection to that involving emergency activity: they stated that a hospital with large fixed costs could and should carry this type of recurrent expenditure as part of its 'bread and butter' activity; and should have in place processes to deal with unanticipated events. (No contrary view was stated at the other sites, or by other respondents.)

However, although the intention was to write complete contracts, transferring financial risk to providers, there was evidence in all study sites of flexibility beyond that envisaged in the contractual documents. This suggests that the contracts were not in fact complete: if they had been, the allocation of financial risk would be complete. It would be agreed at the time the contract was made, and no further applications would be made to the purchasers during the financial year, save in accordance with any explicit contractual provisions.

Although all purchasers stated that they intended transferring financial risk to providers and this is consistent with the formal contracts, most Health Authority managers said that they would in practice share the financial risk if it could be shown that the Trust was not at fault and if the true marginal costs, due to the outbreak of infection, could be identified. In the event of large-scale financial problems concerning infectious disease, purchasers said they would be prepared to share financial risk with providers, or to join with them to apply for additional resources from higher tiers of the NHS hierarchy, being the regional offices of the NHS Executive. This is consistent with general NHS practice with respect to emergency admissions. Some Health Authorities did concede that they had a contingency fund. All said that, if absolutely necessary, they would be prepared to accept a reduction in elective activity caused by a major outbreak of HAI.

Professional networks

As discussed above, if formal contracts are incomplete, personal relationships between individuals may be able to supply missing information. Both the national survey and the case studies suggest that professional networks were important in many local areas. However, in addition to the results reported below concerning the sporadic way in which professional networks dealt with the allocation of financial risk, it was not always the case that professional networks were able to compensate for incomplete contracts.

Almost all CsCDC and ICNs, and the majority of ICDs believed that professional networks were important in conducting negotiation, specification and monitoring between Health Authority and Trusts. Moreover, each group was more likely to see professional networks as important than they were to see contracts as important.

Individuals were likely to see professional networks as more important than contracts, but contracts were also viewed as important. Respondents' views of the role of contracts will be discussed below.

We asked respondents to the national survey a free text question about the extent and nature of non-contractual relationships. A number of the respondents to this question said they had no arrangements (11% of ICDs, 26% of ICNs and, interestingly, only 3% of CsCDC). The remainder referred to the District Infection Control Committee, the Hospital Infection Control Committee [to which ICD, ICNs, and CsCDC are all supposed to belong (50)], outbreak teams or various *ad hoc* groups to deal with specific issues, such as human immunodeficiency virus (HIV). A large number of responding

ICDs (49%) and ICNs (43%) also referred to informal professional contact with members of the Health Authority, and 53% of CsCDC referred to this type of contact with individuals in Trusts.

All of the professionals interviewed in the case study sites viewed personal, professional relationships as vital to managing infectious diseases. They used personal relationships to trace the contacts of an infected person throughout the community. They also stated that, in the event of an outbreak, they cooperated across organizational boundaries. All stated that, with respect to the management of infection, they would not be affected by 'financial considerations' and would not refer to the contract.

At least some CsCDC were in a position to gain information about Trust practices, in other words to monitor infection control procedures and the management of outbreaks. They were members of the Hospital Infection Control Committee, and a number referred to informal relationships as a means of gaining information on Trust practices. In one case study site, the CCDC had been in post for 20 years, and stated that this meant that he knew 'most people' and could use this to find out what was going on within Trusts and to influence practice.

However, networks were not viewed as satisfactory by all respondents, indicating that effective relational contracts had not evolved in those areas. Some implied that they would benefit from more completely specified and enforceable contracts, since they did not have recourse to effective networks. For example, one CCDC stated that having 'no provision for communicable disease issues regularly causes problems with refusal to cooperate—adverse publicity is the only sanction'.

Others stated that the contract was 'inadequate', 'not specific enough' and that it did not 'impose a system for monitoring', features which other respondents, with functioning networks, had seen as at least not problematic or as positively advantageous. Moreover, a substantial minority of ICNs and ICDs said they had no non-contractual arrangements with the Health Authority, implying that professional networks were not universally used to overcome the limits of contracts and provide information across organizational boundaries.

Financial risk and professional networks

Professional networks certainly facilitated pooling risk between organizations, insofar as they facilitated interagency cooperation over outbreak management and tracing contacts, with no concern for financial responsibility. As discussed above, all of the CsCDC, ICDs and ICNs interviewed in the case study sites said that they would manage outbreaks without reference to costs or to contracts. In this sense, professional networks provided the basis for interorganizational networks, in other words, for risk sharing virtual firms. Moreover, the discussion about incomplete contracts suggested a degree of shared responsibility for unanticipated costs.

However, in practice, we did not find evidence of universal, fully developed risk pooling between organizations. There are frequent instances of *ex post* haggling between organizations over who should meet costs. For example, in two sites, there were problems with assigning responsibility for the costs of screening for MRSA: one interviewee argued that this resulted from the failure to identify whether screening was necessary for the optimal management of individual patients (in which case it should be paid for by the provider), or was part of routine disease prevention, making it the Health Authority's responsibility. He contrasted controversies over who should bear costs in the internal market with the 'grey old days' when organizational boundaries were irrelevant.

Other problems with assigning responsibility resulted from another characteristic of infectious disease: its failure to respect organizational boundaries and the poor definition of property rights over infection-free space. Three of the Trusts interviewed in the case study sites argued that they should not bear responsibility for the costs of MRSA, since they blamed outbreaks on poor infection control procedures in local nursing homes.

The dual roles of formal contracts and networks

It should be remembered that the socio-legal theory of relational contracts does not imply that contractual documents have no use. If personal relationships evolve between the contracting parties, which enable them to deal with some of the issues in respect of which the contract cannot be complete, this does not mean that there is no role for formal contractual documents. A mixed use of informal and formal methods is likely to evolve. The results demonstrate that this was the case in respect of infection control in some local areas.

The results suggest that, despite the fact that networks were seen as important by most respondents to the national survey, they also believed contracts had a role. A large number of respondents believed both contracts and networks to be important, and some placed greater emphasis on contracts than networks. These results also show that a small number believed neither was important.

Responses to other questions suggest that at least some respondents believed that networks and contracts played complementary roles. One CCDC, for example, said she/he refers to the contract only 'if there are serious concerns and the issue needs to be raised with senior management. More of my CCDC work is non-contractual and operated due to good professional relationships. Good liaison and personal/professional relationships are the key to success'.

Another stated that, 'About four years ago, I agreed detailed IC specification with three trusts, but those were since dropped by the HA given the style of contracting. However, that initial work helped secure and confirm IC arrangements locally'.

In one of the case study sites, the Health Authority contract managers saw the *process* of negotiating the contract and of involving clinical staff in that process as more important than the final document, as a way of raising the profile of infection control within the trust.

These results provide evidence to support the contention of some commentators who have studied commercial contracts that the process of agreeing contracts can be useful in building trusting relationships. However, it should be noted that the contrary view was also advanced: in one case study site, a manager saw contracts as directly harmful, stating that they could 'de-motivate' individuals.

Infection control as an externality

As discussed above, the characteristics of infectious disease mean that there is a danger that infection control may not be adequately funded. Many infections are costly to monitor (Haley *et al.* 1985). It is also costly to monitor infection control activities, since this would require detailed observation of the behaviour of individuals, including clinical and domestic staff (Handwashing Liaison Group 1999). High monitoring costs mean that if individual hospital directorates or wards are responsible for infection control expenditure, they have an incentive to free-ride on each other by underinvesting in infection control (Cornes and Sandler 1996). In other words, undetected lax practice in one ward may impose costs on other wards as infections spread between wards. The formal arrangements advocated by the Department of Health, which place responsibility for direct infection control activities with the hospital infection control team and central Trust management, may be insufficient to mitigate the tendency for individual directorates to behave opportunistically with regard to infection control since effective infection control requires appropriate purchasing decisions and management across a wide range of areas, many of which continue to be controlled at directorate level.

It follows from the foregoing that infection control might be expected to be adversely affected by decentralized budgeting within hospitals. The role of decentralized budgets was investigated. A substantial minority of ICNs (39%) and ICDs (27%) believed that they did have an impact. Analysis of their responses, however, suggests that when budget managers experienced resource constraints, they were reluctant to allocate resources to infection control activities. Some respondents noted that when budgets were tight, managers did not regard infection control as a priority, making it difficult to implement infection control policy. One ICD stated that 'no-one wants to spend any money on basic things which have an impact on infection control, e.g. waste bins etc'.

The existence of internal budgets *per se* caused problems for infection control because the budget holders were able to use their discretion when purchasing consumables and equipment. In some hospitals, they were able to do so because there was no internal policy governing purchasing. In other hospitals, with a policy, budget holders nonetheless had discretion because the infection control team believed they had neither a mandate nor the resources to implement the policy. The effect of this was a tendency by budget holders in these hospitals to purchase cheap rather than safe equipment and consumables, or to reuse disposable items. The problem is illustrated by the following responses from three different ICNs:

> 'In one directorate they cannot afford any chairs for visitors so we are constantly asking them not to sit on the bed. No one can afford waste bins – so they are all broken. They buy the cheapest soap and towels so people don't like washing their hands.'
>
> 'Need to be alert for tendency to use cheaper but not necessarily cost-effective products. Need to be alert for re-use of single-use items.'
>
> 'Maternity unit – saved money by using cot sheets in the kitchen to dry up cups, etc. instead of disposable paper roll [(describing the circumstances surrounding a gastro- infection of SRSV) outbreak: 77 staff, 18 mothers].'

Conclusion

As economic theory predicts, the boundaries erected by contracts and devolved budgets, whilst they may or may not have advantages in the overall management of health care resources, are singularly inappropriate as a method of coping with infectious disease control. Contracts do not appear to be an effective mechanism for the governance of infectious disease. Internal budgeting systems in hospitals mitigated against the introduction of effective infection control programmes.

It may be that hierarchical governance structures would be more effective than contractual arrangements. The financial incentives and boundaries produced by contractual relationships would become less apparent. However, many of the issues identified in this chapter, such as uncertainty, agency problems and the problems of asymmetrical information, would not disappear. What is clear is that while some formal structures can militate against effective governance systems for infection control, 'informal' personal relationships are also vital to the complex processes required to run a control of infection system.

References

Acheson, D. (1998) *Report of the Committee of Enquiry into the Future Development of the Public Health Function*. HMSO, London.

Allen, P., Croxson, B., Roberts, J., Archibald, K., Crawshaw, S. and Taylor, L. (2002) The use of contracts in the management of infection disease related risk in the NHS internal market. *Health Policy* **59**, 257–281

Allison, S. (1991) Winter pressure on hospital beds. *British Medical Journal* **303**, 508–509.

Benenson, A.S. (1994) *Control of Communicable Diseases Manual*, 16th edn. An official Report of the American Public Health Association. American Public Health Association, Washington, DC.

Bartlett, W. (1991) Quasi markets and contracts: a markets and hierarchies perspective on NHS reforms. *Public Money and Management* **11** (3), 53–61.

Beale, H. and Dugdale, T. (1975) Contracts between businessmen. *British Journal of Law and Society* **2**, 45–60.

Bradach, J. and Eccles, R. (1991) Markets versus hierarchies: from ideal types to plural forms. In: Thompson G., Frances, J., Levacic, R. and Mitchell, J. (eds), *Markets, Hierarchies and Networks*. The Open University Press and Sage, London.

Burt, R. (1992) *Structural Holes*. Harvard University Press, Cambridge, MA.

Campbell, D. and Harris, D. (1993) Flexibility in long term contractual relationships: the role of co-operation. *Journal of Law and Society* **20**, 166–191.

Coase, R. (1987) On the nature of the firm after 50 years. Unpublished manuscript in Marshall Library of Economics, University of Cambridge.

Cooke Report (1995) *Hospital Infection Control, Guidance on the Control of Infection in Hospitals*. Hospital Infection Working Group of the Department of Health and Public Health Laboratory Service.

Cornes, R. and Sandler, T. (1996) *The Theory of Externalities, Public Goods and Club Goods*, 2nd edn. Cambridge University Press, Cambridge.

Crawshaw, S., Allen, P. and Roberts, J.A. (2000) Managing the risk of infectious disease: the context of organisational accountability. *Journal of Health, Risk and Society* **2**, 125–141.

Croxson, B. (1999) *Organisational Costs in the New NHS: An Introduction to the Transaction Costs and Internal Costs of Delivering Health Care*. Office Of Health Economics, London.

Daintith, T. (1986) The design and performance of long term contracts. In: Daintith, T. and Teubner, G. (eds), *Contract and Organization: Legal Analysis in the Light of Economic and Social Theory*. Gruter, New York.

Deakin, S., Lane, C.F. and Wilkinson (1994) Trust or law? Towards an integrated theory of contractual relations between firms. *Journal of Law and Society* **21**, 329–349.

Department of Health (1989) *Working for Patients*. Secretaries of State for Health, Wales, Northern Ireland, Scotland Cm 555, HMSO, London.

Granovetter, M. (1985) Economic action and social structure: the problem of imbeddedness. *American Journal of Sociology* **91**, 481–510.

Haley, R.W., White, J.W., Culver, D.H., Meade Morgan, W., Emori, T.G., Munn, V.P. and Hooton, T.M. (1985) The efficacy of infection surveillance and central programs in preventing nosocomial infections in US hospitals (SENIC). *American Journal of Epidemiology* **121**, 182–205.

Handwashing Liaison Group (1999) Handwashing: a modest measure with big effects. *British Medical Journal* **318**, 686.

Humphreys, D. and Duckworth, G. (1997) Editorial. *Hospital Infection* 1.

Jensen, M. and Meckling, W. (1976) The theory of the firm: managerial behaviour, agency costs and ownership structure. *Journal of Financial Economics* **3**, 305–360.

Lorenz, E. (1999) Trust, contract and economic cooperation. *Cambridge Journal of Economics* **23**, 301–315.

Lyons, B. and Mehta, J. (1992) Why do firms write (or not write) contracts? Mimeo

Macneil, I. (1981) Economic analysis of contractual relations: its shortfalls and the need for a rich classificatory apparatus' *Northwestern University Law Review* 75.

Macaulay, S. (1963) Non contractual relations in business. *American Sociological Review* **28**, 55–70.

North, D.C. (1990) *Institutions, Institutional Change and Economic Performance*. Cambridge University Press, Cambridge.

Organization for Economic Co-operation and Development (1992) *The Reform of Health Care: A Comparative Analysis of 7 OECD Countries*. OECD, Paris.

Ouchi, W. (1979) A conceptual framework for the design of organisational control mechanisms. *Management Science* **25**, 833–846.

Pennington Report (1997) *Report on the Circumstances Leading to the 1996 Outbreak of Infection with E. coli O157 in Central Scotland, the Implications for Food Safety and the Lessons to be Learnt*. The Stationery Office, Edinburgh.

Plowman, R., Graves, N. and Roberts, J. (1997) *Hospital Acquired Infection*. Office of Health Economics, London.

Roberts, J.A. and Upton, P.A. (2000) *E. coli O157 An Economic Assessment of an Outbreak*. Lothian Health and London School of Hygiene and Tropical Medicine, Edinburgh.

Sabel, C. (1991) Studied trust: building new forms of co-operation in a volatile economy. In: Pyke, F., Beccatini, G. and Sengenberger, W. (eds), *Industrial Districts and Local Economic Regeneration*.

Sako, M. (1992) *Prices, Quality and Trust: Interfirm Relations in Britain and Japan*. Cambridge University Press, Cambridge.

Williamson, O. (1975) *Markets and Hierarchies: Analysis and Anti Trust Implications*. The Free Press, New York.

Williamson, O. (1985) *The Economic Institutions of Capitalism*. Free Press, New York.

Chapter 16

Evaluating US food safety regulations which use benefit and cost information

Jean Buzby, Felix Spinelli and Clark Nardinelli[1]

Introduction

This chapter highlights some of the key challenges and common themes in economic analyses for US food safety regulations. After a brief overview of economic analyses for US regulations, this chapter discusses three food safety rules which have incorporated the costs of food-borne illnesses in their economic analyses: (i) the 1996 Pathogen Reduction/Hazard Analysis and Critical Control Point (PR/HACCP) rule for meat and poultry; (ii) the 2000 *Salmonella enteritidis* rule for shell eggs; and (iii) the proposed rule for ready-to-eat (RTE) meat and poultry products (MPPs). One particular focus here is the valuation of premature deaths from food-borne illness because it can be a large component of the total costs of Federal food safety regulations. The discussion explains and illustrates how the economic methodology to handle the valuation of premature death is evolving. The chapter concludes with a forward-looking discussion about private and public incentives to improve food safety.

Each year in the USA, there are an estimated 76 million food-borne illnesses, 325 000 associated hospitalizations and 5000 deaths (Mead *et al.* 1999). The bulk of these illnesses, or 62 million, are from *unknown* pathogens or agents that have not been identified and thus cannot be diagnosed. Knowledge about known and emerging food-borne pathogens and their food vehicles is limited, though expanding with advances in pathogen detection and identification techniques such as DNA fingerprinting and more rapid microbial tests.

US firms that make or distribute food products have a variety of incentives to produce safe food products. A system of market, regulatory and legal components provides these incentives to firms (Garber 1998a, b, extended to

---

[1] The views expressed in this Chapter are those of the authors and do not represent the views of the Economic Research Service, the US Department of Agriculture or the Food and Drug Administration.

food safety). These incentives generally take the form of adverse consequences for firms responsible for selling pathogen-contaminated food. The following are the three basic components of this incentive system.

1. Market forces: firms risk losing business reputation, market share and sales revenue if consumers become aware of safety problems with a firm's products.

2. Food safety laws and regulations: firms that violate Federal, State or local food safety laws or regulations may be subject to various penalties imposed by courts or government agencies, including fines, product recalls and temporary or permanent plant closures.

3. Product liability law: firms found responsible under product liability law for contaminated food products that made people ill may have to pay financial compensation to the plaintiffs as well as punitive damages (Buzby *et al.* 2001). Firms also pay court costs and legal fees, regardless of most outcomes.

Of the three components of the food safety incentive system, this chapter focuses on food safety regulations. In the USA, there are three main agencies with regulatory jurisdiction over food safety. The Department of Health and Human Services' (DHHS) Food and Drug Administration (FDA) has oversight over animal feeds, medicines and all domestic and imported food intended for human consumption (except for meat and poultry and some egg products). The US Department of Agriculture (USDA)'s Food Safety and Inspection Service (FSIS) has jurisdiction over these other food products. Meanwhile, the Environmental Protection Agency (EPA) has oversight of drinking water, pesticides, and toxic substances and wastes.

These three agencies have instituted many food safety regulations, some dating back nearly 100 years. In 1997, there was an expanded food safety effort called 'A National Food Safety Initiative', which was coordinated by these three agencies plus the US Centers for Disease Control and Prevention (CDC) in the DHHS. As part of this effort, there was a discussion about organizational options for restructuring the US Federal food safety system (see http://www.foodsafety.gov/~fsg/cstrpl-4.html). To date, there has not been a major realignment of food safety agencies or functions as there have been in some other countries.

Executive Order 12866 directs agencies to conduct an economic analysis of all proposed or existing regulations, which meet certain conditions, to inform decision makers of the consequences of alternative regulatory actions. In particular, according to Office of Management and Budget (OMB) Circular A-4 (2003), the economic analysis should provide sufficient information to decision makers so that they can determine whether:

◆ there is adequate information indicating the need for regulation and that government intervention is likely to do more good than harm

- the potential benefits to society justify the potential costs, recognizing that not all benefits and costs can be described in monetary or even in quantitative terms, unless a statute requires another regulatory approach
- the proposed action will maximize net benefits to society (including potential economic, environmental, public health and safety, and other advantages; distributional impacts; and equity), compared with other regulatory options
- where a statute requires a specific regulatory approach, the proposed action will be the most cost-effective, including reliance on performance objectives wherever feasible
- agency decisions are based on the best reasonably obtainable scientific, technical, economic and other information (Office of Management and Budget 2003).

While most economic analyses should include these elements, variations may be warranted when a potential regulation raises novel legal or policy issues, has a highly unequal distribution of effects or has large but non-measurable human health implications. The economic analysis should also satisfy the 'Unfunded Mandates Reform Act of 1995' (P.L. 104–4) requirements. Under this Act, agencies must provide a quantitative and qualitative assessment of the anticipated benefits and costs of all Federal mandates resulting in annual expenditures of US$100 million or more (in 1995 US dollars), including the benefits and costs to State, local and tribal governments or private sector businesses. Additionally, Federal agencies must give special consideration to the impact of the regulation on small businesses in accordance with the Regulatory Flexibility Act (P.L. 96–354). The OMB reviews these economic analyses. Typically, when the rule is finalized, implementation is phased in over time, though emergency measures may become effective immediately or shortly after the rule is finalized.

General principles of economic analysis for US regulations

There is no blueprint for conducting an economic analysis (EA) and different regulations may call for different analytical approaches and emphases (Office of Management and Budget 2003). For example, the crucial question in one proposed regulation may be whether a market failure exists, and much of the analysis may be devoted to answering this question. In another case, it may be clear that a market failure exists and the main emphasis in the analysis might be to determine the anticipated magnitude of the benefits of the proposed regulation.

An EA of an economically significant rule contains three elements. The first element is the statement of the need for a proposed action. This element addresses whether the problem constitutes a market failure or presents a compelling public need such as to address a distributional concern or improve a governmental process. The second element is an examination of alternative approaches and the agency's rationale for selecting the proposed action over other alternatives. The third component of an EA is a cost-benefit analysis (CBA), which is a weighing of the pros and cons of a proposed regulation against a baseline (i.e. the best assessment of the current state without the regulation). To the fullest extent possible, benefits and costs should be expressed in terms of the discounted currency (in this case, in constant dollars). Expressing both benefits and costs in dollars makes it easy to calculate net benefits. Positive net benefits mean that the regulation may be a good use of public spending, whereas negative net benefits mean that it is not. Additionally, expressing net benefits in dollars means that the cost of the proposed regulation can be compared with other options for public expenditures. OMB recommends that if benefits and costs occur over time, regulatory and other analyses should discount the streams of benefits and costs using real (i.e. adjusted for changes in the price level) annual discount rates of both 3 and 7%. The 3% is an estimate of the real rate of time preference for health-related benefits and costs; the 7% rate is an estimate of the average before-tax real rate of return to incremental private investment. Monetization of both the major benefits and costs is preferred. When monetization is not possible, and when there is no dispute over the existence of substantial benefits, a cost-effectiveness analysis may be used (a comparison of costs with the 'number' of physical benefits, for example) to identify the most cost-effective means to attain those benefits. In addition, OMB recommends that agencies carry out cost-effectiveness analyses for all major rulemakings for which it is possible to develop measures of effectiveness for the expected health and safety outcomes (Office of Management and Budget 2003).

Usually, the impacts of regulatory actions are not known with certainty but are more appropriately estimated in terms of the probability of their occurrence. For food-borne illness, the term 'risk' generally refers to a probability distribution over a set of outcomes such as the probability that individuals will be hospitalized or die prematurely because of their illness (i.e. 'premature death'). Estimating the benefits and costs of regulations includes two components: (i) a *risk assessment*, part of which characterizes the probabilities of occurrence of the different outcomes; and (ii) a *valuation of the levels and changes in risk* experienced by the populations that the regulation affects. Both of these components need to be conceptually consistent and the risk assessment should be conducted so that the results can be used within a cost-benefit framework. The risk assessment used in a CBA analysis is not a safety assessment; it does not tell us whether a food is 'safe', only what the probabilities are.

Analysts never have complete information and therefore they must be attentive to the quality and reliability of data, models, assumptions, scientific inferences and other information. Sensitivity analyses may be conducted to cover a wider range of plausible model specifications and values of key parameters. Properly calibrated, CBA provides information that helps risk managers make rational decisions about which risks are most amenable to reduction, given various financial and other constraints facing government, individuals and food companies. Additionally, CBA can help risk managers modify policies so as to increase net benefits.

Valuing food safety benefits and costs

If government regulations improve the safety of the food supply, consumers benefit by having fewer food-borne illnesses and associated premature deaths. Benefits can be measured by the reduction in the present value of the anticipated stream of medical costs, productivity losses and other costs that would result from averting these illnesses and deaths. Alternatively, benefits can be measured by the value consumers place on the reduction of risk. Meanwhile, new regulations may raise producer costs for items such as new equipment, training programmes, or research and development. Firms may also face higher costs from changes in production processes such as increased heating temperatures and/or holding times. Other costs may include reduced consumer choice of products and/or quality, and new costs for the government. Economists have developed three primary methodologies for valuing the benefits of a proposed policy.

1. Cost of illness. The cost of illness (COI) approach tallies the dollars spent on medical expenses and the dollars of employment compensation that are forgone as a result of illness, accidents or premature deaths.

2. Willingness to pay. The willingness to pay (WTP) approach measures the resources (dollars) individuals are willing and able to give up for a reduction in the probability of encountering a hazard that will compromise their health. The two most common measures of WTP assign dollar values to the 'benefits' of life and health based on either (i) direct consumer surveys (stated preference); or (ii) inferences from consumers' market behaviour (revealed preference).

3. Quality-adjusted life years. The quality-adjusted life years (QALYs) approach assigns values to health outcomes on a 0–1 scale, with 0 indicating

death and 1 indicating good health. With a QALY scale, adverse health outcomes that compromise both lifespan and functional ability are converted to a common unit of account (Golan and Kuchler 2001). QALY scales were developed for use in cost-effectiveness analyses. They can, however, be used to estimate monetary benefits if the QALY values are converted to monetary measures using a dollar value per QALY conversion factor.

The cost of illness method

Although the WTP approach is theoretically superior to other approaches because it reflects the observation that individual preferences are unique and that individual demands for risk reduction vary (Kuchler and Golan 1999), agencies may prefer other approaches because of measurement difficulties. In particular, for food safety regulations, the COI approach has been used frequently to provide estimates of the present value of lifetime costs to society averted because of a reduction in illness and premature death due to a regulation under review. For that reason, the COI approach is emphasized in this chapter. In essence, these averted food-borne illness costs can be used to represent the benefits of the regulation in a CBA. The primary advantages of the COI approach are that it presents economic costs in a straightforward manner easily understood by policy makers, and that it represents real costs to society. Kuchler and Golan (1999) provide details about the strengths and weaknesses of the COI and WTP approaches.

A detailed description of the mechanics of a COI analysis is beyond the scope of this chapter. However, a COI analysis traditionally starts with the estimates of the annual number of food-borne illness cases for a particular pathogen under study and then divides this number into severity groups, such as those who: (i) only had mild illnesses; (ii) sought the advice of a physician; (ii) were hospitalized; and (iv) died prematurely because of their illness (see Buzby et al. 1996 for detailed food safety examples). Those who develop chronic complications may be analysed in a separate severity category. The bulk of the analysis entails calculating the corresponding medical costs, lost productivity costs, value of premature deaths and other illness-specific costs, such as special education, for a particular pathogen. These COI calculations may incorporate estimates from other approaches, such as QALYs and WTP. Subsequent steps in the analysis identify what portion of these costs could potentially be averted by a proposed regulation.

Estimating these costs in a COI analysis may be complex due to several challenges. For example, direct medical expenses are often difficult to determine and interpret because of the intricacies of disease coding and insurance arrangements. Meanwhile, lost productivity costs may also be difficult to ascertain because of the various forms of compensation that are available to employees and because large portions of the US population are not in the workforce, such as children, retirees, or homemakers and home caregivers. Also, COI analyses face data limitations and require decisions about which secondary chronic complications should or can be included given current medical knowledge and data.

One challenge in a COI analysis for a proposed food safety rule is to determine what portion of illnesses from a particular pathogen are caused by the consumption of the particular food groups covered by a proposed regulation, such as what portion of all listeriosis cases are due to RTE meat. Another challenge is to establish the anticipated cause and effect of the proposed rule and its effectiveness in reducing food-borne illnesses.

Perhaps most importantly, there is no consensus among economists or among agencies concerning how best to estimate the value of a premature death [i.e. value of a statistical life (VOSL)]. This is a particularly crucial challenge because the valuation of death can be the largest component of total estimated costs. Because of this lack of consensus, the methodology for how economists value premature deaths continues to evolve over time, and members of different parts of the Federal government have convened periodically to work towards greater consistency in valuing fatality risks. For example, a conference titled 'Valuing the Health Benefits of Food Safety' was held at the University of Maryland in September 2000 (http://www.ers.usda.gov/publications/mp1570). Most agencies, however, use values that fall within a moderate range. The OMB 'best practices' document (Office of Management and Budget 2003) states that the WTP approach is preferred when valuing reductions in fatality risks that are expected by implementing a proposed regulation. In essence, the WTP approach provides estimates of the value of relatively small changes in the risk of death aggregated over a population, and the resulting estimates are not associated with an identifiable individual. The following discussion presents two recent US food safety regulations and one proposed food safety regulation with special emphasis on how fatalities were valued. The valuation of fatalities is emphasized because of the prominence of these estimates in economic analyses of government regulations.

The PR/HACCP meat and poultry rule

In July 1996, a new rule that published as a proposal in February 1995, required Federal- and State-inspected meat and poultry processors and slaughterhouses to adopt a Pathogen Reduction/Hazard Analysis and Critical Control Point (PR/HACCP) system to identify potential sources of food safety hazards and establish procedures to prevent, eliminate, control or reduce these hazards. HACCP plans generally follow a systematic approach involving seven principles, which are to: (i) conduct a hazard analysis; (ii) identify critical control points (CCPs) for physical, biological and chemical hazards; (iii) establish critical limits for preventative measures associated with each CCP; (iv) establish CCP monitoring requirements; (v) determine and perform corrective actions; (vi) establish record-keeping systems; and (vii) conduct verification procedures.

While the July 1996 rule covered biological, chemical and physical hazards, the emphasis was on controlling contamination from microbial pathogens. In particular, these establishments were required to: (i) develop a HACCP plan to identify and control food safety hazards in their products; (ii) meet applicable pathogen reduction standards; (iii) conduct microbial testing to determine adequacy of sanitary dressing procedures used in slaughter operations; and (iv) establish and follow written sanitary standard operating procedures.

The COI method was used to estimate the benefits of this proposed rule. This COI analysis included medical costs, costs of lost productivity and the value of premature deaths. In particular, the estimates for the value of premature deaths in this July 1996 regulation were estimated using the human capital approach developed by Landefeld and Seskin (1982). This now outdated approach generated the present value of expected lifetime after-tax income and housekeeping services at a 3% real rate of return, adjusted for an annual 1% increase in labour productivity and a risk aversion factor of 1.6. The risk aversion factor essentially adjusts the accounting of estimated lost productivity with a WTP component and was based on the ratio of life insurance premium payments to life insurance loss payments. In most cases, life insurance premiums represent what households would be willing to pay 'for potential losses associated with the death of an income-earning household member' (Landefeld and Seskin 1982, p. 562). The Landefeld and Seskin (1982) (LS) value of a statistical life lost is:

$$VOSL = [\sum_{t}^{T} \frac{Y_t}{(1+r)^t}]\alpha$$

where T = remaining lifetime, t = a particular age, Y_t = after-tax income including labour and non-labour income, r = household's opportunity cost of investing in risk-reducing activities and α = risk aversion factor. The major limitation of this approach is that it did not fully consider the value that individuals may place on (and pay for) feeling healthy, avoiding pain and suffering, or using their free time for utility-enhancing activities. Because the approach does not cover all of these valuable aspects of health, the approach is now thought to understate the true societal costs of illness and is no longer used for economic analyses of food safety regulations.

In the CBA for this rule, one key assumption necessary in estimating the benefits of the rule was the extent that the rule would reduce pathogen contamination and subsequent illnesses. There was some concern about the February 1995 proposed rule's assumption that the rule would eliminate essentially 100% of those pathogens that enter the meat and poultry supply at inspected processing establishments and about how the cost-benefit ratio would change with different effectiveness rates. Therefore, the final rule (*Federal Register* 1996) included a sensitivity analysis using different effectiveness rates in reducing pathogens.

Additionally, USDA's Economic Research Service (ERS) performed a more detailed sensitivity analysis that evaluated the benefits and costs of this rule under three pathogen reduction rates (20, 50 and 90%) and two approaches to value premature deaths (Crutchfield *et al.* 1997). (The final rule occurred prior to OMB's 1996 recommendation that the WTP approach be used to value the premature deaths.) The analysis assumed that the benefits of pathogen reduction would begin in 2000 (when the rule was to be fully implemented) and would extend for 20 years. The scenarios in the first two rows of benefits in Table 16.1 used the Landefeld and Seskin approach which gave estimated values of a premature death ranging from US$15 000 to US$2 million, depending on how many years of life are lost. The latter two benefit scenarios called mid-range II and high-range, used a flat US$5 million WTP value for each statistical life lost based on Viscusi's review of the risk premium revealed in labour markets. Viscusi (1993) compared wage differentials in 24 wage-risk studies and inferred that the extra wages associated with the increased overall hazard of one death from risky jobs are clustered between US$3 million and US$7 million (in 1990 dollars). Several regulatory agencies use either Viscusi's range of estimates or the US$5 million mid-point when analysing the benefits of proposed public safety rules. More recent COI estimates from ERS now use this US$5 million value after adjusting it for age and updating it to current dollars; and FDA has used this estimate in some of their QALY calculations.

This example illustrates the importance of assumptions on the final benefit and cost estimates. Benefits varied widely depending on the choice of pathogen reduction rates and valuation method for premature deaths. The benefits of reducing pathogens, which include lower costs of illness and death, ranged from US$2 billion to US$172 billion over 20 years, depending upon the assumed level of pathogen control and the VOSL. For the analysis, ERS used costs estimated by FSIS of HACCP of US$1.1 billion and US$1.3 billion over 20 years. This means that irrespective of which level of pathogen reduction or which VOSL was assumed here, the benefits are likely to exceed the costs of

Table 16.1 Scenarios used to evaluate HACCP rule and benefits assumptions

Scenario/description	Pathogen reduction (%)	Discount rate (%)	Valuation method for premature death/disability	Annualized benefits[1]		Annualized costs	Net benefits
				Low	High		
Low-range benefits	20	7	Landefeld and Seskin	1.9	9.3	1.1–1.3	0.8–8.0
Mid-range benefits I	50	7	Landefeld and Seskin	4.7	23.4	1.1–1.3	3.6–22.1
Mid-range benefits II	50	3	Viscusi, VOSL = US$5 million	26.2	95.4	1.1–1.3	25.1–94.1
High-range benefits	90	3	Viscusi, VOSL = US$5 million	47.2	171.8	1.1–1.3	46.1–170.5

[1] Benefits begin to accrue 5 years after the HACCP rule is enacted, and extend over 20 years [US$ billion (1995)].

[2] Landefeld and Seskin VOSL (value of a statistical life) estimates after averaging across gender and updating to 1995 dollars using BLS usual weekly earnings.

Source: Crutchfield *et al.* (1997). See http://www.ers.usda.gov/briefing/FoodSafetyPolicy/features.htm for updated estimates.

HACCP. In this analysis, the cut-off point for costs to outweigh the benefits would occur if 17% of meat and poultry-related food-borne illnesses could be prevented by the rule. Since this rule, other HACCP rules have been proposed or instituted for the food commodities of fish and fishery products, and juice.

Salmonella enteritidis in shell eggs

In the 1980s and 1990s, *S.enteritidis* emerged as a leading food-borne pathogen in the USA. The number of *S.enteritidis* isolates and *S.enteritidis* outbreaks reported to the CDC both increased rapidly. Evidence from the outbreaks pointed to the consumption of raw or undercooked eggs as the likely cause of the increase; the CDC found that 80% of the *S.enteritidis* outbreaks traced to a known food vehicle were associated with eggs. As a result, the FDA and FSIS initiated a series of rulemakings aimed at reducing the incidence of *S.enteritidis* in shell eggs and egg products. The challenge that faced the FDA rather than the FSIS in the late 1990s was to design a rule that could quickly make a substantial contribution to the goal of reducing *S.enteritidis* illness associated with shell eggs. The FSIS was not similarly challenged as was the FDA because the processed eggs regulated by the FSIS were not then associated with *S.enteritidis* illnesses.

The agency considered several possible regulations, including: (i) safe handling labels; (ii) refrigeration of shell eggs held at retail at 7.2°C (45°F); (iii) refrigeration at 5°C (41°F); (iv) HACCP programmes for shell eggs; (v) in-shell pasteurization; (vi) limited retail sell-by periods; (vii) combinations of two or more of the above options; and (viii) no new regulatory action.

The final rule the FDA published in December 2000 combined options (i) and (ii) (*Federal Register* 2000). It required the following safe handling label on cartons of shell eggs that had not been treated with heat (or something equally effective) to destroy *Salmonella*:

> SAFE HANDLING INSTRUCTIONS: To prevent illness from bacteria: keep eggs refrigerated, cook eggs until yolks are firm, and cook foods containing eggs thoroughly.

The provision for a safe handling statement would reduce illnesses by increasing the proportion of eggs that were cooked enough to eliminate the risk, even if the eggs were contaminated before cooking. Safe handling statements work by providing information that leads to changes in behaviour, but nothing in safe handling statements forces changes in the preparation of shell eggs. The FDA assumed that the safe handling statement would decrease the probability that people would consume raw or undercooked eggs, but would not eliminate undercooking.

The rule also required that, when held by retail establishments, shell eggs must be stored and displayed at a temperature of 7.2°C (45°F) or lower. The temperature provision of the rule would reduce the illnesses associated with *S.enteritidis* in shell eggs at retail because refrigeration slows the growth of pathogens in contaminated eggs.

The FDA selected the labelling and refrigeration option in part because the CBA showed that this option generated higher estimated net benefits than the alternatives. In what follows, we will describe how the FDA estimated the benefits and costs of the shell eggs rule.

The FDA combined the USDA *S.enteritidis* risk assessment of 1998 and the CDC estimates of the incidence of egg-related *S.enteritidis* (Mead *et al.* 1999) to obtain the initial estimates of the incidence of illness from contaminated eggs. The *S.enteritidis* risk assessment estimated that of the 47 billion shell eggs consumed annually, 2.3 million were *S.enteritidis* positive. According to the 1999 estimates from the CDC, *S.enteritidis* in shell eggs caused more than 112 000 illnesses per year (see Table 16.2). The FDA used the *S.enteritidis* risk assessment model to determine the proportional decline in illnesses likely to occur as a result of the labelling and refrigeration rule, then applied that result to the CDC illness numbers to determine the likely decline in the number of *S.enteritidis* illnesses.

Because costs per case differ by the severity and duration of the illnesses, the FDA needed to estimate the severity distribution of the roughly 15 000 preventable annual cases to estimate the benefits of the rule. Table 16.2 shows the estimated effects of the refrigeration and safe handling labels mandated by the FDA rule in preventing illnesses, arthritis and premature deaths. The CDC surveillance results indicated that 92% of victims do not seek medical attention. The FDA assumed that these cases were mild. The surveillance result showed that 15% of those who sought medical attention for *S.enteritidis* would be hospitalized. Of those who were hospitalized, about 5% would die prematurely because of their illness. The case-fatality rate equalled the probability of seeking medical attention (8%) multiplied by the conditional probability of hospitalization (15%) multiplied by the conditional probability of death given hospitalization (5%), or about 0.06% for a total of nine preventable deaths. Various studies have found the proportion of acute cases that lead to post-*Salmonella* reactive arthritis to be from 2 to 6.4%. The USDA *S.enteritidis* risk assessment used a 2–4% range, with the mean equal to roughly 3%. The FDA assumed that slightly less than 3% of acute salmonellosis cases led to reactive arthritis.

The benefits of the rule equal the value of the illnesses and deaths prevented. The FDA assumed that the health benefits associated with preventing

Table 16.2 Effects of the FDA Shell Egg Labelling and Refrigeration Rule

	No. of illnesses	Reactive arthritis	Deaths
Baseline from *S.enteritidis* in shell eggs	112 138	3011	66
Number likely to be prevented[1]	14 958	410	9

[1] Estimated numbers prevented are median results from simulations of distributions with a long right tail.

The views expressed in this chapter are not official policy of the US Department of Agriculture or the US Department of Health and Human Services.

salmonellosis included reduced: (i) loss of functional status (including mobility, physical, activity and social activity); (ii) pain and suffering; and (iii) expenditures on medical treatment. The FDA measured the losses suffered by victims of salmonellosis with a QALY index. The QALY approach uses a daily scale of well being—called a quality-adjusted life day—which varies from 1 for good health to 0 for death. The loss per day is the difference between 1 and the quality-adjusted life day. For example, with the scale used by the FDA in the analysis, people with mild salmonellosis (diarrhoea, nausea, vomiting, fever and headache) have an estimated quality-adjusted life day equal to 0.527, which implies a daily loss of 0.473. Mild cases last about 2 days, for a total loss in quality-adjusted life days of 0.946 (2 × 0.473) and a loss of QALYs of about 0.003 (0.946 ÷ 365). In contrast, post-*Salmonella* reactive arthritis causes a daily loss of 0.21 per day and per year and may last for the rest of the victim's life. The FDA used a distribution for the age of onset for salmonellosis, based on CDC surveillance results, that implied that the average chronic case of post-*Salmonella* reactive arthritis lasts about 13 years, for a total loss of 2.7 QALYs (13 × 0.21).

To perform the CBA of the rule, the FDA put the loss of QALYs in monetary terms. The agency assumed that the most likely value of a small reduction in the probability of death, commonly called the VOSL, was US$5 million (Viscusi 1993). The average number of life years lost in the studies that generated the US$5 million estimate was 36 years. With a discount rate of 3%, the average discounted numbers of life years lost was 21.8 years. The value of a single QALY was therefore about US$230 000 (US$5 million = 21.8). The value of QALYs lost for cases of salmonellosis would equal the number of years lost multiplied by US$230 000.

For fatal cases, the FDA multiplied the value of a QALY (US$230 000) by the discounted number of life years lost per fatality. Most of the deaths attributed to *S.enteritidis* are of elderly persons. Of the 27 deaths linked to food-borne *S.enteritidis* disease outbreaks from 1988 to 1992, 23 (85%) fatalities occurred in nursing homes (Bean *et al.* 1997). To estimate benefits from preventing deaths, the FDA assumed that the probability that the victim was aged 75 or older was 80%. The loss of QALYs is much less for victims aged 75 and older than for victims from the rest of the population. The agency estimated that the average loss of discounted QALYs would be about 6 years for victims aged 75 and older and about 26 years for other victims. The benefits of preventing death from acute salmonellosis, then, were estimated as US$1.4 million for elderly victims and US$6 million for all others. The difference between the two values reflects the difference in life expectancy of elderly and non-elderly victims.

Although the FDA did not include medical costs associated with deaths from acute salmonellosis in the total costs, direct medical expenditures for non-fatal cases and cases that developed reactive arthritis were included. Medical costs tend to be a relatively small component of per person costs. For example, the medical costs of acute salmonellosis vary from nothing for a mild case to over US$9000 for severe cases (Buzby *et al.* 1996).

The total health costs per case are the sum of monetary value of lost QALYs (which include lost functional status and pain and suffering) and medical expenditures. The FDA estimates the total health benefits from its food safety rules with the following general formula:

Total health benefits = (number of non-fatal cases prevented × QALY per case × US$ per QALY) + (number of non-fatal cases prevented × US$ medical costs per case) + (number of deaths prevented × US$ per death)

To estimate the benefits of the shell egg labelling and refrigeration rule, the FDA used a more complicated version of the general formula. The more complicated formula classified non-fatal illnesses into subcategories based on severity and duration, and used two values (US$1.4 million for elderly victims and US$6 million for all others) for fatal illnesses. The calculation generated an estimated annual benefit from the rule of US$260 million.

Labelling retail cartons of shell eggs and increasing the amount of refrigeration generates costs as well as benefits. The FDA concluded that the main cost of the refrigeration provision would be the cost of purchasing or upgrading commercial refrigerators used in retail establishments. The agency assumed that the requirement for a safe handling statement on the label would generate two different costs. One cost would be the one-time cost of redesigning and changing the plates used to print labels on egg cartons. The other cost would be the continuing loss of consumer surplus associated with changes in the way eggs were prepared. The agency assumed that people who, in response to the safe handling label, changed the way they cooked and consumed eggs would lose consumer surplus from giving up soft-boiled, poached, runny scrambled or other types of undercooked eggs. The agency estimated that the sum of these costs (more refrigeration, new label plates for egg carton, lost consumer surplus) would be US$56 million in the first year the rule became effective, and US$10 million (continued lost consumer surplus and some increase in energy costs) in all later years.

The estimated benefits clearly outweighed the estimated costs of the rule: the best estimate of US$260 million in benefits per year greatly exceeds costs of US$56 million in the first year and US$10 million thereafter. What is more, none of the other regulatory options generated net benefits that were as high. Because both benefits and costs were uncertain, however, the FDA tested the robustness of the results with computer simulations that replaced point estimates with probability distributions to estimate benefits and costs. The computer simulations generated ranges of both benefits and costs, but the low end of the distribution of benefits easily exceeded costs.

The final rule on labelling and refrigeration of shell eggs demonstrates how a public health agency can use information from a risk assessment and a CBA to design a regulation to mitigate an emerging public health problem. The rule came about as part of a general goal of reducing *S.enteritidis* from shell eggs, as articulated in President's Council on Food Safety's Egg Safety Action Plan. The risk assessment and CDC surveillance estimates established a baseline and provided a means to estimate the effectiveness of policy options. Various specialists within the FDA, including labelling experts, commercial refrigeration experts and behavioural scientists, looked at how different rules might work in retail stores, and how they might affect consumers. Finally, the CBA of the various regulatory alternatives identified the labelling and refrigeration rule as the regulatory alternative with the highest net benefits.

Proposed rule for ready-to-eat meat and poultry products

Over the past decade, food safety concerns have increased about RTE MPPs, particularly with respect to potential contamination by the subtype of *Listeria* called *Listeria monocytogenes*. In North America and Western Europe, listeriosis has an estimated incidence rate in the range of 4–8 cases per 1 000 000 individuals (US Department of Health and Human Services, Center for Food Safety and Applied Nutrition, Food and Drug Administration, and the US Department of Agriculture, Food Safety and Inspection Service 2001). In the USA, this rate translates into approximately 2500 persons becoming seriously ill each year. Although most listeriosis symptoms are limited to flu-like conditions, it can pose significant adverse health consequences such as death for persons with incomplete or compromised immune systems [including infants, the elderly with underlying health problems, cancer and kidney patients, and acquired immune deficiency syndrome (AIDS) patients] and spontaneous, late-term abortions in pregnant women. As a result, listeriosis has the highest case-fatality rate of the major food-borne diseases.

Listeria contamination is difficult to detect and control. *Listeria* can become established in certain sites or niches within the processing environment where it can grow and multiply, sometimes even under refrigerated conditions. The frequency and extent of *L.monocytogenes* in the food at retail outlets appear to be greatly influenced by: the amounts and frequency of certain foods being present; the potential for growth of *L.monocytogenes* in food during refrigerated storage; the refrigerated storage times before consumption; and the temperature at which the food was held during refrigeration. Additionally, the extent of *L.monocytogenes* contamination varies by product and manufacturing process (Doyle 1988).

A recent joint FDA–USDA *L.monocytogenes* risk assessment predicted the relative *L.monocytogenes* potential contamination risk from the 20 most risky food categories and found that frankfurters and deli meats from the RTE MPP class have a high exposure potential (Table 16.3) (US Department of Health and Human Services, Center for Food Safety and Applied Nutrition, Food and Drug Administration, and the US Department of Agriculture, Food Safety and Inspection Service 2001). In particular, on a per serving basis, the baseline analysis found that pâté, meat spreads and fresh soft cheeses had the highest relative risk rankings. However, when frankfurters were subdivided into reheated and non-reheated components, non-reheated frankfurters ranked high in terms of relative risk. An alternate risk ranking is the ranking on a per annum basis where deli meats ranked highest. These findings support the long-standing hypothesis that the further post-processing steps (e.g. slicing, mixing and packaging) taken in the production of frankfurters and deli meats could be directly responsible for their high-risk categorization.

The RTE designation implies that consumers should be able to consume the product without further cooking or other treatment step that would kill any remaining pathogens on the product, meaning that if pathogens are present, illness may result. After the 1996 introduction of PR/HACCP for meat and poultry, the FSIS recommended that plants reassess their HACCP plans to ensure that they are adequately addressing *L.monocytogenes*: if this reassessment revealed that *L.monocytogenes* is a hazard reasonably likely to occur, then the hazard must be addressed in the establishment's HACCP plan (*Federal*

Register 1999). Later in 1998, one outbreak resulting in 80 illnesses, 15 deaths and six stillbirths or miscarriages drew public attention to the link between listeriosis and the consumption of hot dogs and deli meat products (Detroit-Free Press 2001). Also, in some recent years, almost 50% of all FSIS recalls have involved *L.monocytogenes* contaminated product (e.g. 25 of 55 recalls in the 1999 financial year). As part of the set of food safety initiatives and directives defined in autumn 2000, one goal was to achieve a 50% reduction in listeriosis by 2005. According to the CDC in April 2005, this goal is nearly met for 2005. For the year 2004, the estimated illnesses associated with *L.monocytogenes* decreased 40% when comparing 1996–1998 with 2004 (Vugia *et al.* 2005). These and other factors, events and issues compelled USDA's FSIS to take action in February 2001.

The proposed RTE rule

The 'Performance Standards for the Production of Processed Meat and Poultry Products' (*Federal Register* 2001) rule, commonly referred to as the ready-to-eat meat and poultry product rule, actually consists of four provisions and a use-by date labelling policy option. The four provisions were: replacement of two separate existing regulations, one involving canning and another on the assurance of trichina-free pork; extension of existing lethality and stabilization performance standards to those RTE MPPs not previously covered in the so-called roast beef rule (FSIS Docket No. 95–033F; 64 FR 732); and, the main focus of this section, mandatory environmental *Listeria* spp. testing.

The first two provisions fall into 'regulation reform', where the main intent is to replace existing regulations that have a command-and-control orientation with a more HACCP-like regulatory approach. With regulation reform, firms would have the option to continue using current production methods or alter their production practices as long as they can validate that their processes still achieve existing food safety goals. It is likely that establishments would only deviate from current practices if such changes are cost reducing. Accordingly, these two provisions are considered neutral with respect to benefits and neutral to positive in lowering costs: as such, they are not included in this analysis.

The third provision extends existing performance standards (involving *Salmonella* in meat and poultry and *Escherichia coli* O157:H7 in beef) to additional RTE MPPs. Many of these products are produced using traditional methods which have never been scientifically validated to meet any standards, are quite diverse, satisfy only small niche markets and are produced in establishments that have long been monitored by the FSIS and considered adequate to produce safe products. In some cases, where current practices fail to meet the new standards, establishments may have to alter their process, such as

Table 16.3 Predicted relative risk rankings for listeriosis among food categories for three age-based subpopulations using median estimates of predicted relative risks for listeriosis on a per serving and per annum basis

Food category	Per serving basis by subpopulation			Per annum basis by subpopulation		
	Intermediate[1]	Elderly[2]	Prenatal[3]	Intermediate[1]	Elderly[2]	Prenatal[3]
Seafood						
Smoked	3	3	3	6	6	7
Raw	14	14	14	17	20	17
Preserved	7	7	6	13	13	13
Cooked RTE crustaceans	6	5	5	9	8	9
Produce						
Vegetables	17	17	17	11	9	11
Fruits	18	18	18	16	14	14
Dairy						
Soft mould-ripened and blue-veined cheese	9	9	9	14	15	15
Goat, sheep and feta cheese	16	16	16	18	17	18
Fresh soft cheese	2	1	1	7	11	6
Heat-treated natural cheese and processed cheese	15	15	15	10	10	10
Aged cheese	19	19	19	19	18	19
Fluid milk, pasteurized	10	10	10	3	2	2
Fluid milk, unpasteurized	11	11	11	15	16	16
Ice cream and frozen dairy products	20	20	20	20	19	20
Miscellaneous dairy products	12	13	13	5	4	5

Meats						
All frankfurters	8	8	7	4	5	4
[Only reheated frankfurters]	[15]	[15]	[15]			
[Only non-reheated frankfurters]	[1]	[2]	[2]			
Dry/semi-dry fermented sausages	13	12	12	12	12	12
Deli meats	4	4	4	1	1	1
Pâté and meat spreads	1	2	2	8	7	8
Combo foods						
Deli salads	5	6	8	2	3	3

[1] Intermediate = the remaining population after taking account of the elderly and prenatal (no breakdown by health condition).

[2] Elderly = includes people 60 or more years of age.

[3] Prenatal = includes fetuses and newborns from 16 weeks after fertilization to 30 days after birth.

Source: DHHS/USDA (2001, pp. 16 and 18).

increasing processing times and temperatures, or adding new equipment. While the FSIS has full confidence that current processes achieve existing food safety goals (making this provision unable to produce any increase in public health), the FSIS acknowledges that including these products in a more HACCP-like regulatory framework could lead to substantial cost increases for some producers. The FSIS found that expected cost increases from this provision alone represent about two-thirds of the total potential cost impact generated by the entire proposed rule, whereas industry benefited by increased regulatory consistency across products. The breakdown of expected costs by proposed rule provision is presented in the cost section below.

Meanwhile, the use-by date labelling policy option was put forward because preliminary analysis indicated a potentially high impact on public health (12.4 fewer annual listeriosis deaths), but at an unknown though apparently high industry cost, even if applied only to a few certain RTE MPPs. FSIS concluded that more information was necessary to refine the preliminary beneficial impact generated by such labelling further, particularly its ability to raise consumer awareness and alter their behaviour (in handling, storing and preparing RTE MPPs) and its potential impact on industry costs in developing effective labelling systems and on existing product delivery and handling systems. The remainder of this RTE rule section focuses on the costs and benefits expected to result from the proposed mandatory environmental *Listeria* spp. testing provision.

Possible benefits from environmental testing

To calculate the benefits of this proposed provision, an estimate of the preventable illnesses and deaths from listeriosis was needed. The FDA-FSIS risk assessment results coupled with Mead *et al.*'s estimation of the incidence of major pathogens suggests that the consumption of RTE MPPs is responsible for up to 66% of listeriosis cases (or 1660) and deaths (or 332). A similar combination of CDC work on causes of food-borne diseases by Olsen *et al.* (2000) with Mead *et al.*'s work suggests 167 cases and 35 deaths attributable to consumption of RTE MPPs (as discussed in the February 2001 *Federal Register* proposal and at the May 10, 2001 public meeting presentation by Spinelli). These two sets of estimates provide a broad range for the estimate of the number of cases and deaths probably attributable to the consumption of RTE MPPs. In addition, the FDA-FSIS risk assessment identified the most likely products involved and types of consumers affected. Unfortunately, a similar risk assessment was not available to identify the benefits of testing as a means to spur establishments to take measures to control *Listeria* contamination problems when they arise or the effectiveness of such measures. These information gaps (adjustments to account for the effectiveness of FSIS' proposed environmental testing protocol and for the plant measures in lowering their potential to contaminate product) plus other uncertainties forced the FSIS to make rough estimates on potential benefits, without full confidence and with a wide band. The FSIS determined that this provision could potentially result in 25–248 fewer illnesses and 5–50 fewer deaths over 10 years. The assumed listeriosis case and death distribution by age class associated with the above estimates were assumed to be: (i) prenatal, 14% of the cases, but 29% of the deaths; (ii) elderly, 52% of the cases, but 56% of deaths; and (iii) all other age groups, 34% of the cases, but only 19% of the deaths. Further discussion on the uncertainty surrounding these estimates is provided in the proposed rule analysis (*Federal Register* 2001, p. 12626).

The FSIS relied on the USDAs ERSs' previous analytical base to estimate the monetary value of these cases and death estimates. The total numbers of prenatal cases and deaths were excluded from further consideration due to lack of consensus on an appropriate valuation technique. The remaining premature deaths were valued by using a US$5 million estimate as the foundation and then this value was adjusted for different ages at the time of death and updated to current dollars. Specific assumptions were made on survival rates of reported cases and medical costs. Of the 25–248 cases, 20–198 are expected to survive and incur US$10 300 for mild cases and US$28 300 for severe cases. In total, the medical costs for such hospitalizations over 10 years totalled US$2.9 million–US$29.3 million in constant dollars for each respective case level. Of the 25–248 cases, 5–50 are expected to result in death and subsequent lost productivity. The avoidance of such premature deaths over 10 years was calculated at US$36.5 million and US$500.1 million, in constant dollars. Adding the value of the expected prevented cases and avoided deaths due to increased environmental testing produced a total potential increase in social welfare of US$39.4 million to US$529.4 million, respectively, for the low and high case/death levels indicated above.

Potential industry costs

As indicated previously, performance standards contribute roughly two-thirds of all 10 year costs (US$33.5 million out of US$49.3 million in constant terms) expected to be generated by the proposed rule. Most of these costs involved higher input use associated with increased processing times and temperatures (which could result in higher costs of US$4.41 million annually). First year costs would consist of these costs, plus process validation costs (US$2.72 million) for a total first year cost of US$7.13 million. This expected first year cost impact compares with the proposed mandatory environmental testing provision's estimated impact of US$5.53 million (first year costs of US$1.29 million in HACCP modification costs and US$2.49 million in expected compliance costs plus US$1.75 million in annual recurring testing costs). The expected compliance costs consist of the estimated cost impact of physical modifications in facilities or production processes to remedy contamination problems and, for some establishments, the exit from RTE MPP production. The low recurring costs associated with the mandatory environmental *Listeria* spp. testing provision, relative to the performance standard provision, produce an expected 10 year cost impact of US$15.8 million in constant dollars.

Comparison of benefits with costs

Estimated benefits of the proposed rule reflect only those generated by environmental testing. The only benefit generated by extending performance standards can only be made in qualitative terms: they allow the FSIS to have greater confidence that these products meet existing food safety goals and spread the HACCP-like regulatory framework to a greater number of establishments under their jurisdiction. If one deducts the US$33.5 million in costs associated with performance standards, expected benefits outweigh expected costs for both the low and high estimates of case and death reductions (US$36.5 and US$500.1 are both more than US$15.8). Weighing the cost of the entire proposed rule to benefits fails to meet this test in the low reduction scenario (US$36.5 < US$49.3), but still passes in the high reduction scenario (US$500.1 > US$49.3).

This section and its results highlight three key issues in the economic analysis of food-borne diseases. The first issue is the role and importance of risk assessments in identifying policy options and evaluating their effectiveness in lowering food-borne illnesses and deaths in economic impact analyses. The FDA-FSIS risk assessment identified the most likely products to be contaminated with *Listeria*. Such information helps to focus attention on the likely source(s) of contamination and most effective control measures in those instances. The FSIS is currently investigating the kinds of risk assessments needed to address these issues. Specifically, the FSIS would like to quantify: (i) the role of testing in identifying *Listeria* contamination and the effectiveness of testing as a means of identifying control measures; and (ii) the number of prevented listeriosis cases and deaths that could be expected if such measures were taken. Perhaps the risk assessment effort should best be viewed as an iterative process —a way to focus in on the most relevant questions after earlier information is acquired and analysed. The important contribution that a risk assessment can make is made obvious in the *S.enteritidis* in shell egg analysis. A second— and, in this case, related—issue is the role of environmental testing in a HACCP regulatory framework and its potential to lower public health risk in this particular instance. Several sources in the literature question the role of testing when HACCP plans are properly validated and compare pathogen testing as a HACCP verification tool with 'looking for the proverbial needle in the haystack'. Others contend that environmental testing is essential to ensure that the processing facility is not causing *incidental* contamination that could easily go undetected in finished product tests (Swanson and Anderson 2000). FSIS' interest in environmental testing explicitly recognizes the *incidental* nature in most cases of *Listeria* contamination as well as addresses a specific request in a citizen petition by the Center for Science in the Public Interest (CSPI) calling for increased environmental testing (Public Petition by CSPI, January 13, 2000). A final issue brought out in this section is the need to re-consider how cases and deaths in the fetal/newborn category should be treated. This is especially evident in the case of listeriosis, which has a disproportionate impact on this population subgroup. Not only would this refinement potentially increase estimated benefits in the present analysis, but it would more adequately address this public health concern in other instances where such impacts occur.

What is ahead?

Several aspects of the economic analyses of regulations are evolving, particularly the valuation of premature deaths used in COI analyses that support food safety regulations. As we have seen, the 1996 PR/HACCP regulation incorporated the Landefeld and Seskin method, a now outdated method largely based on human capital. Despite the use of more sophisticated approaches in more recent and proposed regulations such as QALYs for *S.enteritidis* regulation and age-adjusted WTP for the *Listeria* testing regulation, there is no consensus as to the best approach. In the PR/HACCP example, estimated benefits varied widely depending on the choice of valuation method for premature deaths, illustrating the importance of this assumption on the final benefit and cost estimates. Estimated benefits also varied depending on the choice of pathogen reduction rates

All aspects of the economic analyses for food safety regulations could benefit from better data. One substantial information gap concerns the epidemiology of and economics behind the estimated 62 million annual food-borne illnesses whose cause is unknown. Perhaps a method could be developed to estimate the likely economic effects of the emergence of new or newly identified food-borne pathogens. The final rule on labelling and refrigeration of shell eggs is one example of how a public health agency can use information from a risk assessment and a CBA to design a regulation to mitigate an emerging public health problem. Additionally, with more information and data, COI and economic analyses could incorporate more chronic sequelae from food-borne illnesses, such as reactive arthritis, liver disease, Guillain–Barré syndrome and others.

Also evolving is the system of regulatory, legal and market components that provides incentives to firms to produce safe food products. In the US regulatory arena, new food safety regulations have been added while older regulations have been fine-tuned. Meanwhile, efforts are underway to strengthen the government's ability to enforce food safety regulations. There will probably be continued use of COI estimates in CBA for food safety regulations, particularly for HACCP regulations applied to other categories of foods and food products.

Currently, legal incentives to firms to produce safer food are limited partly because of high information and transaction costs necessary to prevail in court (Buzby et al. 2001). Much of the costs of food-borne illnesses caused by firms are borne by ill consumers or their households, shifted to other parties such as employers, private health insurers and governments (and, in turn, taxpayers), or borne by some combination of these groups. If food firms have sufficient product liability insurance to cover a lawsuit, the full financial impact may not be felt by the firm, though their premiums and those of similar firms may increase in the future. One implication of the current social allocation of food-borne illness costs is that food firms receive only limited feedback to produce safer food and therefore probably underinvest in food safety. It is unclear whether food-borne illness litigation will become more common in the future. Food-borne illness—and the reasons for litigation—may decrease if firms continue to improve quality control practices to ensure safer food. In contrast, improvements in pathogen detection and identification techniques may increase the chances that food-borne illnesses will be detected and linked to specific food products and firms.

Some people may consider that market incentives are the most powerful of the three components in the incentive system because firms cannot ignore major market incentives and remain profitable or viable. If consumers become concerned about the safety of a firm's products, consumers may avoid the implicated products, in turn decreasing sales revenue and potentially causing serious financial difficulties for the firm. Market share and stock prices may fall (see Salin and Hooker 2001).

The complexity of the food safety system and the interconnectedness of the three components are shown by the 1996 US outbreak of food-borne illness due to E.coli O157:H7 contamination of unpasteurized apple juice manufactured by Odwalla, Inc. This outbreak raised consumer concerns nationwide about the safety of fresh juice, and this market pressure prompted many juice manufacturers voluntarily to begin pasteurizing juice products previously sold as unpasteurized. Meanwhile, the increasing number of food-borne illness outbreaks due to *E.coli* O157:H7 contamination of unpasteurized juice products led the FDA to propose new regulations for juice products. The adverse consequences of this outbreak on Odwalla from the mixture of market forces, government actions and product liability included a voluntary product recall costing US$12.5 million, a 17% drop in revenue during the first 6 months after the outbreak, a record US$1.5 million Federal fine for interstate shipment of an adulterated food product, and over 20 personal injury lawsuits (Munarriz 1997; Buzby and Crutchfield 1999; Roach 1999).

As with food safety regulations, private system approaches to reduce food safety risks are becoming more widespread and stringent (Caswell and Henson 1997). Private system approaches include self-regulation, vertical integration (to ensure quality/safety of inputs, for example), voluntary or mandatory HACCP systems, and third party certification such as the International Organization for Standardization (such as the ISO 9000 series or 'EN 29000' in Europe). Effective implementation of these private sector approaches is key to enhance food safety. These private sector approaches are often intertwined with each other [e.g. ISO standards often use HACCP and statistical process control principles with multilateral coordination mechanisms (such as Codex HACCP standards)]. Statistical Process Control (SPC), another internationally recognized innovation, also shows promise for reducing food safety risks (Bisaillon *et al.* 1997). SPC uses standardized sampling procedures to reject or accept lots to reach a desired level of quality or safety.

In short, the incentive system and the public and private actions to ensure safer food are complex and intertwined. Food safety regulations, and the economic analyses that support these regulations, are evolving alongside the precedents from food poisoning litigation and the development of new private approaches.

References

American Meat Institute (2001) *Listeria monocytogenes*: Introduction and Basis for Control, Section 3. In: *Listeria monocytogenes* Briefing by the AMI, July 30, 2001.

Bisaillon, J.R., Charlebois, R., Feltmate, T. and Labbé, Y. (1997) HACCP, statistical process control applied to post-mortem inspection and risk analysis in Canadian abattoirs. *Dairy, Food, and Environmental Sanitation* 17, 150–155.

Bean, N.H., Goulding, J.S., Daniels, M.T. and Angulo, F.J. (1997) Surveillance for foodborne disease outbreaks—United States, 1988–1992. *Journal of Food Protection* 60, 1265–1286.

Buzby, J.C. and Crutchfield, S. (1999) New juice regulations underway. US Department of Agriculture, Economic Research Service. *FoodReview* 22, 23–25.

Buzby, J.C., Roberts, T., Lin, C.-T.J. and MacDonald, J.M. (1996) bacterial foodborne disease: medical costs and productivity losses. US Department of Agriculture, Economic Research Service. http://www.ers.usda.gov/publications/Aer741/index.htm, as accessed July 18, 2001.

Buzby, J.C., Frenzen, P.D. and Rasco, B. (2001) Product liability and microbial foodborne illness. US Department of Agriculture, Economic Research Service. http://www.ers.usda.gov/publications/aer799/, accessed July 6, 2001.

Caswell, J.A. and Henson, S.J. (1997) Interaction of private and public food quality control systems in global markets. In: Loader, R.J., Henson, S.J. and Traill, W.B. *Proceedings of Globilisation of the Food Industry: Policy Implications.* pp. 217–234.

Crutchfield, S.R., Buzby, J.C., Roberts, T., Ollinger, M. and Lin, C.-T.J. (1997) An economic assessment of food safety regulations. US Department of Agriculture, Economic Research Service. http://www.ers.usda.gov/publications/aer755/, as accessed June 11, 2001.

Detroit-Free Press (2001) Sara Lee pleads guilty in recall, Plant's contaminated meat killed 15, sickened 80. June 23.

Doyle, M. (1988) Effect of environmental and processing conditions on *Listeria monocytogenes. Food Technology* 42, 169–171.

Federal Register (1995) Pathogen reduction; hazard analysis and critical control point (HACCP) systems; preliminary regulatory impact assessment for Docket No. 93–016P, 60, 6774–6889.

Federal Register (1996) Pathogen Reduction; Hazard Analysis and Critical Control Point (HACCP) systems; final rule. US Department of Agriculture, Food Safety and Inspection Service. 61, 38805–38989.

Federal Register (1998a) Egg Products Inspection Act regulations; final rule. 63, 69967–69972.

Federal Register (1998b) Refrigeration and labeling requirements for shell eggs. 63 45663–45675.

Federal Register (1999) *Listeria monocytogenes* contamination of ready-to-eat products. 64, 28351–28353. 9 CFR Parts 416 and 417, Docket No. 99–025N.

Federal Register (2000) Food labeling, safe handling statements, labeling of shell eggs; refrigeration of shell eggs held for retail distribution; final rule. 65, 76092–76114.

Federal Register (2001) Performance standards for the production of processed meat and poultry products. 66, 12590–12636.

Garber, S. (1998a) Product liability, punitive damages, business decisions, and economic outcomes. *Wisconsin Law Review* 1998, 1237–295.

Garber, S. (1998b) Good deterrence, bad deterrence and challenges in product liability reform. Rand Institute for Civil Justice http://www.rand.org/centers/icj/garber.html, as accessed July 31, 1998.

Golan, E. and Kuchler, F. (2001) *Economists, economics, and food safety policy.* Presented at the Association for Public Policy Analysis and Management Annual Research Conference Washington, DC, November 1–3, 2001.

Kuchler, F. and Golan, E. (1999) Assigning values to life: comparing methods for valuing health risks. US Department of Agriculture, Economic Research Service, Agricultural Economic Report Number 784, November 1999, http://www.ers.usda.gov/publications/aer784/

Landefeld, J.S. and Seskin, E.P. (1982) The economic value of life: linking theory to practice. *American Journal of Public Health* **6**, 555–566.

Mead, P.S., Slutsker, L., Dietz, V., McCaig, L.F., Bresee, J.S., Shapiro, C., Griffin, P.M. and Tauxe, R.V. (1999) Food-related illness and death in the United States. *Emerging Infectious Diseases* **5**, 607–625.

Munarriz, R.A. (1997) Odwalla, Inc. *Daily Trouble* November 25. http://www.fool.com/DTrouble/1997/DTrouble971125.htm, accessed October 14, 1998.

Office of Management and Budget (1996) Economic analysis of Federal regulations Under Executive Order 12866. January 11. http://www.whitehouse.gov/omb/inforeg/riaguide.html, accessed June 11, 2001.

Office of Management and Budget (2003) Circular A-4, regulatory analysis. September 17. http://www.whitehouse.gov/omb/circulars/a004/a-4.html.

Olsen, S., MacKinon, L., Goulding, J., Bean, N. and Slutsker, L. (2000) Surveillance of foodborne disease outbreaks, United States—1993–97. *Morbidity and Mortality Weekly Reports, Surveillance Summary* **49**, (SS01), 1–51.

Roach, J. (1999) Odwalla makes a comeback. *Environmental News Network* September 21. http://www.enn.com/enn-features-archive/1999/09/092199/odwalla_5157.asp, accessed November 1.

Salin, V. and Hooker, N.H. (2001) Stock market reaction to food recalls. *Review of Agricultural Ecnomics* **23**, 33–46.

Swanson, K. and Anderson, J. (2000) Industry perspectives on the use of microbial data for hazard analysis and critical control point validation and verification. *Journal of Food Protection* **6**, 815–818.

Roberts, T., Buzby, J. and Ollinger, M. (1996) Using benefit and cost information to evaluate a food safety regulation: HACCP for meat and poultry. *American Journal of Agricultural Economics* **78**, 1297–1301.

US Department of Health and Human Services, Center for Food Safety and Applied Nutrition, Food and Drug Administration, and the US Department of Agriculture, Food Safety and Inspection Service (2001) *Interpretive Summary: Draft Assessment of the Relative Risk to Public Health From Foodborne Listeria monocytogenes Among Selected Categories of Ready-to-eat Foods.* January 2001.

Viscusi, W.K. (1993) The value of risks to life and health. *Journal of Economic Literature* **31**, 1912–1946.

Viscusi, W.K. and Aldy, J.E. (2004) The value of a statistical life: a critical review of market estimates throughout the world. *Journal of Risk and Uncertainty* **27**, 5–76.

Vugia, D., Cronquist, A., Hadler, J., Tobin-D'Angelo, M., Blythe, D. *et al.* (2005) Preliminary FoodNet data on the incidence of infection with pathogens transmitted commonly through food-10 sites, United States, 2004. *Morbidity and Mortality Weekly Reports* **54**, 352–356.

Chapter 17

Global governance of international public health: the role of international regulatory cooperation

Lilani Kumaranayake

Introduction

Public health has emerged as a critical issue globally. The human immunodeficiency virus (HIV)/acquired immune deficiency virus (AIDS) pandemic is devastating many countries, reducing life expectancy and rolling back decades of economic progress (UNAIDS 2004). Other infectious diseases such as tuberculosis and malaria are growing as global public health threats (World Health Organization 2004). The severe acute respiratory syndrome (SARS) epidemic demonstrated the extent of global interconnectedness and the need for rapid responses. New public health regimes, such as the Global Fund to fight AIDS, Tuberculosis and Malaria (GFATM), are leveraging and distributing large flows of funding (Brugha *et al.* 2004). Global civil society, including international non-governmental organizations (NGOs), play a significant role in delivering public health services and advocacy, raising issues related to accountability and transparency (Kumaranayake and Lake 2002; Spar and Dail 2002; Spiro 2002; Wapner 2002). The severity and extent of the disease burden have resulted in greater scrutiny of national and international governance of public health as well as increasing involvement of international law (Fidler 2002). A key focus has been on the Trade Related-aspects of Intellectual Property Rights (TRIPS) agreement that has been very controversial with respect to its application to pharmaceuticals (Reichman 2000; Dreyfuss 2001; Correa 2002; Sykes 2002; t'Hoen 2002).

Regulation occurs when government or authority controls or influences the activities of individuals or organizations to affect changes in behaviour (Maynard 1982; Kumaranayake 1997; Raustiala 2000). International regulatory cooperation (IRC) can be defined as cooperation (either bilaterally or multilaterally) between governments, agencies or organizations, on regulatory activities, where this may include the development of legislation, regulation or standards, and any related activities, e.g. the development of harmonized regulatory processes, the establishment, recognition and application, by at least two governments, agencies or organizations having identified a mutual benefit in working together, with common regulatory processes or standards applied in determining compliance with regulation. Regulatory cooperation therefore covers a range of activities including, but not limited to: information sharing; laboratory collaborations; joint review; parallel review; development of memoranda of understanding; preparation of mutual recognition agreements; and harmonization of data requirements or scientific assessment processes.

IRC is a growing phenomena in a number of areas (Raustiala 2000; Guzman 2002), including health (Indech 2000; Silverglade 2000; Ward 2000, Abraham and Reed 2001). There has been limited consideration of what and how IRC may be used to achieve objectives on the international public health and humanitarian assistance agendas. Traditionally, international actors have played a role in ensuring standard setting. The World Health Organization (WHO) has been predominant in this. Whether this model is appropriate or feasible for IRC development in the context of international public health is questionable. A number of issues arise with the consideration of IRC for health, including the role of supranational regulators, the role of institutions and global civil society, and whether interests between resource-rich and resource-poor countries are sufficiently convergent for IRC within the context of international public health. With HIV/AIDS declared a global public health emergency by the WHO in 2003 and the United Nations focus upon HIV/AIDS (UNGASS 2001), the issues of how IRC can be more effective in addressing priority concerns takes on ever greater importance.

This chapter examines the role of supranational regulators in IRC examining the World Trade Organization (WTO) and the WHO, in particular looking at the WTO with respect to the case of HIV/AIDS drugs and the conflict and relationship between Canada and the WHO during the SARS crises. The chapter starts by considering the various theoretical models of regulatory development and then examining them in practice.

The economics of regulation and international regulatory cooperation

There are two basic economic theories that try to explain why regulation exists and the rationale for government intervention. The key distinction between the two theories is in the way government or supraregulator is assumed to behave. The *Public Interest approach* or *Welfarist approach* to government behaviour visualizes the government or state as seeking to promote the general interests of the society and thus will choose policies to further this. Alternatively, a *Public Choice* approach predicts that the behaviour of the government is the resulting interaction of individual choices made by voters, politicians and bureaucrats. Based on these two approaches to government behaviour, there are two competing theories to explain the presence of regulation.

The public interest approach was the earliest school of thought regarding regulation. Regulation was provided by the government in response to the public demand for the correction of inefficient or inequitable market practices (Posner 1974). This explanation of regulatory action is rooted in the analysis of markets and reasons for market failure. A public interest perspective towards regulation predicts that the government will take action to correct inefficient or inequitable market practices. Many are uncomfortable with the notion of the government as an efficient and costless intervenor in the market. Secondly, the theory allows for no apparent mechanism to link 'public interest' with legislative action that maximizes public welfare (Posner 1974). It is clear that markets within the health sector are largely imperfect. These markets have many characteristics (such as asymmetric information, moral hazard and uncertainty) which lead to market failure. Thus *a priori*, there is a strong public interest rationale for government involvement in the health sector. The more difficult question is just what form this intervention should take.

The self-interest view of regulation is based on the idea that regulation is supplied by the government in response to demands by various interest groups (whose motivation is to maximize the benefits/incomes of their members). The theory, first discussed by Stigler (1971) and later by Peltzmann (1976) and Becker (1983), suggests that regulation is the result of the interaction of special interest groups who provide financial and political support in return for favourable legislation. The key idea behind this theory is that the cost of a regulatory intervention is quite high. Thus the amount of effort and resources that a special interest group will expend will depend on the probable gains (rents) that will arise from the legislation.

The model predicts that the possible impact of regulation is to redistribute wealth away from the general public and towards the special interest groups; and that as the power of special interest groups changes, legislation will change over time. The model allows for the possibility of government failure, whereby the interaction between voters, special interest groups, politicians and bureaucrats leads to public choices which will not improve efficiency or equity relative to an unregulated market.

The effectiveness of IRC will to some extent be determined by the manner in which IRC is developed and implemented. Of particular interest to international public health is the role of the supranational actors—in particular the WTO and WHO.

IRC is becoming more common as regulatory authorities around the world must deal with issues that transcend a single population or jurisdiction. Other driving forces for a move toward increased IRC include globalization, the attendant increased movement of products and services, and, in the health context, the need to address rapid advances in technology. The desire for efficiency and transparency in regulatory approaches is also an important driver for increased IRC. IRC poses a number of challenges crossing geographical, legal and cultural boundaries. In the absence of IRC, domestic laws will impinge on international activity with the potential for overlapping jurisdictions, conflicting legal regimes and over-regulation (Guzman 2002).

Within the context of IRC and international public health, a broader set of questions arises. This is due to the global nature of health and service delivery, flows of financing and information that are both bilateral and multilateral, and the often emergency nature of activity. In a majority of the cases, these flows are from resource-rich to resource-poor countries. The scope for more formal and legally binding IRC within this global context is contingent on a number of factors, including the feasibility of establishing regulatory structures and rules in the broader context of global governance, as well as considerations relating to the implementation of those rules.

There is a range of possible IRC engagement among countries for various goods and services. The simplest is for individual countries to take unilateral action, but the issue is to what extent this can lead to the desired outcomes. The next level of cooperation is harmonization, with the challenge being to achieve agreements and establish common standards (Indech 2000; Silverglade 2000; Ward 2000; Abraham and Reed 2001). The final level of cooperation is supranational regulation which is the most intense and difficult level of engagement. Higher levels of cooperation may potentially lead to higher levels of effectiveness, but are accompanied by increasing transaction and compliance costs, accountability, transparency, information and monitoring complexities (Raustiala 2000; Rothstein 2003).

There is an emerging sense that in order to promote and protect people's health in the global economy, effective rules and regulatory frameworks are needed (Turmen 1999). However, the implementation of regulatory interventions is also highly dependent on global governance structures. There remains considerable debate about which structures are needed, ranging from informal regimes of industry self-regulation and voluntary compliance, to supranational

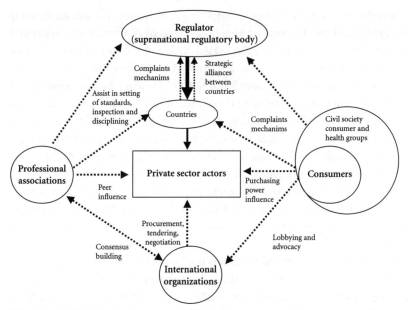

Fig. 17.1 Potential institutional actors and actions to achieve regulatory goals in a global context.

Source: Kumaranayake and Lake (2002).

and binding regulations (Deacon 1997). The creation of the WTO in 1995 is one of the most significant developments, to date, towards establishing supranational regulation, where the WTO enforces a series of multilateral trade agreements.

Regulation has a critical role in structuring positive benefits and minimizing negative consequences. The context of IRC is much more complicated that the standard bilateral regulator–regulatee relationship seen in national level regulatory structures (Kumaranayake *et al.* 2003). Figure 17.1 highlights the potential and (in some cases actual) role that different institutional structures and actors can play in achieving regulatory goals through both formal and non-formal means. The solid lines indicate the traditional regulator–regulatee relationship, and the dashed lines indicate the web of broader relationships that will affect the achievement of regulatory goals. This conceptual framework can be used to highlight the important relationships that can be used to achieve regulatory goals in the context of IRC.

The WTO as a supranational regulator: the case of HIV/AIDS drugs

One of the most significant things affecting essential drugs has been the role of TRIPS within the context of the WTO. The creation of the WTO in 1995 is one of the most significant developments in the movement towards establishing supranational regulation. The Uruguay round of discussion on tariffs and trade led to the creation of a rules-based system of global regulation. One of the core elements was the creation of the WTO to enforce the agreement. The WTO provided the institutional and legal framework for the multilateral trading system (Drager 1999), and was given substantial power to enforce the trade agreements, including the authority to review a country's national policies, settle disputes and impose substantial sanctions on countries who are found to be violating the agreement. The enforcement powers of the WTO are substantially larger than those of previous international organizations. The Uruguay round of trade talks also broadened the scope of the type of commodity that was covered under the WTO, with agreements extending to services such as insurance and intellectual property rights as well as health care (UNDP 1999).

One of the trade agreements emerging from the Uruguay round was the negotiation of a global agreement on intellectual property rights: the agreement on TRIPS. A key component of TRIPs in relation to pharmaceuticals, from the perspective of low- and middle-income countries (LMICs), was the protection of pharmaceutical patents for a period of 20 years. The TRIPS agreement imposed a patent both on the pharmaceutical process and on the final product. Prior to this, only the pharmaceutical process had been patented, allowing domestic companies to use different pharmaceutical processes to produce generic (and much cheaper) versions of brand name drugs. The TRIPS agreement conferred a 20 year global monopoly[1] to pharmaceutical companies through its patent protection, and so enhances a company's ability to charge premiums for new technologies as well ensure that they are not copied (Donald 1999). By 2000, countries, with the exception of least developing countries, had to grant legal protection by patent to pharmaceutical products. The least developing countries have until 2005/2006 to implement these regulations. Products in the pipeline before January 1, 1995 are exempt from TRIPs (Velasquez and Boulet 1999). These intellectual property rights were largely enshrined following initiatives by industrialized countries (World Health Organization 1998). The standards imposed by the TRIPs agreement were similar to that in industrialized countries and were far higher than existing patent protection found in most LMICs. Two exemptions were allowed in the TRIPs agreement: compulsory licencsing (CL) and parallel importing (PI). CL allows for the legal manufacture and use of generic drugs without the agreement of a patent holder. A judicial or administrative authority

---

[1] The monopoly affects all countries who are signatories of the TRIPs.

(e.g. national body) is allowed by law to grant a licence, without permission from the patent holder, on various grounds of public interest. PI occurs when branded drugs are purchased from a third party in another country, rather than directly from the manufacturer, taking advantage of the fact that pharmaceutical companies charge significantly lower prices in one country rather than another.

The debate with respect to drugs to treat HIV/AIDS-related illnesses and the role that TRIPs is seen to be playing provides a good example of the role of regulation at the international level, and the global and national linkages (Kumaranayake and Lake 2002). Several less developed countries have been under pressure from western governments to make changes to their health policy and legislation that would restrict their ability to issue CLs and engage in PI, despite these clauses being consistent with TRIPS (Wilson *et al.* 1999), as they attempted to conform to the WTO deadlines of 2000 and 2005 to be TRIPs compliant. This so-called 'TRIPs-plus' policy has been particularly high-lighted in both Thailand and South Africa (Bond 1999; Wilson *et al.* 1999).

Even before the TRIPs agreement was in place, Thailand upheld product patent protection, as a response to US pressure and the threat of trade sanctions limiting Thailand's ability to import into the lucrative US market. It is apparent that the 'ratcheting-up' of international regulatory standards with respect to pharmaceutical drugs seen in TRIPs was closely linked to the interests of western countries with strong pharmaceutical manufacturers (Braithwaite and Drahos 1999), and consistent with actions trying to achieve these ends prior to TRIPs. Since 1992, only three generic drugs have been produced and released from the SMP (Safety Monitoring Programme) in Thailand (Wibulpoprasert 1999), despite being exempted from TRIPs.

As the deadline approaches for the TRIPs agreement to be enshrined into law, there is tremendous pressure, particularly from the US government, for countries to adopt legislation that is even more restrictive than TRIPS and goes so far as banning CL and PI. Debate on these issues is now being taken up by consumer and advocacy groups, and there have been some reversals in policy positions in light of these activities. The US President's executive order in May 2000 was significant in that it prohibited the office of US Trade Representative from interfering with sub-Saharan African countries who operate in a manner consistent with TRIPs. This action was in response to substantial lobbying and advocacy efforts—and implicitly allows both CL and PI to take place without the threat of trade sanctions for countries in sub-Saharan Africa. Within a week of this order, five of the main pharmaceutical companies announced that they would commence negotiations on price cuts for HIV-related drugs with international agencies.

What has also been striking about the recent activity surrounding the TRIPs agreement is the important role that coalitions of consumer and civil society groups have had in highlighting the case of the WTO and access to essential medicines. Key NGOs which have been involved are Medecins Sans Frontiers (MSF), an international medical aid organization that won the 1999 Nobel peace prize; Health Action International (HAI), an international network of consumer groups concerned with health and development; and the Consumer Project on Technology (CPT) a Washington-based consumer group, part of the Ralph Nader's Public Citizen organization. The combination of international and US NGOs lobbying for change significantly altered the course of events.

The relationship between national and supranational regulators: conflicts and cooperation between Canada and the WHO during the SARS epidemic

One of the key issues for IRC is the role of supranational structures in design, implementation and monitoring. Within international health, a key player is the WHO, but multilateral governance will have tensions with national practices and interests (Aginam 2002). The relationship between the WHO and different countries with respect to the SARS epidemic and the issuance of travel advisories is reflective of some of the underlying power dynamics which can drive IRC. In contrast to the previous discussion of the WTO and the TRIPs policy, the WHO is not formally a supranational regulatory body with legally binding agreements and the threat of punitive actions. Rather, the WHO leads by setting standards and the provision of information and guidelines.

During the SARS crises in the first half of 2003, a critical tool in the global fight to halt its transmission was the limitation of travel to and from infectious areas. The WHO invoked a rarely used travel advisory system. The chronology of events is presented in Table 17.1. The implementation of the travel advisory, which recommends against any non-essential travel to infected areas, was the source of debate as it would also lead to broader implications for national economies due to the restriction in the movement of peoples and also tourism.

The aberration in the time line in Table 17.1 is the short timeframe between the imposition of a WHO travel advisory for Toronto, Canada and its removal within a week (despite it being placed initially for 3 weeks). There was a subsequent local transmission 1 month after the removal of the travel advisory in Toronto. This is in contrast to the US Centers for Disease Control (CDC) which placed Canada on a less severe 'alert' listing which was imposed on April 22 and only repealed on July 8. Canada was the only major SARS-affected country to have had such a short time on the advisory list, in contrast to the

Table 17.1 Chronology of travel advisory events

China	Vietnam	Hong Kong	Singapore	Canada
November16—2002 16 first case of atypical pneumonia reported in Guangdong	February 26 2003 — WHO officer examines patient with unknown form of pneumonia March 10 2003—WHO officer reports unusual outbreak of illness and calls it 'sudden acute respiratory syndrome or SARS' affecting22 health care workers in hospital	March 11 2003 — outbreak similar to Vietnam of respiratory illness reported among health workers	March 13 2003 — Ministry reports three cases of SARS of people recently returning from Hong Kong	February 23 2003— SARS first recognized in Toronto from women returning from Hong Kong

March 12, 2003: WHO issues global alert about new infectious disease of unknown origin for Vietnam and Hong Kong.

March 15, 2003: WHO issues a heightened global alert around SARS and rare emergency travel advisory for travellers, airline crew and airlines.

March 15, 2003: CDC issues travel advisory recommending that non-essential travel be deferred to Hong Kong, Singapore, Vietnam and China.

April 2, 2003: WHO issues its first travel warning recommending that non-essential travel to Hong Kong and Guangdong Province be postponed.

April 22, 2003: CDC issues health alert for travellers to Toronto, Canada which does not advise against travel but informs travellers of a health concern and provides advice about specific precautions.

April 23, 2003: WHO adds Toronto, Beijing and Shanxi province in China to travel advisory recommending non-essential travel be deferred. WHO officials say travel advisory will remain in effect for at least next 3 weeks.

April 28, 2003: WHO removes Vietnam from the list of SARS-affected areas, and removes travel advisory to Vietnam.

April 29, 2003: WHO lifts its warning against non-essential travel to Toronto, effective April 30, citing local measures to stop the spread of SARS, no newly reported cases in 20 days.

May 6, 2003: CDC lifts travel advisory for Singapore as no new cases reported for 20 days.

May 8, 2003: WHO extends travel advisory to include other parts of China including inner Mongolia and Tianjin and Taipei, Taiwan.

May 14, 2003: WHO removes Canada from the list of areas with SARS transmission after 20 days without a reported case.

May 15, 2003: CDC removes travel advisory for Hanoi, Vietnam as no new reported cases in 30 days.

May 17, 2003: WHO extends travel advisory to include Hebei Province, China and other parts of China including inner Mongolia.

May 23, 2003: WHO lifts travel advisory to Hong Kong and Guangdong, China saying SARS situation has significantly improved.

May 26, 2003: WHO changes status of Toronto, Canada as an area where there has been recent local transmission after 26 suspect and eight probable cases reported.

Table 17.1 (continued)

May 31, 2003: WHO removes Singapore from list of areas where SARS is locally transmitted, as 20 days with no reported transmission.

June 13, 2003: WHO lifts travel warning against non-essential travel to several provinces in China.

June 17, 2003: WHO removes travel warning to Taiwan. CDC downgrades travel advisory to travel alert though advisory remains in effect for Beijing from both WHO and CDC.

June 23, 2003: WHO removes Hong Kong from list of areas with local SARS transmission since 20 days passed since last SARS case.

June 24, 2003: WHO removes travel advisory for Beijing as well as from list of SARS-affected areas since 20 days since last case reported.

June 25, 2003: CDC changes Beijing from travel advisory to alert.

July 2, 2003: WHO removes Toronto from list of areas with recent local SARS transmission as no reported cases for 20 days.

July 8, 2003: CDC lifts its SARS travel alert for Toronto as more than 20 days have elapsed since date of onset of symptoms for last SARS case.

July 9, 2003: CDC lifts its travel alert to Hong Kong retroactively to July 1 as last case reported on May 31.

other (Asian) countries. It is argued here that this reflects the relative influence of these countries on the WHO.

The SARS epidemic and the imposition of travel advisories was non-trivial in its impact on the economies of affected countries. For example, it was estimated that the outbreak of SARS in Canada would lead to a reduction of $1.5 billion in real gross domestic product (GDP) (0.15% in 2003), and a lowering of Toronto's GDP by 0.5%. Canada lost nearly 13% of its volume of international visitors compared with 2002, accounting for about $1.1 billion of the loss in economic activity (Conference Board of Canada 2003). Both the SARS-affected Asian countries and Canada have been highly critical of the travel advisory system; however, it was only Canada that was effective in its quick withdrawal by WHO.

The imposition of the travel advisory on April 23 for Toronto by WHO was met by an intense level of ministerial lobbying. Health Canada (the federal Ministry of Health) sent a formal letter of protest to the WHO and there was intensive lobbying for its removal. The Canadian position was buoyed by the CDC's position that such an alert was not valuable.

A week later, the WHO did a turn-around, with the WHO Director-General Gro Harlem Bruntland revoking the Toronto travel advisory saying that Canadian authorities have agreed to implement screening measures for SARS at airports. [Although at the same time, the ASEAN (The Association of Southeast Asian Nations) agreed to a standardized system of screening for all travellers.] In justifying the WHO position, Dr Guenael Rodier, Director of Communicable Disease Surveillance and Response at WHO, wrote that the decision to revoke the ban was based on consideration of three criteria: a decrease to less than 60 prevalent SARS cases and five new cases a day; a period of 20 days since the last case of community transmission and no new confirmed cases of exportation; and that Canada would begin proactive screening at airports (Rodier 2003). He also praised Canada as 'one of our strongest and most valued partners in international public health', which reflects that Canada is a strong proponent (and funder) of WHO. The strong linkages between Canada and WHO no doubt smoothed the way for the amenability of WHO to remove the travel advisory, despite the fact that the 20 day period for the last case of SARS transmission did not occur until May 14, fully 2 weeks after the revocation of the travel advisory. During this period, the CDC travel alert remained in effect.

The question of whether lifting the Canadian travel advisory was premature was more pressing in light of the second wave of cases of SARS in Toronto which were reported at the end of May 2003. An investigation by Health Canada (2003) found that hospitals discontinued SARS expanded precautions in early and mid-May in advance of the end of the 20 day period where no SARS cases had been reported (May 14). While it is hard to attribute direct causal connection between the revocation of the travel advisory and early discontinuation of SARS precautions, the emergency atmosphere related to SARS transmission was certainly dispelled by the revocation of the travel advisory.

Conclusions

It is crucial to recognize the range of state and non-state actors and institutions that interact with a regulatory system, particularly as IRC expands. The case studies above demonstrate that existing power relationships between the supranational bodies and individual countries can significantly influence both the establishment of standards and the way that regulations or standards are implemented. In the case of the WTO, the TRIPs policy represented a 'ratcheting-up' of standards related to patent protection (which many have argued are contrary to international and national public health objectives), reflecting the predominant power of western (primarily the USA) countries as the WTO was established. In the case of the SARS epidemic, international standard setting was not consistent between countries, reflecting the strength of individual country links with the supranational body. As many of the international institutions are funded by western countries, the rise of IRC begs the question of to what extent regulations for international public health will reflect the interests of these funders relative to lower income countries. Further research on the potential role of IRC needs to consider areas where IRC may be more useful (e.g. harmonization of standards between developing and developed countries and whether this means raising or lowering standards) and the capacity of lower income countries to participate in such arrangements. Within the context of globalization of public health issues, IRC in its various forms can potentially play a large role, but the case studies demonstrate that IRC may in itself result in non-optimal outcomes reflecting the relative power relationships between actors.

References

Abraham, J. (2002) A social science framework for the analysis of health regulation technology: the risks and benefits of innovative pharmaceuticals in a comparative context. *Health, Risk and Society* **4** (3).

Abraham, J. and Reed, T. (2001) Trading risks for markets: the international harmonisation of pharmaceutical regulation. *Health, Risk and Society* **3** (1).

Aginam, O. (2002) From the core to the peripheries: multilateral governance of malaria in a multi-cultural world. *Chicago Journal of International Law* **3**.

Braithwaite, J. and Drahos, P. (1999) *Ratcheting up and driving down global regulatory standards*. Presented at the International roundtable 'Responses to Globalisation: Rethinking Equity and Health'. Geneva, July.

Becker, G.S. (1983) A theory of competition among pressure groups for political influence. *Quarterly Journal of Economics* **93**, 371–400.

Brugha, R., Donoghue, M., Starling, M., Ndubani, P., Ssengooba, F., Fernandes, B. and Walt, G. (2004) The Global Fund: managing great expectations. *Lancet* **364**.

Conference Board of Canada (2003) *The Economic Impact of SARS*. Conference Board, Ottawa.

Correa, M.C. (2002) Unfair competition under the TRIPs agreement: protection of data submitted for the registration of pharmaceuticals. *Chicago Journal of International Law* **3**

Deacon, B. (1997) *Global Social Policy, International Organisations and the Future of Welfare*. Sage, London.

Donald, A. (1999) Political economy of technology transfer. *British Medical Journal* **319**, 1298.

Drager, N. (1999) Making trade work for public health. *British Medical Journal* **319**, 1214.

Dreyfuss, R.C. (2001) Coming of age with TRIPS: a comment on J.H. Reichman, The TRIPS agreement comes of age: conflict or cooperation with the developing countries. *Case Western Reserve Journal* **33**.

Fidler, D.P. (2002) Introduction to written symposium on public health and international law. *Chicago Journal of International Law* **3**.

Guzman, A.T. (2002) Introduction—International regulatory harmonization. *Chicago Journal of International Law* **3**.

Health Canada (2003) Update: severe acute respiratory syndrome—Toronto 2003. *Canada Communicable Disease Report* **29** (13).

Indech, B. (2000) The international harmonization of human tissue regulation: regulatory control over human tissue use and tissue banking in select countries and the current state of international harmonization efforts. *Food and Drug Law Journal* **55**.

Kumaranayake, L. (1997) The role of regulation: influencing private sector activity within health sector reform. *Journal of International Development* **9**, 641–649.

Kumaranayake, L. and Lake, S. (2002) Regulations in the context of global markets. In: Lee, K., Buse, K. and Fustkian, S. (eds), *Crossing Boundaries: Health Policy in a Globalising World*. Cambridge University Press, Cambridge.

Kumaranayake, L., Hongoro, C., Lake, S., Mujinja, P. and Mpembeni, R. (2003) Coping with private health markets: regulatory (in)effectiveness in sub-Saharan Africa. In: Soderlund, N. and Mendoza-Arana, P. (eds), *The New Public–Private Mix in Health: Exploring the Changing Landscape*. Alliance for Health Policy and Systems Research/WHO, Geneva.

Maynard, A. (1982) The regulation of public and private health care markets. In: McLachlan, G. and Maynard, A. (eds), *A Public/Private Mix for Health: The Relevance and Effects of Change*. Nuffield Provincial Hospitals Trust, London.

Peltzman, S. (1976) Toward a more general theory of regulation. *Journal of Law and Economics* **19**, 211–240.

Posner, R.A. (1974) Theories of economic regulation. *Bell Journal of Economics and Management Science* **5**, 335–358.

Raustiala, K. (2000) Compliance and effectiveness in international regulatory cooperation. *Case Western Reserve Journal* **32**.

Reichman, J.H. (2000) The TRIPS agreement comes of age: conflict or cooperation with the developing countries. *Case Western Reserve Journal* **32**.

Rodier, G.R.M. (2003) Why was Toronto included in the World Health Organization's SARS-related travel advisory? *Canadian Medical Association Journal* **168** (11).

Rothstein, H.F. (2003) Neglected risk regulation: the institutional attenuation phenomena. *Health, Risk and Society* **5** (1).

Silverglade, B.A. (2000) The WTO agreement on sanitary and phytosanitary measures: weakening on food safety regulations to facilitate trade? *Food and Drug Law Journal* **55**.

Spar, D. and Dail, J. (2002) Of measurement and mission: accounting for performance in non-governmental organizations. *Chicago Journal of International Law* **3**.

Spiro, P. (2002) Accounting for NGOs. *Chicago Journal of International Law* **3**.

Stigler, G.J. (1961) The economics of information. *Journal of Political Economy* **86**, 213–225.

Stone, A. (2002) Microbicides. *Nature Reviews of Drug Discovery* **1**, 977.

Sykes, A.O. (2002). TRIPS, pharmaceuticals, developing countries, and the DOHA solution. *Chicago Journal of International Law* **3**.

t'Hoen, E. (2002) TRIPS, pharmaceutical patents, and access to essential medicines:.. A long way from Seattle to Doha. *Chicago Journal of International Law* **3**.

Turmen T. (1999) Making globalisation work for better health. *Development* **42** (4), 8–11.

UNAIDS (2004) *2004 Report on the Global AIDS Epidemic: 4th Global Report*. UNAIDS, Geneva, Switzerland.

UNGASS (2001) *United Nations General Assembly Special Session on AIDS (UNGASS) Declaration (2001)*. United Nations, New York.

Velasquez, G. and Boulet, P. (1999) Essential drugs in the new international economic environment. *Bulletin of the World Health Organization* **77**, 288–292.

Wapner, P. (2002) Introductory essay—Paradise Lost? NGO and global accountability. *Chicago Journal of International Law* 3

Ward, S.M. (2000) Global harmonization of regulatory of regulatory requirements for premarket approval of autologous cell therapies. *Food and Drug Law Journal* 55.

Wibulpoprasert, S. (1999) *Globalisation and access to essential drugs: case study from Thailand.* Paper presented at Amsterdam meeting on Globalisation and Access to Essential Drugs, November 1999.

Wilson, D., Cawthorne, P., Ford, N. and Aongsonwang, S. (1999) Global trade and access to medicines: AIDS treatment in Thailand. *Lancet* 354, 9193–9195.

World Health Organization (1998) *Globalisation and Access to Drugs: Perspectives on the WHO/TRIPS Agreement.* WHO Action Programme on Essential Drugs, Geneva.

World Health Organization (2004) *The World Health Report—Changing History.* WHO, Geneva

Chapter 18

Trade and infectious disease outbreaks: ensuring public health without compromising free trade

Vasant Narasimhan

Introduction

In today's increasingly interconnected global economy, nations exchange goods and information with terrific speed while people travel with greater frequency and over longer distances. Nations depend now more than ever on international trade and tourism to be key components of their economies. In 2000, the World Trade Organization (WTO) estimated US$5.47 trillion in international merchandise trade and that 1.5 billion air travellers people travelled to other nations (World Trade Organization 2001). In addition to expanding trade and travel, however, the global economy has increased the potential speed and scale of infectious disease movement by destroying geographic containment. The potential now exists for a variety of infectious agents to spread via goods or people to new regions, with serious human health consequences.

Faced with the potential risks of infectious spread, countries increasingly employ trade and travel restrictions to prevent the potential entry of infectious agents from an affected country or region. These measures are aimed at protecting either human populations or domestic livestock and agriculture from the disease in question. Such measures have significant economic consequences for nations suffering from an outbreak, often developing nations. These countries face substantial economic losses as trade and travel revenues fall precipitously and are often slow to recover. For example, India is reported to have suffered an estimated US$2.2 billion dollars in economic losses from the 1994 presumed outbreak of plague in Surat. With the growth of information technology, information spreads quickly and allows countries little opportunity to prevent an adverse international reaction. In the vast majority of cases, the risk of international spread via goods and tourism is extremely low. Thus, for the most part, trade and travel restrictions far exceed a reasonable response based on medical science and international law. Global institutions, particularly the WTO and the World Health Organization (WHO), must now find the set of policies that allow countries to ensure the safety of their citizens without unduly affecting trade and travel.

Balancing the goals of public health and free trade requires an improved understanding of the trade-related costs of outbreaks, when these costs are reasonable, and how they can be mitigated. This chapter will review the relationship between trade and infectious disease in humans, recent cases of trade losses related to outbreaks, and the current international regulations governing interactions between reporting and responding nations. While concerns over the spread of disease among livestock and plant populations also have serious trade-related economic impacts, this chapter will not consider this important issue.

History

Trade and travel provide a potentially straightforward way to move infectious diseases of humans across borders and continents. Travelling individuals can readily move diseases such as tuberculosis, human immunodeficiency virus (HIV) and hepatitis across long distances. Certain infectious agents can move directly with shipments of agricultural and food products such as diarrhoea-causing bacteria with fruits. In other cases, disease affecting animals can potentially 'cross over' into the human population, leading to epidemics. Vectors such as mosquitoes, rats and flies can move with cargo shipments or in transport vehicles. Of utmost concern are highly infectious diseases that could rapidly spread through a recipient country, such as plague, cholera and the haemorrhagic fevers. In order to prevent spread, countries can limit trade and travel either out of the country or into the country until the threat from the outbreak has diminished.

Closely related for centuries, trade and infectious disease have become increasingly interconnected over recent decades. Throughout history, infectious diseases have spread via trade routes and colonial trade networks. During the thirteenth century, the Mongolian empire and Mediterranean traders are thought to have spread plague through much of Eurasia and ultimately to Europe (McNeill 1998). Spanish and Portuguese colonists are believed to have brought malaria to the western hemisphere through their African slave trade. The same colonists also introduced measles and smallpox (Crosby 1972). As travel increased, so did instances of disease movement. Notably, in 1918, the great influenza epidemic spread globally through the movement of people. In recent decades, there has been an even further increase in international spread. The AIDS epidemic rapidly spread globally in part because of improved travel within and between continents (Garrett 1994). Cholera has re-emerged in the western hemisphere because of trade routes between Asia and Latin America (Colwell 1996). There is increasing concern that drug-resistant tuberculosis is spreading via air travel. Today, infectious diseases, common and uncommon, are readily able to cross borders via trade and travel.

Preventing the spread of infectious disease through trade and travel restrictions is not new. The practice of quarantine of ill travellers has been used for centuries. Following the Black Death epidemic of plague in the fourteenth century, Mediterranean ports instituted strict quarantine regulations resulting in suspected ships being placed in seclusion with their crew for 40 days (Rosen 1958). Trade ships in South America suspected of cholera were refused entry in the nineteenth century for fear of contamination. With the growing importance of international trade in the early twentieth century, countries endeavoured to employ a more coordinated approach. The Organisation Internationale d'Hygiene Publique was established in Paris in 1907 to gather information on disease outbreaks for eventual distribution to participating countries. The reporting of cholera and plague was required initially, while yellow fever, typhus and relapsing fever were added later. European countries feared that these diseases would cross their borders from the poorer countries where they principally occurred (World Health Organization Division of Emerging and Other Communicable Disease Surveillance and Control 1996). Such efforts at coordination were hampered by limited surveillance capabilities and fear of negative trade consequences for open reporting of outbreaks.

In the latter half of the twentieth century, the relationship of trade and travel with the spread of infection received increasingly more attention. International regulations began to a play a more critical role in ensuring the balance between efficient trade and public health (discussed further below). In 1951, the WHO issued the International Sanitary Regulations, renamed the International Health Regulations (IHR) in 1969 (revised in 1981), which required member states to notify WHO within 24 h of outbreaks of: cholera, yellow fever and plague. The authors hoped to ensure maximum international security from disease spread with minimal disruption of international traffic (World Health Organization 1983). While WHO possessed no enforcement powers, it hoped countries would comply through persuasion and recommendations. In practice, however, this was not the case. Many countries enforced excessive restrictions on countries reporting an outbreak. This led to massive under-reporting amongst member states. Non-reporting countries justified their fears given the high cost paid by reporting countries. In addition, the IHR pertained only to three diseases, failing to address all other re-emerging and emerging infectious diseases that may have the potential for international spread. WHO officials agreed that because of these two issues, the two goals of maximum security and minimal disruption have not been met (Fidler 1997).

Current regulatory frameworks

In order to address concerns of excessive restrictions to trade and travel, both the WHO IHR and WTO Agreement on the Application of Sanitary and Phyto-sanitary Measures (hereafter called SPS) contain regulations that specify appropriate actions. As discussed above, the original IHR outlined in broad terms the reasonable measures that countries could employ, with specific guidelines for outbreaks of cholera, plague and yellow fever. The IHR provided nations with general rules for arrival and departure of ships and planes, and how to treat imported goods, but were not specific to particular situations (World Health Organization 1983). A revision of the IHR has been approved providing much broader guidelines and mechanisms to ensure appropriate responses are taken by countries (World Health Organization 2005).

WTO currently uses the SPS to provide basic rules on when and to what extent nations can apply measures to restrict the entry of unsafe products that threaten human health; measures that would normally be considered unfair trade practices. The SPS also stipulates that countries have the right to protect their citizens, but should refrain from excessive measures unless based on scientific evidence (World Trade Organization 1995). Countries are more likely to employ such protectionist measures because of the relaxing of trade restrictions following the General Agreement on Trade and Tariffs (GATT 1994) (World Trade Organization 1998). To ensure that this does not occur, the SPS measures provide for members to raise disputed policies before a panel of experts for review and consultation. They also provide for a committee on Sanitary and Phytosanitary measures to 'facilitate ad hoc consultations or negotiations among members on specific sanitary and phytosanitary issues' (World Trade Organization 1995). In order to 'harmonize' the numerous country guidelines, WTO recognizes certain groups, such as the Codex Alimentarius Association and the International Office of Epizootics, as providing an international standard for appropriate action. Because of their common goal of maximum health protection with minimal international traffic disruption, both WHO and WTO plan to work together to prevent conflict between the two regulations while exploring possibilities for collaboration (Table 18.1) (World Health Organization and World Trade Organization 2002).

While no specific agreements exist, there is potential for WHO to assist the WTO in monitoring whether countries take appropriate measures during an outbreak.

Table 18.1 Regulatory frameworks. Adapted from the Revision of the International Health Regulations: Public Health and Trade, WHO (1999)

	International Health Regulations (IHR)—WHO	Sanitary and Phytosanitary Measures (SPS)—WTO
Purpose	Direct and coordinate international public health work, technical cooperation in health, control and eradication of disease	Principle international body for negotiating trade liberalizing agreements and resolving trade disputes
Goals for health and trade	Prevent international spread of disease with minimum interference with world traffic	Help trade flow as freely of possible. Apply trade restricting measures only if scientifically justified
Rights of members	IHR dictates maximum measures that can be taken	Right unilaterally to restrict trade if to protect public health
Response in epidemic events	Can act to support affected nation to contain outbreak	No action without member request
Notification requirements	Must notify WHO of any outbreak specified in the IHR	Obligation to notify WTO of any trade restrictions
Dispute resolution process	Semi-formal process that is rarely used	Comprehensive, structured, dispute resolution process

Because of their common goal of maximum health protection and minimum international traffic disruption, WHO and WTO intend to collaborate in order to prevent conflict between the two sets of regulations. No specific agreements exist between the two organizations, but recent discussions raise the potential for WHO to assist WTO in monitoring whether countries take appropriate public health measures during outbreaks. It will be WTO's role to assess trade practices.

Case studies

Over the last decade, there have been a number of well-documented instances when infectious disease outbreaks have led to substantial trade-related economic losses to reporting countries (summarized in Table 18.2). The most significant among these in monetary terms is the case of Britain's crippled beef industry over concerns over bovine spongiform encephalopathy (BSE). There are probably many more such cases that have occurred on a more limited scale (World Health Organization and World Trade Organization 2002). To date, the

Table 18.2 Recent trade-related outbreaks

Year	Affected Country	Disease	Effect on trade and travel	Estimated trade-related losses (source)
1991	Peru and Chile	Cholera	Trade restrictions across all industries particularly fisheries and agriculture. Travel restrictions and lost tourism	Between US$700 million and US$1.5 billion (Government of Peru)
1995–2000	UK	BSE	Trade restrictions and demand shifts for the beef industry	US$5 billion–US$6 billion (Government of the UK)
1994	India	Pneumonic plague?	Trade restrictions across all industries. Travel restrictions and lost tourism	US$2 billion–US$2.5 billion (Government of India)
1996	Japan	*Escherichia coli* 0157:H7	Trade restrictions on beef industry	US$15 million (Trade Industry)
1996	Guatemala	*Cyclospora*	USA banned raspberry imports for 2 years	US$1 million–US$2 million affecting local farmers (US Government)
1997	Hong Kong	Avian flu	Trade restrictions on poultry industry	US$13 million (Trade Industry)
1997	East Africa	Cholera	EC blocks fish exports	Unknown
1998	Malaysia	Nipah virus	Trade restriction on swine industry with significant losses to local infrastructure (pig stocks, farms, etc.). Minor travel losses.	US$400 million–US$450 million (Malaysian government)
1997–99	Horn of Africa	Rift Valley fever	Middle Eastern countries place restrictions on beef imports	Unknown
2001	UK	Foot and mouth disease	Trade restrictions and lost tourism despite no threat to humans	Not fully calculated

literature in this area has focused on a better understanding of the international legal and regulatory frameworks that govern the use of trade restrictions during outbreaks. Very little work has been done on valuing the trade losses that these outbreaks cause.

Because of the lack of systematic analysis of the trade-related economic effects, examining case studies provides a useful first step to understanding the issues involved. Below, three case studies from developing countries are discussed in detail to help illuminate different dimensions of the trade and infectious disease relationship.

Plague in India

On September 20, 1994, Surat Civil Hospital, Gujurat, admitted seven patients with pneumonia-like symptoms. Despite penicillin treatment, two of the patients died within a day. By September 23, 1994 there were media reports of a plague outbreak in Surat and these reports quickly spread throughout the world. As many as 500 000 people fled Surat and the surrounding area, and this led to fears that plague might be carried to other large Indian cities and beyond (Burns 1994a). The Indian Ministry of Health, in accordance with the IHR, formally notified WHO, examined all persons leaving the country with any plague-like symptoms, and fumigated cargo from all ports of departure against rodents (*New York Times* 1994). On October 3, 1994, India declared that the epidemic was under control and by the end of the month WHO declared the outbreak to be over (World Health Organization 1998).

At the time, official reports indicated 52 deaths in the country from plague and 876 clinically confirmed cases. A subsequent report from the All India Institute of Hygiene and Public Health indicated that not a single case of plague was confirmed on the basis of WHO bacteriological standards (Inter Press Service 1994).

Before the scientific confirmation of the 1994 plague outbreak had been carried out, press releases were giving estimates of the level of disease, and television broadcasts were showing people wearing cloth masks fleeing from the affected area. Within a week of the initial reports, countries throughout Asia and the Eastern Mediterranean stopped flights to and from India (Dahlburg 1994). Before a single case was confirmed in western India, Bangladesh stopped the movement of goods and people at border crossings with India. Bangladesh, Oman, Qatar and the United Arab Emirates stopped importing all foodstuffs from India, and many other countries followed suit. Canada, France, Germany, Italy, the UK and the USA issued warnings to their citizens on travel to India. Italy placed an immediate embargo on all goods from India at all Italian ports, while Sweden, a major trading partner of India, cancelled all textile shipments (Burns 1994b). These measures were taken even though WHO requested that no travel or trade restrictions be imposed on India. Although the reported cases were confined to the poor in defined areas, many people changed their plans for travelling to India at the height of the tourist season (Jain 1994). The outbreak also affected Indians travelling abroad, as they were often held up at airports, placed in quarantine or even sent back to India. Even some Indian citizens resident in other countries were subjected to unwarranted scrutiny. Such measures against citizens of countries suffering from an outbreak are prohibited by the IHR. Because of its historical importance, plague rapidly placed a stigma on India that took months to fade.

Only after the lifting of all sanctions and the normalization of travel and trade patterns did the full cost of the outbreak become clear. In 1994, India's trade deficit rose to more than twice that of the previous year (Fidler *et al.* 1997). In response to the loss of at least 2.2 million tourists during the season, the Ministry of Tourism reduced its hotel prices by 50%. Estimates of quantifiable losses vary, but most reports place total losses associated with the reported outbreak at over US$2 billion (Levy and Gage 1999). Long-term projections of losses will probably prove higher. Both the US Centers for Disease Control (CDC) and WHO concluded that the response was excessive and unnecessary (Inter Press Service 1994). Other countries, observing the price that India paid, will probably be more reluctant to report similar outbreaks in the future.

Cholera in Peru

In January 1991, an epidemic of cholera began in Peru and eventually spread throughout South America. Between January 24 and February 9, 1991 a total of 1859 people in Peru with clinically diagnosed cholera required hospitalization and 66 deaths were reported (UN Food and Agriculture Organization 1998). Subsequently, cholera appeared along the Pacific coast in Chile, Colombia and Ecuador, and spread inland towards the Amazon and Brazil. From January 1991 to September 1994, CDC reported a total of 1 041 422 cases and 9642 deaths, with a case fatality rate of 0.9%. WHO declared the epidemic to be over in 1995.

Because cholera spread through Peru initially, the international response began with actions focused on that country. Bolivia, Chile and Ecuador banned imports of Peruvian perishable foods, and soon afterwards Argentina banned all fish products from Peru (and even suspended an international soccer match). Within 2 weeks of the beginning of the outbreak, the European Community had imposed a complete boycott of all Peruvian fish, thereby crippling one of the country's primary industries (Atwood 1991). The European Community proceeded to ban all imports from Peru, and other countries followed suit. On February 26, the Prime Minister of Peru accused many countries of taking restrictive measures that unfairly blocked the country's export trade (Long 1991). The embargoes continued and were expanded, and other countries introduced specifications on the number of days required between cargoes leaving Peru and arriving in foreign ports, usually well in excess of advice given by WHO. By mid-March 1991, many Peruvian exports were subjected to international embargoes. Certain countries, among them the USA, required all food products from Peru to be tested for cholera, again going beyond WHO recommendations. The President of the Peruvian Chamber of Tourism claimed that news releases led to the cancellation of half the reservations made by foreign travellers to the country. It was estimated that Peru's tourist industry lost US$150million. Even in the tourist centre of Cusco, where few cholera cases had been reported, half the hotels had closed and most of the others were empty (Xinhua General Overseas News Service 1991). Many European countries placed restrictions on Peruvian travellers, some of whom were sent back to Peru on arrival in Europe.

Meanwhile, cholera continued to spread in South America. In April, some European countries widened the ban on fish exports to include Colombia and Ecuador (Inter Press Service 1991). Chile predicted economic losses of over US$300 million, and losses for other countries in the region were expected to be similar. These estimates did not include unmeasured effects on future tourism, trade and overall reputation. For Peru, the economic losses on trade alone in 1991 were estimated at more than US$770million (Long 1991).

Nipah virus in Malaysia

In the winter of 1998, there was an outbreak of a febrile illness affecting persons living in farming regions of Malaysia. Initially downplayed by the Malaysian government, hospitals continued to see cases of the unidentified illness until February 1999. Eventually, as press reports began to increase and with thousands of people fleeing their villages, the Malaysian government disclosed that the outbreak was believed to be an unknown Hendra-like virus that was associated with proximity to swine. The virus would ultimately be known as the Nipah virus. Malaysia immediately instituted a culling programme in which some 1 million pigs were terminated. By the end of the outbreak a few months later, officials estimated there had been 261 cases and 111 persons dead.

Once Malaysia publicly disclosed the outbreak, the international response was swift and substantial. In 1998, the pig farming industry produced goods valued at US$300 million–US$400 million [4% of the gross domestic product (GDP)] with an export value of US$150 million, and government projections suggested that the outbreak would lead to a substantial decline in output. Given that Malaysia was just recovering from the Asian financial crisis, many workers in the country were only returning to reasonable income levels. As soon as the government made its announcements, regional trading partners reacted. Singapore implemented an import ban on all livestock, and Thailand blocked all pork. Other Southeast Asian countries placed limited bans on livestock. Many Malay urban consumers began to demand access to foreign pork to avoid mounting risks. Many travellers cancelled plans despite assurances from the WHO and the CDC that only those with direct contact with pigs had been afflicted. As the Malaysian pork industry began to collapse, Malay authorities publicly claimed that sanction by neighbouring countries were part of a deliberate trade war. Because there are no international guidelines on an appropriate response in this situation, Malaysia had little recourse. The cost of the outbreak to the Malaysian pork industry in 1999 and 2000 is estimated to be at least US$400 million–US$450 million.

Understanding the economic impact

The three cases above and the data in Table 18.1 help illustrate some prevailing issues in the trade-related costs of infectious disease outbreaks. Learning from these case studies can help build the frameworks that will help assess future outbreaks.

Understanding how countries employ trade and travel restrictions is not always straightforward. Countries have a number of interests to contend with including ensuring public health, managing public concerns, protecting domestic industries and perhaps even retaliating for previous trade restrictions it received previously. While in theory trade and travel would only be restricted in so far as it protected the interests of public health, in practice this was often not the case.

Trade in goods

At minimum, responding countries place restrictions on goods directly related to the infectious disease in question. In the majority of cases, this involves the agricultural or animal product industry, as was the case in Malaysia, Peru and the UK. Under the SPS agreement, these restrictions are justified as long as they are based on scientific evidence and are temporary. The revised IHR, now approved (World Health Organization 2005), encourage countries to consult with the WHO and other health authorities before taking action to ensure trade is not unduly affected

In some cases, however, countries place restrictions on goods unrelated to infectious outbreaks. This was the case for both Peru and India where countries placed trade restrictions on industries ranging from textiles to produce, all of which pose no threat of spreading cholera or plague. There are a few reasons why countries might employ such measures. The first is to manage public anxiety and to create the perception that all measures are being taken to ensure public safety. The second is protecting domestic trade interests in which the country is deliberately setting out to protect local producers. The third is a lack of knowledge and guidance on what appropriate measures might be. While the SPS strongly advise against such measures, there is little recourse if the responding country claims they are acting on their public health interests. The existing IHR then should have protected India and Peru from undue economic sanctions; however, the WHO could not enforce the IHR policies so little in effect could be done. Under the revised IHR, these types of responses could be mitigated by WHO's operational support (World Health Organization 2005)

Trade in goods can also be affected outside of formal government actions. As the media rapidly disseminates information about an outbreak, the way consumers and traders view products from the affected country is naturally affected. While such effects are hard to measure, in some cases, such as in the plague epidemic in India, they are probably substantial. Mitigating this response is much more difficult and falls in large part on the media who need to provide accurate information early on in an outbreak.

Travel and tourism

During an outbreak, many countries wait before posting any travel restrictions as in the vast majority of cases there is minimal risk to travellers. In the case of Peru and India, there was an initial response to limit travel that was later removed. Even if governments do not formally institute travel warnings, individual travellers often change travel plans based on media reports. India's tourism industry was devastated by the cancellation of tens of thousands of travel plans over many months even though the risk of plague was minimal. As with the case for goods, governments must be encouraged to take reasonable approaches and the media must provide accurate, high quality information early on in an outbreak.

Assessing economic losses

In each of the cases considered, governments based their economic loss calculations on internal estimates, industry figures, quarterly changes in exports and shifts in tourism reservations. It should be noted that there is no consistent, systematic methodology for assessing the trade-related impact of outbreaks. There are quite obviously a number of biases in relying on government estimates as there may not be clarity on what can be attributed to the outbreak and what may be attributable to other social and economic trends. For this reason, most economic cost estimates are provided with a fairly large range to capture the range of possibly affected economic activities. In some cases, estimates are clearer than others. In the case of Malaysia, estimates primarily involved the swine industry excluding potential losses in tourism and other industries tangentially affected. A similar situation holds for the UK in its estimates of loss from BSE. As the number of cases grows, policy makers will require better methods to assess the impact of outbreaks rapidly. This will ultimately aid the resolution of dispute proceedings if an affected country were to appeal to an international body.

Depth and extent of impact

Trade figures and estimates of yearly losses do not capture the full extent of how outbreaks can cripple trading economies. For most developing countries, individual farmers bear the majority of the economic hardship. When the USA banned Guatemalan raspberries due to concerns over *Cyclospora*, the dollar value to Guatemala was relatively small at US$1 million–US$2 million. The effect on local farmers was probably devastating. Anecdotal evidence suggests similar situations throughout Africa which is often faced with outbreaks that reduce foreign demand even if they do not lead to formal trade restrictions. Poor countries tend to suffer from more outbreaks but cannot afford the trade losses that inevitably follow.

Conclusions: challenges and opportunities

Balancing the needs of public health and the economic interests of countries will be a continuous challenge as countries balance their various competing interests. There are a few issues that need to be addressed to increase the likelihood that a better balance can be achieved.

1. Countries should acquire and release timely and accurate information early in an outbreak. For developing countries, this will require improving diagnostic and surveillance capabilities

2. Clarify and enforce the IHR and the SES regulations, particularly those clauses relating to appropriate conduct in response to disease outbreaks. Engaging regional trade organizations may be a useful approach to improve adherence.

3. Create means to provide substantive support for developing countries economically damaged by disease outbreaks.

4. Educate the media on how to disseminate information appropriately on outbreaks so as to minimize economic damage done to the affected country.

New efforts are underway to improve these issues, including the recent adoption of the revised IHR (World Health Organization 2005) and efforts by regional trade groups such as ASEAN, the Asian regional trading organization, to educate member states on infectious disease and trade. In addition to these policy efforts, the research community should endeavour to clarify the trade-related costs of outbreaks and the impact of different policy efforts on mitigating these costs and improving infectious disease control.

References

Atwood, R. (1991) *Peru Scorns 'Unfair' Trade Practices over Cholera Epidemic*. Reuters North American Wire. February 26.

Burns, J.F. (1994a) Thousands flee indian city in deadly plague outbreak. *New York Times* September 24.

Burns, J. (1994b) Plague in India giving visitors second thoughts. *New York Times* October 9.

CDC (1991) Update: cholera outbreak—Peru, Ecuador, and Colombia; reprint of World Health Organization report 'Small Risk of Cholera Transmission by Food Imports'. *Morbidity and Mortality Weekly Reports* **40**, 225.

Colwell, R.R. (1996) Global climate and infectious disease: the cholera paradigm. *Science* **274**, 2025–2031.

Crosby, A. (1972) *The Columbian Exchange*.

Dahlburg, J. (1994) Plague scars image, economy of modern India; Asia: epidemic reminds trade giant that social change hasn't kept up with business strides. *Los Angeles Times* October 5.

Fidler, D. (1997) Return of the fourth horseman: emerging infectious disease and international law. *Minnesota Law Review* **81**, 771.

Fidler, D., Heymann, D. *et al.* (1997) Emerging and reemerging infectious diseases: challenges for international, national, and state law. *International Lawyer* **31**, 778–799.

Garrett, L. (1994) *The Coming Plague*.

Inter Press Service Chile (1991) Losses from cholera could reach $500 million. May 2.

Inter Press Service India (1994) Plague ending says health group, but world still wary. October 13.

Jain, N. (1994) *India's Trade Deficit Rises*. United Press International, December 6.

Levy, C. and Gage, K. (1999) Plague in the United States, 1995–1997. *Infections in Medicine* January, 54–63.

Long, W. (1991) Market focus: cholera compounds Peru's economic misery: along with the human losses, the epidemic has taken a toll on tourism and exports—two key sectors of the struggling country. *Los Angeles Times* April 23.

McNeill, W. (1998) *Plagues and Peoples*. Doubleday, New York.

New York Times (1994) India says spread of plague is halted. October 4.

Rosen, G. (1958) *A History of Public Health*.

World Health Organization (1983) *International Health Regulations*, 3rd edn. WHO Geneva.

World Health Organization (1998) Human plague in 1996. *Weekly Epidemiological Record* **47**, 366–369.

World Health Organization (2002) *International Health Regulation Revision Project. Global Crises—Global Solutions*. World Health Organization, Geneva.

World Health Organization (2005) Revision of the International Health Regulations May 23, http://www.who.int/mediacentre/news/releases/2005/pr_wha03/en/index.html Accessed June 30, 2005.

World Health Organization Division of Emerging and Other Communicable Disease Surveillance and Control (1996) *Emerging and Other Communicable Diseases Strategic Plan 1996–2000.* WHO/EMC/96.1.

World Health Organization and World Trade Organization (2002) *WTO Agreements and Public Health.*

World Trade Organization (1995) *Agreement on the Application of Sanitary and Phytosanitary Measures.*

World Trade Organization (1998) *Understanding the WTO Agreement on Sanitary and Phytosanitary Measures.* May.

World Trade Organization (2001) *International Trade Statistics.*

UN Food and Agriculture Organization (1998) *Import Ban on Fish Products from Africa Not the Most Appropriate Answer.* FAO Press Release 98/21.

Xinhua General Overseas News Service (1991) *Peru to Go on with Fish Exports Despite Alleged Contamination.* February 16.

Chapter 19

Epilogue: Application to Contemporary Challenges: Avian 'flu and MRSA

Introduction

The purpose of this volume was two fold: to offer those involved in the control of infectious disease an economic perspective and tools that would contribute to their task, and to introduce economists to some of the characteristics of infectious disease that pose interesting challenges for the discipline. The application of economics to the control or management of many of the major infections is provided in this volume and these applications offer insights and templates that might be used to explore other diseases. Economics has a role in placing a disease on the policy agenda. It can help in understanding the incentives and motivations of those involved in reporting and containing the spread of disease. It can evaluate and contribute to the design of cost-effective interventions. Economics can show the implications of poor governance structures and weak contracts for the design and application of guidance and regulations.

There are many threats posed by the resurgence of old and the emergence of new diseases. These should be placed in the context of many diseases that continue to pose problems on a day to day basis and impose considerable disease burdens and absorb scarce resources but attract little media attention. Facets of HIV/AIDs, TB, malaria, hepatitis C, antibiotic resistance, flu, pneumonia and foodborne and zoonotic diseases are considered in previous chapters. In this epilogue we will draw upon the concepts introduced earlier to explore two infectious that are at the forefront of contemporary concern: MRSA and Avian flu.

MRSA

MRSA has become emblematic as a dread disease haunting acute hospital units and taking its toll on mortality and morbidity. In a survey of infectious disease doctors and nurses and public health doctors it came top of the list of threats to infection control in hospitals (Allen *et al.* 2000, Roberts *et al.* 2000). *Staphylococcus aureus* is one of the most common bacteria. It is widespread in the community with an estimated one third of the population 'colonised': carrying it on their skin or in their nose or throat with no adverse affects. It can cause a range of problems from minor skin infections to serious life threatening conditions such septicaemia and pneumonia. MRSA is the drug resistant strain of this bacteria. About 80% of in-patients who acquire MRSA do not suffer any infection. They do, however, provide a reservoir of infection that can spread to others in hospital, to those in residential accommodation for the elderly and increasingly to the wider community; and colonised persons can become infected if their immune system is challenged by other illnesses or medical interventions.

It has been dubbed the 'super bug' for two reasons: it raises the spectre of antibiotic resistance so threatening to a world that believed it had tools to cope with infections and because of the high mortality rates associated with the disease that targets vulnerable people who expect hospitals to cure not infect patients.

Unlike many other infections it has not needed a 'burden of illness' study to place it on the policy agenda. However the intensity of resource use involved with its treatment and control are documented in case studies and anecdotal descriptions by practioners. Expensive drugs are required to treat the disease and because of the potential toxic effects of these drugs they need monitoring intensively. Infection control can absorb many resources; it involves surveillance, laboratory tests for patients and staff and active bed management and possibly cohort nursing, especially if, as is often the case, single rooms are not available. MRSA puts pressure on hospital beds because those who are infected stay in hospital longer. To control its spread it is often necessary to close wards or units. Not a popular option when, as in the UK, beds are needed to meet waiting list targets. It was reported that infectious disease doctors and infectious disease nurses spent 50% of their time on its surveillance and control and 'the MRSA positive patients stayed in ITU six times as long as MRSA negative controls', (Roberts *et al.* 2000).

A number of interventions to prevent MRSA and reduce transmission have been advocated. Evaluation of these interventions is of a rather uneven quality. In a recent systematic review of the impact of isolation few studies yielded generalisable estimates of resource use, (see Cooper *et al.* 2003, and see Kumaranayaka *et al.* Chapter 4 on generalisability). Studies took place at different times in very different contexts and included a different range of resources costed in different ways at different times. Attempts have been made to estimate a cost of a typical case—costs range widely and some cases die early in the disease. Death is difficult to encompass in simple costing studies of the use of resources in hospitals ie. it is cheap in terms of resource use but expensive in terms of lives lost. If a value was placed on risk of loss of life and included in the analysis the returns to interventions would increase many fold, (see Buzby *et al.* Chapter 16). The cost of caring for an average surviving case during the acute phase was estimated as £12 000 at 2002 prices (see Cooper *et al.* 2003).

The calculations to estimate the cost-effectiveness of interventions involve making an assumption about the impact of the intervention on the transmission rate and costing the cases avoided by the intervention. Most estimates suggest that the cost of the illness is so high that many interventions using dynamic models are highly cost effective. Even the costs of constructing single bay units or isolation units discounted over time are dwarfed by the potential costs saved by limiting transmission. Isolation units even if they are insufficient to accommodate all cases play a useful role in reducing the intensity of any outbreak, (See Cooper *et al.* 2003). Although these estimates from dynamic modes rely upon sparse data they appear to be robust when a range of sensitivity tests are carried out.

The evaluation of any intervention depends on accurate measures of the impact before and after the policy is put in place. This implies good surveillance systems. Wilson *et al.* (2005) set up a data base as a basis for evaluating an intervention that involved the infection control team following up all infections arising after surgery and reporting back any infections to surgeons and management. This intervention yielded a many fold rate of return. Systems that rely upon voluntary unstructured reporting of incidents may be manipulated by hospitals keen to maintain their image as safe and reliable. There is clearly scope for opportunistic behaviour; indeed those with good surveillance systems might appear to have higher rates than those who take little care to identify and report infections, (see Riviere-Cinnamond Chapter 12 and Jamasji-Pavri Chapter 14).

The UK government is intent upon tackling any such opportunism. To guard against under reporting of MRSA a *S. aureus* bacteraemia surveillance system has been put in place and has been mandatory since 1st October 2005. All NHS Acute Trusts in England must report each MRSA episode that is detected in their Trust. (HPA 2005). This scheme will provide a data base that can be used to identify risk factors and possibly evaluate interventions later. On average 9000 cases of *Staphylococcus aureus* were reported each six month period since 2001 by NHS acute Trusts in England some 40% were resistant, (HPA 2006). Over 360 patents per year lose their lives to MRSA each year in England according to a recent survey of death certification (National Office of Statistics, 2006).

In order to meet government targets of reducing MRSA rates Trusts must get to grips with managing effective control procedures. There is a substantial problem of agency. Many persons, some potentially colonised, look after a patient who may stay in bed in an environment contaminated with MRSA or may move around the hospital visiting departments for investigations and operations down corridors and in lifts used by many other patients and visitors. If infection does occur it is often difficult without extensive microbial investigations to find the source of infection. Lack of definitive attribution is a problem for agency. If blame cannot be allocated then it is difficult to put in place incentives and penalties to encourage compliance.

Placing accountability for infection control squarely on the chief executive was an extremely important improvement in the governance of infection in hospitals. Previously chief executives had only been responsible for financial probity. (Alford *et al.* 2001). The tighter clinical governance should encourage those who draw up contracts for services to ensure that those with knowledge of infectious disease control are involved in the contracting process. A feature sadly lacking in earlier rounds of contracting, (see Allen and Croxson Chapter 15). This led to moral hazard by contractors who were able in some cases to cut corners with cleaning tasks and contracts that were poorly specified did not allow ward staff to supervise cleaning work or ask for tasks to be done. All communications had to be done by line managers—nurses informing nurse manages who would inform the management in the hospital who would contact the contractors who could then instruct staff—probably too late to be of use to the ward staff. This bad contracting was possibly inevitable as in the early years of the 'purchaser/provider' split in the NHS; contractors lacked experience or had not considered the implications of the contract on the running of the hospital. In one case contractors cut back even on the sparse material that they had agreed to provide and cleaners felt it necessary to bring in their own material, (see Crawshaw *et al.* 2000). Many of these issues could have been dealt with by better contracting.

One strategy that has been adopted in the NHS in Britain is to place greater attention on hand hygiene in the form of 'now wash your hands' campaigns. Placing of antimicrobial scrubs in wards for use by all those in contact with patients, in one compliance with guidelines on hand washing and cleaning, can be hard to maintain (Pittet, 2001), but reduces agency failure, as staff can be observed using antimicrobial scrubs. Indeed the ultimate principal in the agency relationship, the patient, is encouraged to oversee compliance and challenge staff whom they observe not cleaning their hands. Previously the perceived lack of either time or facilities for hand washing had been used to excuse unhygienic practices that had become the norm. However, in introducing more stringent controls and penalties care has to be taken not to erode the trust and goodwill of staff and affect staff-morale leading to a reduction of effort. (McMaster 1998). Studies to evaluate hand cleaning strategies are under way.

Antimicrobial policies in hospitals and in the community no doubt underlie the development of resistant organisms. A study of 300 hospitals throughout Europe found a positive association between MRSA and antibiotic use. It also found that hospitals which under took specific interventions such as isolation of infected patients and surveillance of staff for evidence of colonisation had lower rates of MRSA (HPA 2005). Appropriate prescribing of the right drug at the right time is clearly important. Reductions in inappropriate use of antibiotics to treat viral infections and failures in the proper use of prophylactic remedies, particularly those administered before operations, have contributed to the pressure that leads to the development of resistance. (Schmid 2003, Bratzler 2005)

The development of antibacterial resistance has an intergenerational impact, (see Coast Chapter 10). There is a possibility that some drugs may recover their potency. Cycling of drugs could take place as those that are losing potency can be replaced by ones that have regained potency, (see Laxminarayan in Chapter 4.).

There may well be additional benefits from programmes to reduce infections for, as well as eradicating the target organisms, they may clear the environment of other organisms that cause disease. There will be joint production. The pay off to this joint production is an attractive possibility—and we could achieve economies of scope and utilise our scarce resources more efficiently, an attractive possibility to any economist intent on maximising use of resources. With infectious disease however such ambitions may be thwarted as the removal of the bad organisms can also mop up some of the benign protective organisms allowing scope for the emergence of more virulent organisms to occupy the space suggesting some diseconomies of scope.

Reducing the time exposed to danger is one intervention that may have profound affects on transmission rates. A study is underway to evaluate the benefits of faster testing. Standard tests to identify MRSA can typically take three days or more to achieve a result. New kits are coming online that aim to produce results much quicker. There are two obvious ways in which the faster testing can have an impact on cost effective management of MRSA. It can limit patient's exposure by reducing the transmission time of those admitted to a ward and it can save the time non-infected individuals spend in expensive isolation wards prior to test results being obtained.

In preparation for undertaking the study the time lapse from the taking of swabs to the time the results were transmitted to the ward was tracked. Construction of this time line indicated a number of problems. There were significant delays in transporting and delivering swabs to the laboratory. There were delays as out of hour services were not available in all laboratories to test for MRSA and sometimes tests were left over the weekend. Further delays were encountered in the reporting of negative tests to staff in wards. These were often left to internal paper communication systems whereas positive test results were communicated by phone. This had implications for the use of beds as reporting of negative cases took so long. Information on tests was some times elicited by nurses as part of bed management if there was a capacity problem. This preliminary study indicates that benefits could be achieved by improving the efficiency—removing X-inefficiency- of procedures for testing and reporting even when using the standard tests. (Babad *et al.* 2005)

Exploration of the strategies that were used in the hospitals in the study identified two approaches. One was to isolate if MRSA was suspected and the other was to isolate only if the test result was positive. In the latter case transmission was likely to occur in the ward whilst the test result was awaited. Two models were developed to test the cost effectiveness of faster testing in these scenarios. Benefits of faster testing were found in both scenarios. There was a small saving from the isolate-if-suspect strategy, as increased test costs were more than offset by the fall in costs arising from a reduction in use of isolation bed days. For the isolate-if-positive strategy there was a much bigger reduction in costs, which was driven by reduced 'downstream' transmission costs. Such transmission gains would already have accrued to the isolate-if-suspect group as the transmission rate whilst in isolation was assumed to be small. Thus it would appear that faster testing would lead to a reduction in new MRSA cases with a concomitant health gain. The model's conclusions are highly sensitive to the assumption made about the costs of the faster test.

MRSA is a continuing challenge. Economics has a role in meeting this challenge by assessing the cost effectiveness of interventions and in highlighting the importance of agency relationships in implementing good practice policies. It can contribute to issues of governance and to the adoption of appropriate contracts between the parties.

Avian flu

Avian flu H5N1 casts its long shadow as it migrates with wild birds relentlessly westwards. It is singled out as the most likely candidate to initiate the now over due 'flu pandemic. World agencies including WHO, World Bank, Food and Agriculture Organisation (FAO) and the World Organisation for Animal Health (OIE) have undertaken major initiatives to deal with the problem and have prepared plans of action and guidelines (WHO 2005, World Bank 2005). They have built up stock piles of antiviral drugs and eased regulations to facilitate the rapid development of a human flu vaccine by 'fast-tracking procedures for the development and licensing of a pandemic vaccine' and facilitating rapid production when the strain becomes available. (WHO 2005 p14 and Annex 2).

The World Bank has estimated the cost of a likely pandemic to be $800bn. However, the Lowry Institute for International Policy have estimated that the impact on global output may be as high as $4400bn (Financial Times, 2006). Estimates have also been made of the resources needed to monitor and control the virus (World Bank 2005, Roberts, 2006, BBC 2006). One hundred countries and 20 international agencies sent representatives to a pledging conference sponsored by the People's Republic of China, the European Commission and the World Bank, held in Beijing in January 2006, to raise funds to help countries find the resources to strengthen their veterinary and health services to deal with the potential threat of a pandemic. The World Bank estimated that $1.2 to 1.4bn would be needed but in fact some $1.9bn was pledged. Pledges came from: US $334m, EU $260m, Japan $159m, Russia $45m and Australia $42 and other countries. There was also $30m from Roche to provide 2m doses of Tamiflu. Most of the fund will be allocated to rapid containment, early warning systems and reducing human exposure. It will be spent in high risk countries that have weak surveillance and laboratory facilities. The underlying theme of this unusually strong collaboration is summed up in a statement by Markos Kyprianuo, EU Health Commissioner, 'This is not charity. This is not just solidarity. This is self-defence.' Markos, (Yeh, 2006).

The interdependence of the world facing a pandemic is clear. No one region and certainly no one country can act alone. The public good elements of control of the potential pandemic are clear, exclusion is not possible and there is no potential for rivalry. Any action that controls the emergence or spread of the disease potentially protects all those who might otherwise be affected. The strategies put in place by the international organisations reflect these externalities. A network has been constructed for the purposes of controlling the outbreak that 'formalises the sharing of epidemiological information and provides the operational framework for joint field missions to affected areas,' (WHO 2005, see Kumaranayake, Chapter 17 on cooperative arrangements). This collaboration reflects the sentiment expressed about Avian flu shortly after the SARS outbreak. 'This is a serious global threat to human health,' said WHO Director General Lee Jong-wook. '.... we can possibly control it before it reaches global proportion if we work co-operatively and share needed resources,' (BBC, 2004).

WHO global strategy identifies five critical actions needed to address an influenza pandemic: reduce human exposure, strengthen early warning systems, build capacity, and intensify rapid containment operations, co-ordinate international research and development (WHO 2005). The global strategy of the FAO and OIE was to minimise the global threat and risk in humans and domestic poultry. The three organisations have jointly 'established a Global Early Warning and Response System (GLEWS) for trans-boundary animal diseases. The new mechanism combines the existing outbreak alert, verification, and response capacity of the three agencies and helps ensure that the disease tracking at WHO benefits from the latest information on relevant animal diseases' (WHO 2005, p 7).

Cooperative governance, however, may not occur at all levels. As the progress of the epidemic in poultry stocks has emerged the weakness of governance structures to protect the public health has been all too apparent. Indonesia delayed a cull, although millions of chickens were infected, until they were sure that the H5N1 strain was involved. 'Few decisions to report rely simply on scientific matters. Even infections that should be reported under International Health Regulations have been kept secret to protect trade or tourism. Many of the infected flocks are the property of the poorest members of society who often live in close proximity to poultry and as well as being likely to lose their flocks they are at great risk of catching the infection and providing a mechanism for re-assorting the bacteria and so facilitating the development of a human to human strain and possibly triggering a pandemic. The incentives to hide outbreaks are great. Beijing, for example, experienced a 94% drop in the tourist trade in 2003. But the public health benefit of early intervention is greater. The cull of all the poultry in Hong Kong in 1997, estimated as 1.5 million birds, within three days, reduced opportunities for further direct transmission to humans, and may have averted a pandemic.' (Roberts, 2006).

Control is difficult because the dynamics of the virus are not well understood. It is known that ducks can secrete the virus without themselves succumbing to the disease and that mammals thought not to be at risk from the infection have developed the disease. Eradication of the disease seems increasingly impossible as the disease has been found in wild birds providing vectors of infection locally and along migration routes. Conditions thought conducive to eradication are: effective interruption of transmission; sensitive diagnostic tools to detect infection that can lead to transmission, humans are essential for the life cycle of the agent, and there is no other animal reservoir and no environmental amplification, (Ottesen et al. 1997). Avian flu does not have these properties. It thus poses a problem of long term containment as well as the more immediate threat of initiating a pandemic (WHO 2005).

A number of interventions and preventative strategies are being adopted. The dominant method is culling. Culling is a process that is not without hazards. Even when undertaken by government dictate the culling process will be carried out by contractors or producers themselves. It may not be done well. The specific contracts (or administrative arrangements) for culling can be drawn up but as inspection cannot be made of each cull. It is possible that birds may not all be destroyed, the process of culling may contaminate the environment, and those doing the culling and disposal of the birds might not be properly protected and become infected. The culled birds can be eaten by other animals and birds, or even stolen for human consumption. Culling requires enforcement which is costly.

Compensation is a possible tool that can be used to encourage compliance with regulations relating to reporting and culling. Care has to be taken in designing and implementing compensation schemes. Lack of compensation or meagre compensation may encourage deception and frustrate attempts at control. If the compensation is too high, however, it might encourage trade in infected birds amongst producers who wish to qualify for the subsidy so may amplify the spread of disease. The rate should be carefully balanced to ensure compliance and compliance should be monitored with penalties for fraud. But few countries have the resources for adequate compensation and insurance schemes are still rudimentary.

Culling may be replaced by quarantine that preserves stocks whilst containing the spread of infection. Quarantine like culling can provide a less than perfect barrier against the spread of the disease. Like culling it can be abused and it can be costly to enforce.

Attempts to minimise risk to flocks include taking 'free range' flocks in doors and creating quarantine zones around any outbreak. A strategy that was considered effective until the outbreak amongst penned up turkeys in France. The other dominant intervention is vaccination. Whilst no vaccine against human to human infection can be manufactured until the virus is identified a vaccine against the avian virus is now available. It has been suggested that this should be used to protect large flocks. France and Netherlands have obtained permission from the European Union (EU) to vaccinate birds but the movement of the vaccinated flocks is to be severely restricted, (EU 2006). Vaccination may mask low levels of infection making it impossible to test whether they are disease free or not so the strategy is being widely debated but it may have a role to play in controlling the spread to areas adjacent to an outbreak but not subject to culling.

On the whisper of a likely new threat the domestic trade lobby is quickly activated. We see examples of economic reactions to outbreaks similar to those described in Chapter 18 by Rasinathan already well established. Italy imposed a ban on feathers imported from eastern neighbours and imposed controls on the transportation of poultry following the detection of five dead swans; it imposed border controls on traffic from Slovenia after a suspect swan, found there, was sent to the EU test centre in Weybridge in England. Japan has restricted imports of French chicken and pate as turkeys succumb to the infection in France. At present human reaction rather than state controls have had the greatest impact on trade. It was reported in The Times 17th February, 2006 (Elliott 2006) that 'cheap chicken is flooding into Britain from the other countries where the arrival of the deadly avian flu virus in wild birds has led to a drop in sales' p16. Fears were expressed about the impact of these imports on British industry in spite of domestic demand holding up. It was reported that sales of chicken were down 70% in Italy and the poultry industry had lost £480m in a week and between 30 000 and 180 000 workers had lost their jobs. The losses encountered in Europe so far palls into insignificance compared to the impact on the industry in East Asia where tens of millions of birds have been slaughtered.

As well as international bodies many local agencies are involved in the control, each with its own chain of command, goals and procedures. Integrated governance mechanisms must be in place, as gaps in the chain of governance may lead to delays in reporting or lack of diligence that can have catastrophic consequences.

The concept of governance is particularly useful in exploring how uncertainty and risk affect the control and subsequent economic impact of the infection, (Roberts, Chapter 13). There are certain stages—critical control points—in any investigation where governance and capacity issues are crucial. These critical control points are points of inflection in the progress of an epidemic. If control is lost at these points, infections may take on a different trajectory and can spread dramatically. Governance issues may impede control activities and together with a lack of human capacity, infrastructure and technical facilities allow an outbreak to become an epidemic or pandemic.

Governance can be enhanced by adopting the HACCP approach to control of infection that has been used for many years in large food producing plants, (see Roberts Chapter 13) and is a tool increasingly adopted to manage and investigate public health procedures. The HACCP approach can indicate points of hazard that if badly handled can lead to serious repercussions not only to the organisation concerned but also to the national and international economy. Estimation of the cost of loss of control at each critical control point can inform decisions about the possible returns to investment to reduce the risk at each control point.

Six stages in disease control are identified and each may be exposed to opportunistic behaviour or compromised by lack of resources. These stages include:

1. recognition of the disease, its pathology and virulence;

2. surveillance to identify new cases;

3. identification of the disease source,

4. transmission routes,

5. treatment of cases and prevention of secondary spread

6. modifications to prevent or limit future spread of disease.

At each stage there will be critical control points that need to be identified and risks quantified. Each stage involves interaction amongst professionals and relationships between principals and agents in public bureaucracies and market structures. These relationships exist in the context of legal and regulatory systems imposed by national governments and international organisations, (see Kumaranayake, Chapter 17). It is essential that at each stage the governance structure is scrutinised to see whether there is scope for opportunistic responses that might affect the control of the epidemic. Failures at each and every stage may also result from lack of resources—including logistical and intellectual capacity. Once the dynamics of transmission are known it should be possible to assess the consequences of failure of governance at each stage. Trade offs between interventions at each control point may become apparent allowing policy priorities to be assessed at each step.

In assessing the impact of control the use of models are very helpful. Indeed in preparing for the plans to control Avian flu modelling is a very important. Modelling has been used to predict the spread of disease, determine the economic burden and resources needed for basic control. Fundamental to the development of simple models is the basic reproduction rate R_0. 'This parameter measures the intrinsic ability of a parasite to invade and persist in specified host populations.' (see Anderson and May 1991). It depends on three basic factors: the natural history of the infection (especially the duration of infectiousness); the route of transmission, the environment and the behaviour of the population, the important aspects of which are determined by the route of transmission. Infectious disease models need to take into account the special characteristics of infection. 'Infectious disease is fundamentally different from non-infectious disease in that the risks of disease to an individual are intrinsically linked to the risk to others in the population; incidence is a function of prevalence.' Medley *et al.* 1997 p 35. Externalities are all encompassing but complex depending on the number exposed, numbers infected and numbers immune, the organism may shift or mutate frequently further complicating the control process. Unlike many factors used in production the impact of resources used to control infections is not linear and continuous, '. . . biological populations are controlled by processes that are nonlinear. For example, doubling the number of vaccine doses given or halving the density of vectors will not result in halving the incidence.' (Medley 1997 p 35). 'Consequently, any control policy adopted will impose selective pressure, which may result in the selection of strains of a pathogen with specific changes that overcome or mitigate the control policy. This is seen most dramatically in terms of development of drug resistance. However there is also the possibility of antigenic changes to circumvent immunity induced by vaccination.' (Medley *et al.* 1997 p 35, see also McLean 1995).

The development of resistance has already threatened the antivirus strategy based on drugs such as oseltamivar marketed by Roche as Tamiflu (House of Lords, 2005). India has invested heavily in a generic drug industry and is well placed to produce stocks of the antiviral drug but this investment along with the stock piles set up in many countries will be threatened if resistance develops. The technological response to the disease may well shift during the epidemic, (see Grieve, Chapter 5). Models will need to be adapted rapidly to take into account such changes. The capacity of the drug industry to produce the potential vaccines on the necessary scale is posing an unexpected constraint in dealing with a pandemic. The productive capacity of the industry has to be addressed. Plans to involve the companies in cooperative work to develop and provide a possible vaccine in the least possible time have been attempted, (see WHO 2005, Kumaranayake Chapter 17).

Human capacity is vital. It is, however, lacking in many parts of the world. Networks of experts working together are required to 'crack' the problem, see for example the collaboration that took place during the SARS epidemic, (WHO 2003). Capacity might become stretched even with extensive use of networks. Some steps have been taken to build capacity. WHO's programme for Health Security Capacity Development aims to improve competence in laboratory and epidemiological disciplines and to develop global surveillance.

Travel is also affected by outbreaks. If the outbreak were to develop into a disease with person-to-person spread there would be precipitous changes in air travel and the tourist trade and business traffic may be affected. This puts strain on the airlines and the tourist trade. Information is very important during outbreaks and WHO and individual countries provided information to travellers on a daily basis during epidemics, (see Kumaranayake Chapter 17 for a discussion of the impact of WHO interventions travel restrictions on Canada during the SARS outbreak). At present the advice is to avoid contact with poultry 'travellers to areas experiencing outbreaks of H5N1 avian infection should avoid contact with live animal markets and poultry farms. Large amounts of the virus are known to be excreted in the droppings from infected birds'. (WHO 2005).

However carefully such international and national announcements are drafted, risks are likely to be portrayed in the popular press in quite stark terms that will amplify the risks. During the SARS outbreak reservations on airlines travelling to the Far East fell dramatically, hotels in Hong Kong and Singapore were empty and international conferences were cancelled in Asia and in Canada.

If cases are identified then treatment and prevention of secondary spread will be of utmost importance. The identification of contacts may be possible but if the disease has a short incubation time and has a high reproduction rate there will hardly be time for contacts to be traced and isolated. Avoiding secondary spread will be difficult but some attempt at limiting social interactions may be useful. Quarantine of certain areas and movement restrictions may be possible. This was used in the SARS outbreak, often accompanied by penalties and threats for non-compliance with the quarantine restrictions.

Capacity to care for sick individuals may quickly become a major issue especially in poor countries. Many developed countries, however, find their hospitals barely able to cope with a seasonal flu epidemic in a predominately fit or vaccinated population. They are hardly likely to be able to cope easily with a new virulent disease in an unprotected population. Plans exist to cope with medical emergencies. These involve stopping any scheduled admissions, moving patients to different units, opening up emergency facilities etc. The opportunity costs of these actions will be very large as sick people waiting for treatment are displaced by flu victims or delayed by ward closures. It is doubtful that capacity in intensive care facilities, in UK for example, could cope with a large epidemic. Physical resources may not be the main concern, however, in an epidemic of such virulence. Staff are likely to be affected. Surge capacity should be in place and human capacity should be resilient, often the knowledge is embodied in just one or two individuals. Firms and organisations have been asked to draw up plans to meet the possible loss through death or sickness of 25% of its staff. Large numbers of sick people affect the wider economy. They cannot participate in the workforce and they may need others to look after them further depleting the workforce. They may generate demands for some products and reduce the demand for others so dislocating the local economy. The local economies could in certain extreme circumstances become paralysed by lack of workers and public utilities may be at risk. Many will die and need mortuary facilities and burial or cremation or other forms of funeral arrangements.

The logistics of the operation will be crucial. The logistics will require an authoritative governance structure to ensure smooth operations and the maximum use of facilities. Establishing a chain of command in advance of any large outbreak is good practical advice. The Canadian experience with Sars demonstrates the problems of having poor local co-ordination between those involved in the outbreak control.

Anxiety about the potential ravages to lives and the global economy is acute. A pandemic, it is estimated, could affect one quarter of the world's population, cause deaths of millions of people and plunge the economy into depression. Investment in effective policies to control Avian flu outbreaks and delay a pandemic would yield a many fold rate of return. If the $2bn fund reduced the epidemic by a mere 1% the returns would be $8bn. 'Whatever resources you put in place—compared to the potential pandemic cost—it is peanuts. It is nothing.' Margaret Chan, quoted by Yeh Financial Times 17th January 2006. Property rights to the benefits are diffuse and thus there is likely to be under investment. The economic problem, however, is not merely one of raising funds it is in deploying them efficiently.

Conclusion

MRSA is now endemic in many hospitals. It is difficult to regain this ground lost to the organism. But many initiatives have been introduced that should if used in a co-ordinated way begin to make some impact on the prevalence of MRSA in hospitals. One of the worrying aspects of control is the growth of the infection in the community that may not only cause problems there but will provide a reservoir of infected persons who will enter the hospitals and undermine the progress made. Governance structures together with targets and penalties are now in place in the UK. These should begin to yield results but given the reservoir of colonised cases now out in the community it may well take sometime to gain control of the problem. Many evaluative studies are underway that will help to design future policy initiatives and technical improvements in testing for the organism are progressing fast.

The saga of Avian flu has barely begun. As the organism, now probably endemic in wild birds, proceeds around the world there is likely to be a rash of outbreaks, culls, calls for compensation and claims of subterfuge and malpractice. If the virus mutates into one that can cause human to human infection then skills and resources and good governance will be essential if the dire predictions are to be avoided. If the efforts are successful and a pandemic is avoided then people will deny there was ever a threat. If there is a pandemic they will certainly ask why more was not done. Economic analysis can contribute to the development of an appropriate and efficient response to the control of the infection.

References

Alford, K., Plowman, R.M., Roberts, J.A., (2001) *The Way Ahead, Progress towards the control of Hospital Acquired Infection*, National Audit Office, London.

Allen, P.A., Croxson, B., Roberts, J.A., Archibald, K., Crawshaw, S., Taylor, L. (2001) Contracts and budgets in the management of infectious disease, *Health Policy*.

Allen, P.A., Croxson, B., Roberts, J.A., Archibald, K. (2000) The use of Contracts in the Management of Infectious Disease Related Risk in the NHS Internal Market. *ESRC Risk and Human Behaviour Programme* Newsletter No.7.

Anderson, R.M. and May, R.M. (1991) *Infectious Diseases in Humans* Oxford University Press, Oxford.

Arnold, M. and Studemann, F. (2006) France confirms first case of virus *Financial Times* 20th February p6, London.

Babad, H., Jacklin, P. and Roberts, J.A. (2005) Faster testing for MRSA *Capital Doctor* 48/49 41–43. Oxford.

Barber, T. (2006) Italy imposes controls after bird flu discovery, *Financial Times* 13th February p 10, London.

BBC News (2004) January 27th.

BBC News (2006) Funding Capacity January 18th.

Cooper, B.S., Stone, S.P., Kibbler, C.C., Cookson, B.D., Roberts, J.A., Medley, G.F., Duckworth, G.J., Lai, R., Ebrahim, S. (2003) *Systematic Review of isolation policies in the hospital management of methicillin resisitant Staphlyococcus aureua: a review of the literature with epidemiological and economic modeling*. HTA.

Crawshaw, S.C., Allen, P., Roberts, J.A. (2000) Managing the risk of infectious disease: the context of organisational accountability, *Health, Risk and Society* **2** (2): 125–141.

Dowdle, W.R. and Hopkins, D.R. (1997) ed *The Eradication of Infectious Diseases Dahlem Workshop Reports*, Wiley.

Elliott, V. (2006) Flu-scare chicken hits British Market *The Times* Feb 17th London.

Financial Times, (2006) January 19th p. 10.

Health Protection Agency (2005) Antibiotic Resistance, prevention and control (ARPAC) EU funded project. Reported 13th September.

House of Lords (2004) Select Committee Report Antimicrobial Resistance.

House of Lords (2005) Report on resistance in Tamiflu.

Jain, A. India calls for calm as it fights bird flu outbreak, *Financial Times* 20th February p.6, London.

McLean, A.R. (1995) Vaccination, evolution and changes in the efficacy of vaccines— A theoretical framework *Proceedings of the Royal Society*, B **261**: 389–393, London.

McMaster, R. (1998) The X-efficiency properties of competitive tendering, in Bartlett W., Roberts, J.A., Le Grand, J. eds *Revolution in Social Policy*, Policy Press, Bristol.

Medley, G.F., Nokes, D.J. and Edmunds, W.J. (1997) The Role of Mathematical Models in Eradication of Infectious Disease in Dowdle, W.R. and Hopkins, D.R. ed *The Eradication of Infectious Diseases* Dahlem Workshop Reports, Wiley Chichester.

Ottesen, E.A., Dowdle, W.R., Fenner, F., Habermehl, K.-O., John, T.J., Koch, M.A., Medley, G.F., Muller, A.S., Ostroff, S.M., Zeichardt, H. (1997) Group Report: How is eradication to be defined a what are biological criteria? In Dowdle WR and Hopkins DR ed *The Eradication of Infectious Diseases* Dahlem Workshop Reports, Wiley, Chichester.

Pittet, D. (2001) Compliance with hand disinfection and its impact on hospital acquired infection, *Journal of Hospital Infection* 48 S40–46.

Roberts, J.A., Archibald, K., Taylor, L., Crawshaw, S., Allen, P., Croxson, B. (2000) MRSA and Meningitis: Perceptions of Risk to the Public's Health. *ESRC Risk and Human Behaviour Programme* Newsletter No.8, 2000.

Roberts, J.A. (2006) Funding of global control of bird flu, *BMJ* 332 189–90. London

The Times (2006) 17th February, London.

Wilson, A.P.R., Hodgson, B., Liu, M., Plummer, D., Taylor, I., Roberts, J.A., Jit, M. Sherlow-Johnson (2005) Wound surveillance with post discharge follow up and feed back in a UK teaching hospital *British Journal of Surgery*, in press.

World Bank (2005) *Avian and Human Influenza: financing needs and gaps* 21st December, Washington.

World Bank (2006) *Avian and human influenza: Multidonor Financing Framework*, World Bank Washington.

World Health Organisation (2005) *Responding to the avian influenza pandemic threat, Recommended strategic actions* , WHO, Geneva.

World Health Organisation (2006) *International Pledging Conference on Avian and Human Pandemic Influenza*, WHO Geneva.

World Health Organisation (2006) *Ten things you need to know about pandemic influenza*, Washington.

Yeh, A. (2006) International community pledges $1.9bn for bird flu'self-defence', Financial Times January 19th p7 London.

Yeh, A. (2006) Roche in £20m bird flu donation Financial Times 18th January p.7, London.

Index

DATE DUE

JUN 2 3 2010		
JUN 0 4 2010		

c. 38-293